JENIS FR

Nutritional Supplements

What Works...And Why

A Review
From A to Zinc—and Beyond!

Joe Cannon, MS

Copyright © 2006 by Joe Cannon

ISBN 0-7414-3097-5

Published by:

INFI∞ITY
PUBLISHING.COM

1094 New DeHaven Street, Suite 100
West Conshohocken, PA 19428-2713
Info@buybooksontheweb.com
www.buybooksontheweb.com
Toll-free (877) BUY BOOK
Local Phone (610) 941-9999
Fax (610) 941-9959

Printed in the United States of America

Printed on Recycled Paper

Published May 2006

For my teachers...
All of you who have touched my life over the years.
Some of you know who you are.
Others do not...
Each of you has impacted my life in so many positive ways.
If not for all of you, my life would be much different and these words would not have been written.

Acknowledgments

In an effort to explain the apparent orderly workings of the cosmos, Albert Einstein once quipped that *God does not play dice with the universe*. Similarly, I likewise have come to the conclusion that God doesn't play dice with us either. It really does appear to me that for some reason even the people we meet are on some level preordained and help guide and shape us into the individuals we are today. Take this book for instance. While my name appears on the cover, it might never have been written if it were not for others who helped me in various ways over the years. I would like to take a moment to formally thank some of those important people here.

Thank you Kelly Bixler. You are not only my editor but my niece and valued friend! Thanks for your patience and for working with me. Your unique insights as a consumer and supplement advocate enabled me to write a better book than I could have on my own. I would also like to thank Kelly's husband, *Kyle*, for his patience during the times when Kelly was spending all those hours helping me with this project.

Thank you Bob Fox. As my brother, you have been a role model of what I might aspire to be. As my *spiritual advisor,* you helped me expand my horizons.

Thank you Jami Appenzeller, By giving me my first editorial position, you helped foster my interest in supplements and for that I am forever grateful.

Thank you Nora Anderson. Presenting for AAAI/ISMA all these years has indeed been a pleasure and has helped give me the luxury of researching and writing this book.

Thank you Tim DiFelice and Adam Freedman. What friends I have in both of you. Thank you both for your friendship and support over the years, especially during my *darkest* hours.

Thank you cherished friends and colleagues. Your suggestions about what supplements you wanted to know about were invaluable and helped me lay the foundation for many of the topics presented in this book.

Thank you Mom and Dad. While I never said it, I always appreciated your never questioning my resolve to take the road less traveled. It is my hope that a copy of this book gets up to you both in heaven.

Lastly, thanks to God, the masterful Chess Player of the universe, who continues to guide me to this very day and reveals to each of us how much more we can be, if we only try...

Table of Contents

Section 2: A Review of Supplements From A to Zinc and Beyond... 27

viii

Start Reading Here!

If you are reading these words, there is a darn good chance you are taking vitamins, herbs or other supplements or are thinking about how they might help you. It is for you that this book was written.

It has been over 10 years since I was first bitten by the bug of curiosity that lead me to start investigating supplements, delving into which ones lived up to their reported claims and which ones didn't. Since that time so long ago, many things have changed; supplements have come and gone from the public eye—and have come back again. Commercials, touting the merits of various nutritional supplements now permeate the airwaves of both TV and radio. Every day, our computers are bombarded with emails for products purporting to do everything from help our immune systems to those even boasting that they can slow the very aging process itself! Today, Internet searches return over one million hits from the phrase *nutritional supplement*. Ironically, in this age of information, it seems that it's harder than ever to get honest answers to make sense of it all. Fortunately though, one thing that has dramatically changed from days past is the quantity of scientific investigations that have been performed on these products. Throughout this book, I will use scientific evidence and rational thinking as my *litmus tests* when reviewing supplements. No testimonials or hype will be included anywhere in this book. Rather, I will endeavor to provide you with *just the facts, in plain English*. While personal testimonials of the effectiveness of a product may indeed in some cases be based on fact, focusing on the clinical research generally provides a more complete description of the supplement's properties.

Section one of this book provides a good review of a variety of topics related to nutritional supplements as well as addresses many questions you may have asked yourself in the past. Issues such as what supplements are, as well as the government's role in regulating them, are reviewed here. This section is very important and will help you get the most out of this book.

In section two, I will review some of the best known (and some of the least known) supplements available today. I will review what the supplement is, what its major claims are and summarize the clinical evidence that's available for that supplement. Throughout this book, I will also tackle the very challenging task of trying to answer *your* questions. While I may not know you personally, over the years, I've talked to thousands of people and have noticed that many ask similar questions when it comes to supplements. I will use their questions as my guide when I review each topic in this book.

Also included in each section are known and suspected side effects and drug interactions—areas which I personally feel are often neglected when discussing supplements. They are, however, very important things to be aware of, especially for those who may have special needs or conditions.

Much of the information you will see is referenced to scientific studies and other credible sources that are listed at the end of the book. I do this because deep down inside, I'm basically a nerd; I personally like books that are referenced because they help me to dig deeper when I do my own research. Supplements can be a very controversial topic and everybody has their own opinions. I know there will be those who will not agree with what I have written. In fact, I'm confident that some will vehemently disagree with me! For those who have other ideas, I hope the providing of references will be of help.

At the end of each review are *My Thoughts,* which is essentially my gut reaction to the topic in question. Here I'll list my opinions and impressions and whether or not I think the supplement is worth your hard-earned money or not.

Writing this book has truly been a labor of love for me. It is my sincere hope that what I have created here will be of help to you as you conduct your own investigations into this most intriguing area of study.

Section 1

Things Not Often Talked About

What Are Nutritional Supplements?

In addition to the multivitamins that practically everybody has taken at one time or another, nutritional supplements refer to a wide variety of compounds such as vitamins, minerals, herbs, amino acids, and parts of plants, as well as combinations of any of the above. In addition, byproducts that are created during the normal breakdown of these substances may also be referred to as supplements. Under current US laws, even some hormones may be categorized as nutritional supplements. Nutritional supplements are referred to as *supplements* because they are meant to supplement or complement a person's daily, healthy diet. A phrase which often goes hand-in-hand with nutritional supplement is *dietary supplement.* These terms mean the same thing and are often used interchangeably.

As mentioned above, various parts of plants are also labeled as supplements. These are sometimes referred to as *phytonutrients* or *phytochemicals* (the prefix *phyto* means *plant*). Examples of phytonutrients include beta carotene, lutein and lycopene—to name a few.

Nutritional supplements that are said to help people become stronger, faster or jump higher are usually grouped into a special class called *ergogenic aids.* For example, scientific studies confirm that creatine—arguably the most researched supplement in history—may enhance strength and power in some individuals. Other reputed ergogenic aids include boron, chromium and zinc. The following table summarizes some of the major types of supplements and gives examples of each.

Examples of Supplements

Vitamins	Minerals	Protein	Herbs	Phytonutrients	Ergogenic Aids
Vitamin B12	Chromium	Soy	Ginkgo	Beta-carotene	Creatine
Vitamin C	Iron	Whey	Ginseng	Lutein	Ginseng

So by now you may be saying to yourself that there is a lot more to supplements than just the multivitamins that sit quietly in your kitchen cupboard. You may also be wondering how things got to where they are today. In my opinion, things really started to change in the late 1980s when newspapers started reporting on a mysterious, rare blood disorder called *eosinophilia myalgia syndrome*. All of the people who had this illness seemed to have one thing in common—they were all using the amino acid, tryptophan, which was a popular natural alternative to sleeping pills. In the end, 37 people died from the disease. While a tainted batch of tryptophan manufactured in Japan was linked to the EMS outbreak, the Food and Drug Administration (FDA) also found that the disease occurred in people who used tryptophan which did not originate in Japan.[586] Based on this information, the FDA pulled tryptophan from the US market. In response to fears that the government might soon regulate all supplements, some in the supplement industry started to rally public support. Pamphlets contending that a doctor's prescription might soon be required for vitamins and other supplements were distributed to the public. Some health food stores also had petitions which patrons could sign, opposing the alleged government interventions. These actions, along with government statistics showing that a very large percentage of Americans regularly consumed nutritional supplements, were ultimately responsible for the passage of a piece of legislation which would revolutionize everything—the Dietary Supplement Health and Education Act of 1994, or *DSHEA* for short. Under DSHEA, nutritional supplements are classified as foods, not drugs and prevented strict government regulations which might curtail their sale. According to DSHEA (pronounced "D-Shay"), the official definition of nutritional supplements is as follows:[1]

- a product (other than tobacco) intended to supplement the diet that bears or contains one or more of the following dietary ingredients: a vitamin, mineral, amino acid, herb or other botanical
  OR
- a dietary substance used to supplement the diet by increasing the total dietary intake
  OR
- a concentrate, metabolite, constituent, extract, or combination of any ingredient described above **AND**
- intended for ingestion in the form of a capsule, powder, softgel, or gelcap, and not represented as a conventional food or as a sole item of a meal or the diet
  AND
- is labeled a "dietary supplement".

This rather wordy definition essentially allows for a much wider variety of substances to be listed as supplements. For example, byproducts (metabolites) created during the normal metabolism of amino acids, vitamins, minerals, etc. can be defined as a supplement. One such metabolite which has received much attention over the past few years in the fitness community is a product called *HMB*—a byproduct that is created during the normal metabolism of the amino acid leucine. We will discuss the claims and evidence for HMB later in this book.

What Claims for Supplements Are Allowed?

Another stipulation of the Dietary Supplement Heath and Education Act of 1994 refers to the labeling of nutritional supplements. Under DSHEA regulations, the makers of dietary supplements cannot make specific claims regarding the preventing, curing or treatment of any disease or condition—unless the claim has been approved by the Food and Drug Administration (FDA).[1] For example, manufacturers cannot claim that a supplement can prevent or treat cancer. What is allowed are referred to as *structure/function* claims. Structure/function claims refer to statements pertaining to how a nutritional supplement might support the structure of the body or the function of a bodily process. For example, the statement that calcium helps build strong bones is a structure/function claim. In contrast, the claim that a fiber supplement can reduce your risk of colon cancer is not allowed. That would be making a disease claim which is not legal under current law. Structure/function claims are pretty easy to recognize because they usually contain words such as *supports*, *aids*, *maintains* or *provides*. The following table is a list of structure/function claims which you may see on nutritional supplement labels and advertisements.

Examples of Structure/Function Claims
• Helps maintain normal cholesterol levels
• Maintains healthy lung function
• Supports the immune system
• Aids digestion

Another regulation under DSHEA is that the labels of dietary supplements must contain the following disclaimer: *These statements have not been evaluated by the Food and Drug Administration. This product is not intended to diagnose, treat, cure or prevent any disease.* This is the government's way of saying to the consumer that the US government is not endorsing the claims made on the supplement in question. It's also reminding the consumer that in spite of the structure/function claim, the supplement should not be used in place of any conventional medical treatment.

Does the Government Regulate Supplements?

Considering the complex definition of nutritional supplements described by DSHEA above, one might imagine that the US government regulates their creation, safety and effectiveness. Well, the answer to this question is both yes and no. Yes, there is some government regulation of supplements but it is much less than is required for prescription drugs. One aspect of all of this that many people may not know is that manufacturers of nutritional supplements usually do not need to notify the FDA or get prior FDA approval before a new supplement is created or marketed to the public. Likewise, supplement manufacturers do not have to submit their products to the FDA or any government agency to prove they are effective or safe before they are sold to the public. The FDA can take legal action against the makers of supplements that are deemed unsafe or which make illegal claims.

The advertising of nutritional supplements usually comes under the jurisdiction of the Federal Trade Commission (FTC). Together, the FDA and FTC can and sometimes do take legal action against nutritional supplements which they feel are in violation of DSHEA regulations. On the downside, this intervention sometimes occurs after a product has made its way in the hands of consumers. So in other words, nutritional supplement manufacturers are on the honor system. We have to take their word as to the effectiveness, safety and quality of the products they produce.

Is the Government Going to Take Away My Right To Buy Supplements?

The odds are this occurring are very remote. Contrary to the editorials that sometimes appear in some magazines, DSHEA has been settled law since 1994 and the FDA has not issued any public statements that it desires to stop the sale of supplements in the US. Furthermore, evidence continues to accumulate that some supplements have beneficial effects on health. Dietary supplements are here to stay—as they should be. That being said, all societies must have rules and laws in place to protect people from harm. The laws governing the sale of dietary supplements in the US are part of that system of laws. While capitalism and free enterprise are two of the engines that power our democracy, the unrestricted sale of dietary supplements helps nobody. In other words, how much faith would we have in any product if quality supplements, made by honest companies, could be sold alongside those that are not only useless but dangerous? The bottom line is that DSHEA, as well as education on the part of consumers, helps minimize the usage and sale of sub par supplements.

What About the Quality of Supplements?

The FDA does require supplement manufacturers to accurately report the ingredients on the label of the product. Unfortunately, though, this does not always happen. For example, investigations do sometimes find discrepancies between what some supplement labels indicate and what the product actually contains.[2,265] This means that a product might contain less or even more than the label indicates. These discrepancies could be due to a number of reasons ranging from the use of inexpensive ingredients, to the lack of proper manufacturing facilities needed to ensure a superior supplement. While some may liken scientific investigations of supplement quality to Big Brother looking over ones shoulder, such reviews are necessary because they help weed out the bad from the good and overall assist the nutritional supplement industry. On the down side, this also forces you, the consumer, to do your homework on the supplements you use. One of the reasons this book was written was to give people a reference to help them do that homework.

Does *Natural* Equal *Safe?*

It seems as though people have been conditioned to believe that just because something is natural or made in nature that it automatically has to be safe to use. A classic example is the commonly used phrase, "a safe, natural alternative" that is found in so many supplement advertisements. But, are all naturally occurring things automatically safe for human consumption? The answer, of course, is no. Many things exist in nature that if ingested by humans, could cause sickness or worse. Mistletoe is a good example. While best known for helping amorous men and women catch a smooch from their loved ones at Christmas, mistletoe is also an herb which some have advocated for ailments ranging from heart disease to cancer. It turns out that mistletoe is quite toxic when ingested and might result in seizures and even death![266] In pregnant women, the consumption of mistletoe might cause women to give birth too early.[30] Other examples of natural-yet-toxic-substances include cyanide and hemlock, both deadly poisons! These are of course, very extreme examples and are only used to highlight the fallacy of *natural equals safe*. While you are probably saying to yourself that you would never eat mistletoe, cyanide or hemlock, the fact remains that some supplements could, in theory, have negative effects. This is one of the reasons why you might see warnings that are specific to children, pregnant and/or nursing women on supplement labels.

Because *natural* does not automatically mean *safe* for human consumption or safe for everybody, readers will always be advised to discuss their supplement usage with a trained medical professional like their physician, pharmacist or dietitian.

Can Supplements Interact with Medications?

Yes, it is possible for a supplement to interact with medications you are taking. These interactions could result in a variety of scenarios including:

1. the supplement *decreasing* the absorption of the medication.

2. the supplement *increasing* the absorption of the medication.
3. the supplement combining with the medication, producing a greater effect than the medication alone.
4. the medication decreases the absorption of the supplement.

Because it is unethical to purposely expose people to potentially dangerous situations in medical research, much of the evidence we currently have on supplement-drug interactions stems from test tube studies, animal research, theoretical thought (in other words, worst-case scenarios) and reports of lone individuals who have experienced problems with supplements. A short list of possible supplement-drug interactions is provided below.

Supplement	Possible Drug Interaction
Kava	anti-seizure drugs & sedatives
St John's wort	antidepressant medications; tissue rejection drugs; heart drugs; HIV drugs; oral contraceptives
Glutamine	anti-seizure medications
Yohimbe	high blood pressure medications
Echinacea	drugs that decrease the immune system
Garlic	blood thinners; HIV drugs
Ginkgo Biloba	aspirin; blood thinner medications

The supplement-drug interactions listed above are by no means the only such reactions that are known or thought to occur. Others exist and we will discuss many more throughout this book. Because of factors ranging from variations in brand potency, shelf-life issues, and even subtle differences between medications, it is possible that people reading these words may be using some of the very medications and nutritional supplements listed above—yet have never suffered any adverse reactions. Other people conversely may experience problems. This is what makes this a tricky issue. By confiding in your physician about the supplements you take, you will be helping to minimize the risk of any adverse reactions which might occur.

The Grapefruit Effect

Grapefruit is a healthy, natural food that is consumed by millions of people every day. Research is emerging that grapefruit may inhibit some forms of cancer as well as help reduce the risk of heart disease.[3] That being said, caution should be exercised by some who use grapefruit, grapefruit juice or grapefruit-extract dietary supplements. Studies show that grapefruit may negatively interact with a number of medications such as drugs used to treat AIDS, heart disease and high blood pressure to name a few.[4] Depending on the drug in question, grapefruit may either decrease or increase the absorption of the medication.[3] Grapefruit definitely is a wholesome food however people with medical issues should talk to their physician before consuming grapefruit so that their medications and their love for health foods can live in harmony.

Who Ya' Gonna Call?

People who experience negative side effects resulting from the use of supplements (as well as medications, medical equipment, cosmetics etc.) are encouraged to report the problem to the Food and Drug Administration

(FDA). The FDA maintains an *Adverse Event* database that catalogs all negative reports on supplements, medications, cosmetics and medical equipment. You can contact the FDA directly by calling 1-800-FDA-1088. You can also submit your report on the Internet by going to www.fda.gov/medwatch.com. On the website, visitors can also opt to sign up to the FDA's free email list which keeps people informed periodically about recalls and other action taken by the FDA.

Can Supplements Interact with Other Supplements?

This is possible. Nutritional supplements that have similar properties could, in theory, produce a larger effect than either supplement could if used by itself. While this might seem desirable, in reality, it may not be. Take, for example, vitamin E and ginkgo. Both supplements have anti-blood clotting ("blood thinning") properties. The additive effect of combining vitamin E and ginkgo might result in the blood becoming too thin and theoretically could produce internal bleeding. Combining supplements that possess anti-clotting properties with prescription medications which also thin the blood might enhance this effect even more.

Can Supplements Help Me?

Maybe. Many clinical studies exist showing that some nutritional supplements promote positive effects in the body. For example, research indicates that folic acid, a member of the B complex family of vitamins, can reduce levels of a compound called *homocysteine*, which has been linked to heart disease.[5,6,7]

Niacin, another B vitamin, has been shown to lower cholesterol levels. High-dose niacin is sometimes even prescribed by doctors for this purpose.

Another supplement is creatine. Creatine is made in the body and is also present in meat. Hundreds of well-designed clinical studies have found that creatine supplementation can enhance strength and power in humans.[8] For this reason creatine is very popular among bodybuilders and other athletes.

Glucosamine sulfate is a compound made naturally in the body. Studies generally find that supplementing with glucosamine may reduce the pain associated with *osteoarthritis.*

Saw palmetto is an herbal remedy with much evidence supporting its use by men with enlarged prostate glands.

These are by no means the only supplements for which research finds positive effects. Others exist and we will discuss them throughout this book.

Disclaimer About the Amounts Mentioned In This Book

This book provides approximations of amounts of ingredients which help might support the effects people are looking for. As a disclaimer, it cannot be stressed enough that the amounts mentioned for the various supplements are *not* endorsements of what you should use. On the contrary, the amounts listed should be viewed as points of reference upon which you, after speaking with your physician, can determine if a supplement is right for you. For the most part, clinical research is the basis for the amounts mentioned in this book. As more research is conducted, these amounts may change over time. To be on the safe side, a wise choice is to start with a lesser amount to see how you react. Because everybody is unique with different health concerns and biochemistries, no one can guarantee that the amounts mentioned in these pages are appropriate for you. Your individual needs and side effects may differ significantly from those mentioned in this book. It is for this reason that that you will be repeatedly reminded to consult your personal physician before undertaking any supplement program. Only your physician can best take into account your health and individual needs and weigh those against whether or not a supplement is right for you.

Who Should Avoid Supplements?

As a general rule, women who are pregnant should avoid supplements unless they are prescribed by their physician. The reason for this is that few clinical studies have gauged the safety or effectiveness of nutritional supplements in pregnant woman. This is for ethical reasons, of course. In other words, it's unethical (and prohibited by scientific rules of conduct) to recruit pregnant women and expose them to a substance which may turn out to be harmful to them and their unborn children.

Small children and teenagers are another group who are often cautioned against using nutritional supplements. The reasons are the same as for pregnant women. Little supplement research is ever conducted on children or teenagers. Also, it's unethical to conduct research on individuals who cannot legally accept the risks that may be involved and who may not fully understand the consequences of their participation in research. Lastly, it is important to note that children are not miniature adults. In other words, results obtained from studies involving adults does not automatically mean the same results would be found using children. This is food for thought for any kids who might be reading these words.

Individuals with medical conditions are also usually cautioned against using nutritional supplements. While studies have found that some supplements may help those with various medical conditions, the plain truth is that for the most part, we do not yet fully understand how many supplements interact with disease states. The risks of using ephedra if you have heart or kidney disease or high blood pressure is well documented.[23] However, the effects—both positive and negative—of many other supplements is less clear. Thus, to be on the safe side, it is generally recommended that those suffering from medical conditions steer clear of supplements unless there is good proof of benefit and most importantly, if it is approved by one's physician.

Doctors and Supplements

As a rule, doctors know about diseases and the treatment of diseases. In the past, the amount of schooling in nutrition and supplements that doctors received was limited. While times are changing, some people still mention that their physicians are not able to answer the questions they have about supplements. There are no easy answers when it comes to this issue. Some colleges now require medical students to take nutrition classes. Online resources are also available to help doctors after they leave medical school. Physicians may also consult with other members of the healthcare continuum such as dietitians, pharmacists, and maybe even—dare I say it—people who write books on supplements. As a general rule of thumb, it has been my personal experience that DOs (doctors of osteopathic medicine) tend to be more familiar with supplements than MDs; however this may not always be the case. Don't assume that your doctor isn't familiar with supplements because he or she is a physician. If you have a question, ask. What they know may surprise you.

Who Should Generally Avoid Supplements?

Who	Reason
Pregnant women	We do not have a lot of evidence on the effects supplements might have on developing babies.
Children	We do not have a lot of evidence of the effects of nutritional supplements in children.
People with medical issues	We do not fully understand how some supplements interact with different medical conditions.
People using medications	We do not fully understand how nutritional supplements interact with the medications that people may be taking.

What About Research?

Research has been and continues to be conducted on nutritional supplements. Some of this research finds, as we discussed briefly above, that various supplements do appear to promote positive effects. Conversely, other research on supplements finds either no beneficial effect or negative side effects. When researching nutritional supplements, consumers must remember the *unwritten rule of science*—that one study finding a positive effect (or a negative effect) doesn't matter a hill of beans. People make mistakes and scientists are no different. So, for this reason, scientists are usually cautious when viewing the results from a single or brand new experiment. It is only after the same results are found from repeated experiments, under the same conditions, that the outcomes of studies are taken seriously. Throughout this book I will use terms like *preliminary* or phrases such as *more research is needed* to alert you that something interesting has been observed with respect to a supplement but that it is not yet taken as gospel truth until more studies are done to confirm those findings.

The subjects used in research are also important. For example, if research finds that middle-aged women who took *supplement X* showed improvement in some area, does this automatically mean that men would obtain the same benefit? Not necessarily. Women and men are different—not only on the *outside* but on the *inside* as well. The classic example of this occurred with the mineral boron, which many bodybuilders and fitness enthusiasts used in the 1990s because of research showing that it might increase testosterone levels. The problem was that the research was conducted on older, postmenopausal women who consumed a boron-deficient diet.[237] There is a big difference between a bodybuilder, who normally eats very well and a 55-year old woman who may not exercise and who purposely eats a non-healthy diet. Boron does not raise testosterone levels in healthy, well-nourished men or women and the people who purchased boron supplements for this purpose wasted their money. Likewise, research conducted on bacteria or animals may not be applicable to humans. When confronted with research supporting a nutritional supplement (or anything for that matter) people should look at who the experiment was conducted on (men vs. women, lab rats, bacteria, etc.) as well as the number of studies finding the same effect. In essence, the more studies that find the same results, the more those results can be believed.

How Old is the Research?

I must admit that I am biased when it comes to clinical research. I like studies that are relatively new and no more than ten years old. One of the potential pitfalls of research is that if you dig deep enough you can probably find studies concluding that the earth is flat!

What About "Clinically Proven"?

Sometimes the phrase *clinically proven* is used as evidence for the effectiveness of nutritional supplements. The phrase "clinically proven" is actually a very generic statement that could mean almost anything. Technically, an experiment conducted by a college freshman in a university laboratory setting could be called a "clinical study". The thing to ask yourself when you encounter this statement is whether or not the *clinically proven* evidence is also a *published, peer-reviewed* study, which we will now discuss next.

What is Peer-Reviewed Research?

Peer-reviewed research is, in my opinion, the best research. To have a study that is peer-reviewed means that before the study was published in a scientific journal, it was first reviewed by other competent scientists (the "peers") whose job is to look for mistakes or flaws in the experiment. Any errors in research that are discovered during the peer-review process must be fixed before the study is accepted for publication. Essentially, having a study published that is peer-reviewed means that you did your homework and dotted all of your I's and crossed all of your T's. The scientific journals in which peer-reviewed research is published are generally not found in the magazine section of your local supermarket. You must subscribe to them and subscriptions may cost hundreds of dollars a year! Articles appearing in popular magazines are generally not peer-reviewed, but they sometimes are based on peer-reviewed research studies. If you have an internet connection, the summaries of millions of peer-reviewed studies can be viewed online at www.pubmed.com. Just go to this web site and type in the word or words you want to research and hit the enter button. The summaries of the studies will then pop up. A word of caution though: reading research summaries is about as exciting as watching the grass grow. They also usually contain lots of numbers which may confuse you. If you are looking to save time, I suggest that you skip down to the last two or three sentences of the summary. That's where you will find the *conclusions* of the study. The more studies you find that come to similar conclusions, the more credibility the observed effect has.

Examples of Peer-Reviewed Journals

• *Journal of Nutrition*	• *Medicine and Science in Sports and Exercise*
• *Pharmacotherapy*	• *Physician and Sports Medicine*
• *Journal of Strength and Conditioning Research*	• *Journal of the American Nutraceutical Association*
• *American Journal of Clinical Nutrition*	• *International Journal of Sports Nutrition and Exercise Metabolism*

What Are Abstracts?

Abstracts are summaries of experiments that are presented at science conventions and are sometimes published in the back of peer-reviewed medical and science journals. Occasionally, abstracts are cited as *evidence* for the usefulness of nutritional supplements. While abstracts are valuable and usually do correspond to clinical studies, this may not always be the case. For example, a study performed at a university may or may not be published in a peer-reviewed publication but rather appear only as an abstract. A non-peer-reviewed abstract can sometimes be spotted by looking at the page numbers listed in the reference for the study in question. A reference that is only one page long could be a tip-off that it's a non-peer-reviewed abstract. In contrast, the abstracts that are listed in the National Library of Medicine (www.pubmed.com) are peer-reviewed because they correspond to complete multiple-page scientific investigations that are published in respected journals.

What About Products That Are Patented?

Sometimes the makers of a supplement will obtain a United States patent to protect their product from being duplicated by others. In the case of supplements, patents might protect stuff like how the supplement was made, the unique blend of ingredients or anything else that the company wishes to protect. This could be particularly important if research begins to accumulate that a proprietary blend of ingredients proved beneficial to people. In that case the company holding the patent could corner the market! It's important to remember, though, that obtaining a US patent does not necessarily guarantee that a supplement works. The best way that we have to determine this is to test it scientifically.

Products vs. Ingredients

If you've skipped ahead and started looking though the supplements that are reviewed in this book you may have wondered why I did not list the brand names of the supplements you may be taking. I did this for two reasons. First, many brands of nutritional supplements will not have published peer-reviewed evidence supporting their effectiveness. Rarely will clinical testing occur first because this could take years to accomplish. Second—and most importantly—as time goes by, products will come and go, but the ingredients of those products will usually stay the same. So, if you know the research behind the ingredients, then you can use that information to interpret the claims for almost any product!

Nutritional Supplement Checklist

Questions to Ask When Researching Supplements	Answer
Is there research on the product showing that it works?	
If yes, was the research conducted on the *product* or the *ingredients* in the product?	
On whom was the research conducted (women, bacteria, etc.)?	
Is the research published in respected scientific publications?	
Is the research published as an abstract, which is not peer reviewed?	
How many other studies find the same effect?	
Have any side effects been observed?	

Joe. Are You Anti-Supplement?

Because I tend to pose tough questions, I am occasionally asked if I am against people using supplements. For the record, I am not. Quite the opposite, I feel there are quality-made supplements and products that can make a fine addition to a healthy diet. Related to this is my belief that people should know the facts about the products they use—both positive *and* negative. Everything has risks and benefits. For some things, the risks outweigh the benefits while in others, the opposite is true. The fact of the matter is that there are supplements that I use myself. So, claims that I am against people using supplements are completely baseless and do not hold any water.

Section 2

A Review of Supplements From A to Zinc and Beyond...

Acidophilus

Believe it or not, bacteria actually live inside of you! Acidophilus, or Lactobacillus acidophilus as it is also called, is one of the many "friendly" bacteria that colonize our digestive and urinary systems shortly after birth and live within us during our lives. Collectively, these friendly bacteria are also called *probiotics*, which literally means *pro-life*, making reference again to the helpful nature of these microorganisms. These bacteria are thought to be friendly because they crowd out other, less-friendly organisms which might cause disease. Sometimes antibiotics kill off these friendly bacteria, which then should be replaced to prevent the growth of harmful microorganisms. While there are many different types of friendly bacteria, most of them can be recognized by having the word lactobacillus (pronounced lack-toe-ba-sill-us) or simply the letter "L" somewhere in the name. For example, you may see *lactobacillus acidophilus* or *L acidophilus* as a component of a probiotic supplement.

Examples of Friendly, Probiotic Bacteria

• Lactobacillus acidophilus	• Lactobacillus amylovorus
• Lactobacillus brevis	• Lactobacillus bulgaricus
• Lactobacillus plantarum	• Lactobacillus sporogenes
• Lactobacillus rhamnosus	• Lactobacillus fermentum

Acidophilus and Diarrhea

While acidophilus and other probiotic bacteria may be touted to treat a wide variety of syndromes and conditions, the bulk of the evidence for them has to do with their role in reducing the symptoms of various forms of diarrhea. For example, a type of lactobacillus—lactobacillus GG—has been shown to reduce diarrhea in children.[247,248] Other research finds that lactobacillus GG may help reduce "traveler's diarrhea"—the type of diarrhea so named because it tends to affect people who travel a lot from one area to another.[248,249] Other studies have also found acidophilus to be helpful at reducing not only the symptoms but duration of diarrhea as well.[250,251]

Acidophilus and Ulcers

Another interesting line of acidophilus research involves ulcers. Many ulcers, it turns out, are caused not by stress but rather by a bacteria called *Helicobacter pylori*.[252] Usually the medical treatment is to give a type of antibiotic which kills the bacteria and eliminates the ulcer. Sometimes, though, the bacteria you want to get rid of doesn't want to go. Some research finds that the use of freeze-dried, inactivated acidophilus cultures combined with traditional ulcer therapy improves the killing of the harmful helicobacter pylori.[253] More research in humans is needed before the use of acidophilus is fully accepted as a co-treatment for ulcers. So far, there isn't much good evidence that acidophilus alone effects ulcers.

Acidophilus and IBS

Irritable bowel syndrome, or IBS for short, is a medical condition of the intestines that usually results in abdominal pain, constipation, diarrhea and bloating. Some research finds that non-living acidophilus supplements may reduce IBS pain in some individuals.[254] Other investigations find that related types of lactobacillus bacteria (Lactobacillus plantarum) may also help IBS sufferers as well.[255] Keep in mind that not all studies find that probiotic bacteria help IBS symptoms. Acidophilus and other probiotics may prove most beneficial as additional steps one can take alongside more traditional therapies which include exercise and reducing the harmful stresses in your life.

Acidophilus and Urinary Tract Infections

A bacterial infection of the urinary tract can lead to a variety of symptoms including painful urination, an almost constant urge to urinate, back pain, fever and possibly vomiting.[256] It seems to be common thought by some that acidophilus and other probiotic bacteria are the treatment of choice for preventing urinary tract infections. Currently though the investigations are mixed with some finding positive improvement and others finding no improvement.[257,258,259] Because some of the warning signs of urinary tract infections may be similar to other more serious conditions, persons experiencing symptoms such as those described here should consult their physician before experimenting with probiotic bacteria.

What are Prebiotics?

Prebiotics are different from probiotics and refer to various substances that support the growth of friendly bacteria (probiotics). One such example of prebiotics is fructo-oligosaccharides (FOS for short). Prebiotics are basically fancy sugar molecules that we humans cannot digest. Since we can't digest them, they pass into our intestinal track where our friendly bacteria consume them. You can think of prebiotics as the *food* for probiotics. While there are many claims made for prebiotics, most are based on preliminary evidence and are deserving of more research.

Acidophilus and the Immune System

Preliminary research finds that some forms of probiotic bacteria may stimulate antibody production and other cells of the immune system following intentional infection with microorganisms.[260,261] Other evidence suggests that some strains of probiotics may even reduce cancer risk by inactivating cancer-causing agents.[262] However, the types of probiotics, the dosages which might help and the cancers they may affect need more research.

How Probiotics are Measured

Probiotic supplements are measured not in milligrams or grams but rather by the number of live bacteria that the supplement contains. For example, a supplement label might report to contain 1 billion bacteria per capsule. The amount of probiotics in a supplement is sometimes reported in terms of *colony forming units* or

CFUs. Thus, a supplement that has 1 billion bacteria per capsule may list it as 1 billion CFUs. Supplements will vary in the amount of probiotic bacteria they contain. Currently, there is little evidence that greater dosages are better than lesser.

One possible consequence of using live bacteria in a supplement could be that the bacteria might die off the longer the product sits on store shelves. Consumers should make certain that the number of live bacteria indicated on the label represents the number of bacteria in the supplement *at the time of purchase*— and not the number of live bacteria present when the supplement was created. This is an important concept to remember when evaluating probiotic supplements. Recent independent analysis of probiotic supplements have noted that as many as 33% of the products tested contained less than 1% of the number of live bacteria they were supposed to contain.[267] In short, do your homework before your buy.

Side Effects and Concerns

In healthy people, acidophilus is pretty safe with flatulence usually reported. Theoretically, taking acidophilus and other probiotics at the same time as antibiotics might kill off the friendly bacteria as well as those causing infection. To minimize this don't take probiotics when using antibiotics or take them several hours apart.

Some concern has been raised over the use of probiotics by persons with poor immune systems. In theory, even friendly bacteria might cause infection in those whose immune system is weakened by disease. Currently, there is at least one person who reportedly died following the use of yogurt while his immune system was impaired by disease.[263] To be on the safe side, people who have received new organs, or who are taking drugs to suppress the immune system or those who have any diseases of the immune system whatsoever should consult their physician before using acidophilus or any probiotic supplement.

Quick Tips for Buying Probiotic Supplements

• What types of bacteria does the product contain?

• How many bacteria are in the supplement?

• Does the number of bacteria per supplement refer to the number of live bacteria when the product is purchased?

• What is the expiration date?

My Thoughts

Studies find that some forms of probiotic supplements including acidophilus may have beneficial effects. Currently, the most positive research on these products is derived from their effects on various forms of diarrhea. Many different types of probiotic bacteria exist and results from one type can't necessarily be extrapolated to other types until more research is done to confirm this. Because it may be difficult to get a quality probiotic supplement, consumers should investigate companies first so they know who they are dealing with. As a rule, I do not recommend buying probiotic supplements off the Internet, from companies you don't know because you may be dealing with people in other countries where quality control may be lacking. Keeping probiotic supplements in the refrigerator should increase their shelf life. Because some bacteria may be destroyed during the digestion process, using an enteric coated brand may improve the delivery of probiotics into the body.

Alpha-ketoglutarate

Alpha-ketoglutarate—or AKG for short—is a compound formed during the Krebs cycle. The Krebs cycle is one of our body's energy-generating metabolic pathways. If that sounds technical, think of it this way: every time you exercise aerobically—such as jogging, bicycling or walking—you are using the Krebs cycle to help power your muscles. AKG is also a precursor to the amino acid *glutamine*, which will be reviewed later in this book. It is well known that muscle tissue loss often accompanies recuperation from surgery.[268] This loss of muscle can decrease a person's strength and lengthen the time it takes people to return to their normal, daily activities. It turns out that when physicians inject AKG into someone who is recovering from surgery, they tend to lose less muscle.[172] Other names that can also refer to AKG is *alpha KG* and *2-Oxoglutaric acid.*

AKG and Exercise

Very intense exercise is a stress that, like surgery, can lead to the loss of muscle proteins. Because of this fact, some fitness enthusiasts and athletes are attracted to AKG supplements in the hopes that it will help them preserve muscle as it does following surgery.[172] The problem with this is that *injections* of alpha-ketoglutarate have been shown to help reduce muscle loss. Limited evidence exists for orally-taken AKG supplements in healthy people. Exercise can elevate ammonia levels in the body which might hinder exercise performance. Some people may use AKG because of research finding that it can reduce the toxic effects of ammonia. In theory, this might be good for exercisers although most of the evidence for this stems from giving AKG to people with kidney disease.[269] Very little exercise-related research currently exists on AKG supplements.

Side Effects and Concerns

AKG appears to be relatively safe in healthy adults. Currently there appear to be no known side effects or drug interactions associated with AKG supplements.

My Thoughts

While intravenous injections of AKG may be helpful to some people in the hospital, the advantage of orally taken AKG supplements in healthy individuals has not been adequately studied. Athletes are sometimes interested in AKG supplements despite a lack of good proof it improves exercise ability.

Androstenedione

Androstenedione (pronounced "an-dro-steen-die-own") is actually a hormone. It is mostly made within the adrenal glands of your body with smaller amounts also made in the testes of men and ovaries of women. Androstenedione (or "andro" for short) first gained widespread public attention when baseball player Mark McGuire admitted that he used it during the 1998 baseball season when he hit an unprecedented 70 homeruns. After that, andro quickly became one of the most popular products of its time because people believed it would make them stronger and more muscular. The rationale behind this belief was the commonly repeated mantra that androstenedione was just one chemical step from being converted to testosterone, the *king* of all male hormones. Thus, andro is thought by some to be a natural alternative to steroids. In the world of strength training and bodybuilding, anything that could be considered a safe, natural alternative to steroids would be like finding the holy grail of fitness. Other names that also refer to Andro include *4-androstene-3,17-dione* and *Androstene.*

Can Andro Raise Testosterone Levels?

While it is absolutely true that androstenedione really is only one chemical step away from being converted to testosterone, it is also true that it is just one step away from being converted to the female hormone, estrogen.[173] In other words, andro can go in either direction; one direction leads to testosterone while the other direction leads to estrogen. So, in theory, yes, andro can be converted to testosterone. In reality however, this doesn't seem to be happening and in fact, it appears that when men take it, andro is more often converted to estrogen.

For example, one study investigated the effects of 200mg of androstenedione in those who lifted weights.[174] The people who participated in the study were 50 men between the ages of 35 and 65. After three months of use it was found that 200mg of andro per day significantly raised estrogen levels. While this particular study also found that testosterone levels did increase by about 16% after the first month of andro use, by the end of the study, testosterone levels had returned to normal. Other research studies also confirm that andro will elevate estrogen levels in men.[175,176,177] In another study, 30 men between the ages of 19 and 29 used 100mg of andro once a day for two months along with a strength training program.[176] The results of this study indicated no change in testosterone levels but a significant increase in estrogen was observed. Another study found an 83% increase in estrogen in men after just two days of using andro at 200mg per day.[181] Based on these and other reports, it is now believed by most experts that andro raises estrogen levels in men.

Some nutritional alchemists try to get around andro's elevation of estrogen by combining it with other ingredients. For example, one study investigated if the combination of andro and supplements such as tribulus terrestris, DHEA, and saw palmetto would prevent andro from raising estrogen levels.[177] Unfortunately, the addition of these ingredients not only was ineffective at increasing testosterone but was also unsuccessful at preventing elevated estrogen levels. Interestingly, some research hints that these ingredients when combined with andro may be effective at raising testosterone levels in older men, who, because of age, may have lower levels of this male hormone.[178] However, estrogen levels were also elevated.

What Are Glandulars?

Before andro and all of the other pro-hormones out there today, there were glandulars. "Glandulars" is a generic term that basically means *ground-up* body parts. Ancient Chinese beliefs held that eating ground-up monkey testes could restore sexual vitality by raising testosterone. This is an example of seeing the bottom left-hand corner of the big picture. This practice doesn't work because there isn't a lot of testosterone in ground up testes to begin with and any elevation in testosterone from external sources shuts down our natural hormone production. Some websites sell ground-up brain parts like pituitary and hypothalamus glands in the hopes that these will boost testosterone production. Again, this won't work either because glands in general are nothing more than protein molecules, and just like any other protein that is eaten, they are quickly broken down to amino acids and never reach the blood as intact hormones. In other words, your body treats glandulars just like it would a turkey sandwich! In this age of mad cow and other diseases, I'd steer clear of glandulars. The bottom line is that they are an expensive—and gross—way to get your protein.

Can Andro Increase Strength?

Most of the scientific evidence conducted thus far indicates that andro does not increase strength in men—even when men participate in a strength training exercise program.[174,176,177,180,181] This may also mean that andro does not help people run faster, jump higher or enhance any amateur or professional sport-related performance. Most of the studies to date have used between 100-300mg of androstenedione per day. Whether or not using more than this amount would have a different effect is unknown.

Can Andro Decrease Body Fat?

Andro seems to strike out again on the matter of decreasing body fat. Thus far the studies conducted have not found that andro reduces body fat or alters the amount of fat to muscle in the body.[46,174,176,177,180]

Andro and Heart Health

Many of the studies conducted have found that andro *lowers* HDL levels. HDL is also known as "good" cholesterol because it removes excess cholesterol from the blood and thus reduces the risk of heart disease. Because HDL is a factor that helps protect the heart, anything that lowers HDL could, in theory, elevate the risk of heart disease. Some speculate that andro may raise the risk of heart disease by at least 10-15%.[179] At this point nobody is certain how much andro causes or contributes to heart disease, but the fact that it lowers HDL levels should be a significant concern for anyone who experiments with this compound.

What about Androstenediol?

Androstenediol is a hormone-like compound that is similar to androstenedione and thought in some circles to be more potent than androstenedione. However, some research notes that androstenediol is not only ineffective at raising testosterone levels but also raises estrogen, lowers HDL (good cholesterol), increases LDL (bad cholesterol) and produces no changes in strength.[174] Until more is known, assume that the side effects for androstenedione also apply to androstenediol.

Side Effects and Concerns

Androstenedione is not without risks. The almost universal finding that andro lowers HDL levels makes its long term use a possible contributor to heart disease. Those individuals who have heart disease, elevated levels of cholesterol or other blood fats should not use androstenedione. Other side effects in men may include male pattern baldness, testicle shrinkage, decreases in sex drive and male breast enlargement.

Because of preliminary evidence that it may stimulate the development of prostate cancer, androstenedione should not be used by those who have a personal or family history of prostate cancer—or any cancer for that matter.[182]

Women who use androstenedione are theoretically also at risk for such undesirable side effects as male pattern baldness, facial hair and acne, to name a few. To date, androstenedione research has been conducted mostly on men. Thus, how this hormone affects women is unclear. There is preliminary evidence that depressed women may have higher levels of androstenedione.[183] Because of a lack of research, it is currently unknown if androstenedione supplements would worsen depression in women.

My Thoughts

The FDA recognizes andro as a steroid hormone and not a nutritional supplement and has sent warning letters to companies informing them to stop marketing it as a supplement or face criminal prosecution. Regardless, of whether it's classified as a hormone or a supplement, andro doesn't seem to make people stronger, improve sports performance or increase muscle-building testosterone levels. What andro does appear to do is raise estrogen levels and decrease HDL in men. So how did Mark McGuire hit 70 homeruns while using andro? Major League Baseball steroid abuse allegations notwithstanding, in my opinion, the bulk of this achievement stemmed from sheer talent and most importantly, hard work. No supplement or steroid will improve your athletic performance without hard work. As proof of this, I am reminded of an old TV news interview with Sammy Sosa who was also hitting unprecedented numbers of homeruns that year. When asked what supplements he used, Sammy replied, "a Flintstones vitamin." I've always been partial to the ones that looked like Betty Rubble myself...

Antioxidants

If you have ever used a nutritional supplement, chances are you have heard the terms *antioxidant,* along with its partner in crime, *free radical.* Antioxidants do not refer to any one nutritional supplement but rather to a variety of supplements, some of which you may already be using. So, for this reason, I would like to provide this overview of what antioxidants and free radicals are in case this stuff confused you in the past.

Personally, the very first time I ever heard the word antioxidant was as a 13-year-old boy watching the old *Merv Griffin TV Show.* Back then, one of Merv's most popular guests was a leather-clad, long-haired research scientist named Dirk Pearson. Every so often, Dirk would show up, talk about science, vitamins, reversing the aging process, and all sorts of really neat stuff that appealed to inquisitive, science-minded kids like myself. Centered prominently on Dirk's discussions of nutrition and reversing the aging process were these things called antioxidants and free radicals. Since those TV appearances so many years ago, free radicals and antioxidants have ballooned into two of the most frequently used words in the vocabulary of health and nutrition.

What are Free Radicals?

Let's travel back in time for a moment, back to high school biology class. Remember the atom? In a nutshell, atoms are some of the smallest things in the universe and everything—you, me, this book etc.—is made of them. Free radicals are atoms too. However, free radicals are a wee bit different than normal atoms, a difference that makes them capable of causing trouble for neighboring atoms and thus the cells of your body. Here's why: normal atoms have a specific number of electrons (negatively charged particles) that orbit around the atom much like the way planets orbit the sun. This keeps the atoms happy and stable. Free radicals are actually missing one or more of these electrons. While the loss of just a few electrons might not seem like much, this slight change makes free radicals radically different from normal atoms (Get it? Free radicals are *radically* different). As a result of this electron deficiency, free radicals roam around cells freely (Get it? Free radicals roam around our cells *freely*) looking for electrons to make them, once again, complete.

Free radicals, if you ask me, are very rude things, because when they run into some unsuspecting atom, they literally bump into it, take what they want—in this case, electrons—and leave without even asking! It's this *wham-bam thank-you-ma'am* chemistry of free radicals that makes them so potentially dangerous. This is because when a free radical steals an electron from another atom, the atom which lost the electron, now *becomes* a free radical! The original free radical in this story is now happy because it has an electron to replace the one it lost, so it is no longer considered a free radical. However this *new* free radical—tortured soul that it is—now roams around looking for an electron to replace the one that was stolen from it!

Maybe I have an overactive imagination but all this stuff seems to me like some weird sub-atomic Count Dracula tale where the free radicals are the vampires and the unsuspecting atoms and molecules from which they *suck* electrons, are their victims, who, like the victims of vampires are doomed to roam the night looking for new victims.

OK, all kidding aside, free radicals are serious business because if a free radical bumps into a crucial piece of cellular machinery—like, say, a DNA molecule—tragic consequences may result. For example, suppose a free radical steals an electron from an atom which is part of your DNA (DNA is your personal software program that has all the directions needed for you to live). Suppose further, that the area of DNA which was damaged by the collision with the free radical contained the instructions needed by your cells to make copies of themselves. While all cells need a way to make copies so they can replace cells that become worn out, an outcome of a collision with a free radical might result in our cells not knowing how to stop the copying process. This might result in cancer! While the development of cancer from free radical attack is possible, it is speculated that free radicals may play roles in all sorts of different conditions ranging from wrinkles and cataracts to diabetes and maybe even the very aging process itself.

What Do Antioxidants Do?

Basically, the word oxidation means the same thing as the word *rust*. Just as metal rusts, so, too, would we if left to nature. Therefore, in a sense, anti-oxidants literally prevent the *rusting* of our bodies. Antioxidants do this by *donating* or giving their electrons to the free radicals. When they do this, they neutralize the free radicals and prevent them from doing any damage. Personally, I like to think of antioxidants as the *Henny Youngmans* of biology. It's as if they say to the free radicals "take my electrons, please!"

Antioxidants and Free Radicals 101

1. Free radicals *steal* electrons from neighboring atoms and molecules and in the process disturb normal cell operations.

2. Free radicals, by disturbing normal cell operations, are thought to contribute to disease. So, free radicals are usually thought of as the *bad guys*.

3. Antioxidants neutralize free radicals from doing harm. Thus, antioxidants are usually thought of as the *good guys*.

Antioxidant Supplements

Some vitamins, minerals and other compounds also act as antioxidants. Some of the more popular examples of antioxidant supplements are vitamin C, vitamin E, green tea, and the mineral selenium to name a few.

Examples of Antioxidants

Vitamins	Minerals	Phytonutrients	Other Classes
Vitamin E	Magnesium	Lycopene	SOD
Vitamin C	Selenium	Beta Carotene	Ginkgo
Vitamin A	Zinc	Lutein	Coenzyme Q_{10}

The theory behind using these supplements is that they help support your body's natural free radical defenses. This might mean that your body would have even greater protection from free radical attack because the antioxidant supplements you consume would *throw themselves on the grenade,* so to speak, to save you. This sounds plausible and some research finds that antioxidant supplements may help. In reality, though, the role of antioxidants in disease prevention is controversial.[270] There is evidence that antioxidants may help decrease the risk of some diseases and syndromes and there is also some evidence that they don't. This is a complicated issue to say the least. Some of the factors that make this difficult to figure out include the type of antioxidant used, the amount of antioxidant used, how long the study lasted and the subjects used in the study (animals, bacteria, people, etc.). Altering any of these or other factors could result in studies coming to different conclusions.

Another thing to consider when interpreting evidence for antioxidants is whether or not the research was conducted with supplements or food that contained the antioxidant in question. Many times a nutrient—antioxidant or not—is used in supplements because of research finding that when people consumed a particular food, they benefited somehow. For example, lutein, lycopene, and beta carotene are all found in supplements mostly because of research that finds beneficial effects may occur when we eat foods that contain these ingredients. As a rule, food and supplements are not the same thing and as we will see later with the case for beta carotene, this line of thinking may have disastrous consequences.

Do People Who Exercise Need Antioxidant Supplements?

Antioxidants are often marketed to people who exercise. The reason for this is that exercise increases the production of free radicals in the body. Thus, in theory, taking an antioxidant supplement might help protect you from free radical damage during and after exercise. Depending on one's level of physical activity, there may be a case for this but for the moment, this question is open to speculation and there is little evidence that antioxidant supplements are better than eating healthy foods. Another issue to consider is that our bodies also have their own antioxidants that increase naturally when we exercise. So, do exercisers need additional antioxidants? Time will tell as more research is done. Regardless, a quality multivitamin and a healthy diet, containing adequate protein, carbs and fats and rich in fruits and vegetables is sage advice for everybody who works out.

Can Antioxidants *Make* Free Radicals?

One of the things that makes the waters murky is the possibility that under some conditions, antioxidants may actually *cause* the formation of free radicals—the very things that antioxidants are supposed to prevent. This is sometimes referred to as the *pro-oxidant* effect of antioxidants. You see, any antioxidant has the potential to produce free radicals under the right conditions (or wrong conditions, depending on how you look at it).[184] Also, it is almost impossible to control the conditions under which antioxidants might produce free radicals. So, loading up on antioxidants might result in the production of billions of free radicals. In theory, years of creating free radicals from high-dose antioxidant supplementation might overwhelm the body and result in the progression of disease. The big problem with this is that we don't fully understand the conditions which might lead an antioxidant to generate free radicals. We also don't know the implication that this might have in terms of our long-term health. Different health problems may react differently to long-term mega-dosing with antioxidants. Some ailments may be helped while others could be made worse. This is a very controversial area and all of the answers are far from resolved. This is however an issue that you should be familiar with because it is rarely mentioned.

Are Free Radicals Always Bad?

While we normally tend to think of free radicals as the "bad guys", this is not always so. For example, our immune systems can use free radicals to destroy invading microorganisms. Free radicals are also indispensable in making energy from food. It is only when free radicals get out of control that they tend to do damage.

My Thoughts

Antioxidants and free radicals are concepts that nutritional supplement users need to be familiar with. There is no doubt that antioxidants play integral roles in the maintenance of health and wellness and that in excess, free radicals can do us harm. There is also little doubt that antioxidants are not the only players in the game. It would be nice if we had all the answers as to how this subtle dance between antioxidants and free radicals really affects us but, at least for the moment, it seems that the more we learn, the more questions we have. While summaries of these topics can be found on various websites, few tend to give more than the usual surface treatment that antioxidants are *good* and free radicals are *bad*. My hope is that you come away from this discussion with an understanding that things are not always as simple as they may seem.

Aristolochic Acid

Aristolochic acid (pronounced a-ris-toh-LOH-kee-ic acid) is a compound found in some plants that have been used in Chinese medicine for almost a thousand years.[230] In supplements, aristolochic acid is usually touted to help decrease weight, improve sex drive, stimulate the immune system and help regulate the menstrual cycle.[46] It is unlikely that you will find aristolochic acid in any stores in the US because the FDA has standing orders to seize any products that contain this herb because it is deemed unsafe. However, because of possible Internet purchases, you may encounter it inadvertently. Other names that also refer to this herb include *Aristolochia auricularia, Virginia snakewood,* and *birthwort.*

The Food and Drug Administration has concluded that aristolochic-acid-containing supplements are not safe for human consumption because they may cause kidney failure.[231] In the early 1990s at least 100 people at a Belgium diet center developed kidney failure after taking supplements containing aristolochic acid.[232] Others in Great Brittan and France have also developed kidney failure after using aristolochic acid products.[232] In some individuals kidney dialysis and kidney transplants were required. In still others, people died. In addition, aristolochic acid is also known to be a potent cancer causing agent.[233,234,235,236] In animals, aristolochic acid is associated with cancers of the kidney, bladder, stomach, lung, and cancers of the lymphatic system (lymphoma). In humans it is associated with cancers of the bladder, ureter and kidney.[46] Aristolochic acid is deemed a human cancer causing agent by the World Health Organization.[234]

Side Effects and Concerns

As was mentioned previously, aristolochic acid is thought to promote the formation of cancer and be toxic to the kidneys. It is not safe for human use. Because of its toxicity, it is not used in any supplements in the US.

Other Names That May Indicate Aristolochic Acid		
• Birthwort	• Virginia Snakeroot	• Texas Snakeroot
• Long Birthwort	• Snakeroot	• Virginia Serpentary
• Pelican Flower	• Serpentaria	• Snakeweed
• Sangrel	• Pelican Flower	• Red River Snakeroot

My Thoughts

The risks are too great to even consider using supplements containing aristolochic acid. Many countries including Germany, Japan, Belgium, Great Britain, Australia, France, Venezuela and Egypt have banned the sale of aristolochic acid. In America, the FDA does not permit aristolochic acid to be incorporated into nutritional supplements and does its best to prevent the importation of this compound into the US.

Arginine

Arginine is a non-essential amino acid, which means your body has the ability to make arginine on its own. Food sources of arginine include dairy products, meat, chicken, fish, nuts, and even *chocolate!* Arginine is also referred to as *L-arginine*, where the "L" refers to the fact that the arginine molecule is *left-handed*. In fact, all of the muscle-building amino acids in the body are left-handed. For this reason, you are likely to see the letter L displayed on all amino acid supplements. On supplement labels, arginine is usually referred to as just that—arginine. Most other terms that refer to this amino acid also include the word arginine which makes recognizing it pretty easy.

Arginine and Growth Hormone

Arginine used to be popular among bodybuilders and other fitness enthusiasts because it was felt that this amino acid could stimulate the release of growth hormone, one of the hormones involved in making muscles bigger. Unfortunately, the research on this subject finds that the amounts of arginine in most supplements do not result in the release of significant amounts of growth hormone. While very large doses of arginine may result in a small increase in growth hormone, it might also be accompanied by such unwanted side effects as bloating, cramping and diarrhea. In addition, it's never been demonstrated that any small, transitory increase in growth hormone that might result from a large dose of arginine has any impact on muscle size or exercise performance. So, based on the majority of clinical evidence, arginine supplements used for the purpose of increasing growth hormone levels are probably useless.[186]

What About Ornithine?

Ornithine is another nonessential amino that the body makes as it needs it. Ornithine, is actually created when arginine is metabolized and was once thought to act synergistically with arginine to boost growth hormone and testosterone levels. The majority of research however does not show that ornithine, alone or in combination with arginine, confers any significant increases in anabolic hormone.[762]

Arginine and Heart Disease

Arginine is a hot topic among researchers who find that when used along with traditional medications, it might help improve congestive heart failure—a type of heart failure where fluid builds up around the heart, reducing its ability to function properly.[187,188] This may be due in part to arginine's role in the production of nitric oxide (NO), a gas that is made in the body which expands blood vessels. Studies have used between 6-20 grams of arginine over the course of the day for heart disease.[46] Because it can alter blood pressure, arginine should not be used without medical supervision.

Angina refers to heart-disease-related chest pain and occurs when the heart does not get enough oxygen. Angina can occur at rest or during physical exertion. Some research finds that arginine may help decrease the symptoms of some forms of angina as well as reduce those symptoms during physical exertion.[189,190] Studies of arginine for this purpose have used between 3-5 grams spread out over the course of the day.

Other evidence also hints that arginine may help people with intermittent claudication.[198] Intermittent claudication is a syndrome common to those with heart disease where pain is felt in the legs when walking. The pain sometimes subsides during rest.

Arginine should not be used in place of traditional heart disease therapies and individuals with medical issues should consult their physician before using arginine because of possible drug interactions.[191]

There is little evidence that arginine prevents heart disease from developing in the first place.[199,200] That being said, some healthy people may use low-dose arginine as part of their daily supplement regimen for this very reason.

Arginine and Muscle Wasting

Arginine, along with the nutritional supplements HMB and glutamine, have shown some promise at increasing muscle mass and preventing muscle decay associated with HIV infection and cancer.[192,193] Collectively, these supplements are found in the patented product, Juven®, made by Metabolic Technologies, the maker of HMB.[194] Currently it is unknown how arginine, along with HMB and glutamine, cooperate to bring about these effects, although it is thought by the manufacturer that the combination of arginine with glutamine promote protein synthesis and boost the immune system while HMB decreases muscle wasting.[194] So far, the combination of these nutrients has mostly been tested on those with HIV/AIDS and cancer. Little research has been conducted on healthy individuals. Readers should also see the HMB section of this book for more information on this topic.

Arginine and Sex

As was mentioned previously, arginine is involved in the production of nitric oxide (NO), which is a gas that helps expand blood vessels, a process technically called *vasodilatation*. When blood vessels are expanded, more blood moves into an area. In men, erections are due in part to the vasodilatation of blood vessels in the penis. Arginine, given at a dosage of 5 grams per day has been studied with some success in men who have erectile dysfunction.[195] For this reason, arginine is likely to be incorporated into some *male performance enhancement* supplements.

Before the men reading these words start getting excited (no pun intended), they should be aware that not all studies find that arginine is effective at treating erection problems.[196] Everybody is different and erectile dysfunction is a complicated issue that may result from a variety of physical, medical and psychological causes. There is also some evidence that hints that arginine may be most effective in men who have low levels of nitric oxide to begin with.[196] The only way to know your nitric oxide level is to get it tested by your doctor. In addition, it should be remembered that just because arginine might expand blood vessels, does not guarantee it will act on the blood vessels of the penis. Thus far, the sexual-aspect of arginine supplementation has been studied mostly in men. Arginine's effects on women's sexual responsiveness are open to speculation.

Arginine and Migraines

About 28 million Americans suffer from migraine headaches. Preliminary evidence suggests that the combination of arginine and the pain killer ibuprofen may help alleviate some forms of migraine headaches.[197] More research is needed to determine optimal dosages and how effective arginine alone is at impacting migraines.

Arginine and Senility

Because arginine may help expand blood vessels via its role in nitric oxide production, some speculate that it may help alleviate some forms of dementia. While the amount which might prove optimal is still being investigated, at least one study has found positive results with 1.6 grams of arginine per day.[201] Because of the possibility of arginine interacting with various prescription medications, those with senility or their caretakers should speak with their family physician before using arginine. Currently there is no evidence that arginine improves memory in healthy persons or makes people *smarter*.

Arginine and Recovery from Surgery

A few studies find that arginine may help quicken recovery time following surgery by boosting the immune system, reducing the number of after-operation infections and improving the healing of wounds.[201,202,203] Most studies with positive findings on these issues have combined arginine with essential fatty acids and RNA supplements. The contribution of arginine itself requires more study.

Side Effects and Concerns

Arginine is generally considered a safe supplement with few side effects in healthy adults. Because it may be attractive to people with special needs or conditions, a few caveats should be exercised when using this supplement.

In theory, arginine may reduce blood pressure. Because of this possibility, individuals who are using medications to treat high blood pressure should use arginine with caution. Arginine combined with high blood pressure medications might result in blood pressure decreasing too much.

Arginine is likely to be an ingredient in sexual enhancement nutritional supplements. People who are using Viagra or any other similar prescription drug should consult their physician before using arginine or supplements that contain arginine. While little information is available, when used together, they may drastically reduce blood pressure.

Some people may use the amino acid lysine to treat flair-ups of herpes simplex virus infection. Emerging research suggests that arginine might counteract this positive effect of lysine.[204]

My Thoughts

While research is ongoing, arginine may hold promise for some people with heart disease when combined with traditional medications. Studies also show that arginine, along with glutamine and HMB may also improve the quality of life of some afflicted with cancer and HIV. Arginine might also benefit some men who suffer with erectile dysfunction; however, it is not a miracle cure and it probably would not significantly improve the sex drives or performance of healthy individuals.

ATP

When you ate your breakfast today, you probably consumed some variety of carbohydrates, fats and proteins. These foods supply you with the energy you need to continue to live and to perform all of your daily activities. However, a concept that is not often mentioned is that before this can happen, the energy contained in food must be transformed into a type of energy that our bodies can use. For human beings, ultimately, this form of energy is called *adenosine triphosphate* or ATP for short. If this is difficult for you to imagine, let's think of it another way. If you were to drive your car up to an oil field in Texas and fill your gas tank with the stuff that is oozing out of the ground, your car would undoubtedly seize up and die. Before your car can use the oil coming out of the earth, it must be transformed into gasoline. ATP is like your *gasoline!* There is energy contained within the chemical bonds that hold the ATP molecule together and when those bonds are broken, energy is released—and that is the energy that you use! Every activity you can think of—walking the dog, washing the car, jogging, lifting weights, getting up at 3AM to go to the bathroom, keeping your heart beating—is powered by ATP. Because ATP is crucial to all types of physical activity, it is sometimes marketed as a nutritional supplement touted to improve exercise performance.

ATP and Exercise

Because ATP supplies energy to the body and powers all of our activities, some theorize that if we consumed more ATP we would have more energy. This extra energy in turn would help us run faster, lift heavier weights etc. This sounds plausible but the problem is that there isn't much proof that it works.[344] When taken orally, ATP seems to be broken down in the digestive system so it probably doesn't enter the body as intact ATP.[344] Enterically coated ATP, which has an extra thick outer coating allowing it to pass through the stomach undigested, might in theory be a better delivery system to get ATP into the body. However, preliminary research finds that enterically coated ATP does not raise blood levels of ATP.[344] Some research has noted that ATP supplements might produce a small increase in the amount of weight that could be lifted while performing a bench press with an exercise machine.[344] The dosage of ATP used in this study was 225 mg. This is interesting however more research should be conducted to verify these results, determine the optimal amount of ATP which might be best and most importantly, to see if ATP supplementation might help athletes and weightlifters who exercise with barbells and dumbbells as opposed to machines.

Medical Uses of ATP

When ATP is injected into the body, it may help improve some medical conditions. For example, when someone has cancer or other serious illnesses, they often suffer from a muscle wasting syndrome called *cachexia*. Several studies show that intravenous ATP therapy can help improve body weight and appetite in people afflicted with this condition. [341,342,343] It is unknown whether orally-taken ATP supplements would also have these effects.

Side Effects and Concerns

ATP supplements seem to be well-tolerated in healthy adults. Because ATP can be metabolized to uric acid, theoretically, people with a history of gout should avoid ATP supplements. To date, little peer-reviewed studies have been conducted on oral ATP supplements.[344]

My thoughts

The majority of research conducted on ATP has looked at intravenous injections of this compound and not orally taken ATP supplements. Studies do show that when given intravenously, ATP may help some medical conditions but this does not necessarily mean oral supplements would show similar results. With respect to exercise, if ATP supplements do work, results might be best obtained by professional or Olympic athletes as opposed to the other 99% of us. Every so often, I see ATP supplements touted as being better than creatine for improving exercise performance. The rationale is that since creatine helps make ATP during high intensity exercise, why not just skip creatine and use ATP instead? The flaw in this reasoning is that creatine, (unlike ATP) when taken orally, can be used by the muscles. And, there are tons of studies showing that creatine works. While the early exercise research is interesting, I'd hold off on ATP supplements until more studies are completed.

Bee Pollen

Bee pollen is a type of bee food. Bees collect pollen from flowers that they land on. In the beehive, bee pollen, along with honey is consumed by bees as nourishment. Historically, bee pollen has been advocated for almost everything; however, the top two reasons in recent years have been anti-aging and improvement of athletic performance. Other names that might also refer to bee pollen include *Buckwheat Pollen*, *Maize Pollen* and *Pine Pollen*.

Bee Pollen and Exercise Performance

Bee pollen has been advocated for years as an *ergogenic aid*—something that can enhance exercise ability. That being said, multiple studies do not find that bee pollen improves strength, speed, power or improves exercise performance.[205,206,207]

Can Bee Pollen Improve Energy Levels?

It's often claimed that bee pollen improves energy levels and helps get people through long and stressful days. Despite testimonials and Internet advertisements, there is no good scientific proof that bee pollen gives people more pep. Bee pollen contains carbohydrates, protein, vitamins and essential fatty acids.[271] The amounts of each of these in bee pollen though is less than that found in food. If you are a healthy person eating a healthy diet that includes carbohydrates, proteins and fats, bee pollen is unlikely to augment your energy levels.

Can Bee Pollen Reverse the Aging Process?

Absolutely not! No studies have found that bee pollen makes people younger. Bee pollen is not the fountain of youth and claims that it is should be viewed with a healthy dose of skepticism.

What About Royal Jelly?

Royal jelly gets its name from the fact that it is the food that only queen bees eat. Nurse bees make royal jelly, which is a mixture of mostly water with some protein, fats and vitamins.[209] Because queen bees have a much greater lifespan than worker bees, royal jelly is sometimes touted as a supplement that can help people live longer. However, there is extremely little scientific evidence that royal jelly reverses, slows or stops the aging process in humans. One preliminary study has found that royal jelly may extend the average lifespan of mice by about 25%, probably by reducing damage to genetic material.[210] However, this is just one study and there is a big difference between a mouse and you! Another study has also noted that royal jelly might lower cholesterol levels in persons with high cholesterol.[211] If this appeals to you, remember that there is far more evidence showing that regular exercise and weight loss also lower cholesterol levels. As with bee pollen, royal jelly can cause allergic reactions which, in susceptible people, may require immediate medical attention.[212]

Side Effects and Concerns

In healthy persons, bee pollen is unlikely to produce any serious side effects. Persons who have allergies to pollen or who are allergic to bee stings should avoid bee pollen because it may cause allergic reactions. Anaphylaxis, which is a severe, potentially life-threatening allergic reaction, is also possible in susceptible individuals.[208]

My Thoughts

I just don't see any reason why anyone should need to supplement their diet with bee pollen. The studies to date do not show that bee pollen improves exercise ability and the claims that it reverses the aging process or makes people live longer are simply ridiculous. Neither bee pollen nor royal jelly has clinically been shown to alter any disease state. While it is possible that bee pollen contains nutrients and/or factors that may one day be found to impact human health, at this point, all claims are speculative. As such, it's probably nest to wait for more research.

Beta-Carotene

Beta-carotene (β-carotene for short) is a member of the carotenoid family of phytonutrients and is a precursor to vitamin A. In other words, the body can convert β-carotene to vitamin A as it needs it. Because vitamin A has known toxic side effects when used in excess, β-carotene is usually taken to be a safer alternative because the body only uses what it needs. Your multivitamin probably contains β-carotene for this reason. β-carotene is found in a variety of foods such as carrots, sweet potatoes and broccoli to name a few. As a general rule, if the fruit or vegetable is yellow, orange or green, it contains carotenoids and probably β-carotene. Another name that sometimes is used to refer to β-carotene is *Pro-vitamin A*.

β-carotene and the Eyes

Some studies find that β-carotene may take part in helping reduce the incidence of age-related macular degeneration (AMD). This is a condition of the eye where a portion of the retina (called the macula) becomes damaged as we get older. This can result in a partial or total loss of vision.[286] Some evidence suggests that 15mg of β-carotene, combined with vitamin E and zinc may reduce not only the risk of AMD but also slow its progression in people already afflicted with this condition.[287] This effect may be related to the antioxidant properties of β-carotene and/or its unique interaction with both vitamin E and zinc. The addition of zinc to this combination seems crucial because no improvement in AMD is observed when β-carotene and vitamin E alone are administered.[288] Interestingly, there is also evidence that finds less AMD in people who have high intakes of food that contains β-carotene—yet another good reason to eat your fruit and veggies.[289]

β-carotene and Sunburn

In some countries β-carotene is incorporated into supplements designed to reduce sunburn. Truth be told, there is some evidence suggesting that β-carotene, along with other carotenoids and vitamin E may reduce sunburn in some fair-skinned people.[290] Two problems with this are that not all studies uphold this effect and so far, this has not been a particularly popular area of research.[290,291] Another issue to consider is people thinking they are impervious to sun damage if they use these nutrients. This is not true and in fact, the evidence is clear that β-carotene, alone or in combination with other nutrients does not prevent skin cancer or other sun-related damage.[292,293] The best protection against sun damage is to limit exposure to the sun and to use a sun screen with an SPF number in the double digits.

B-carotene and Heart Disease

Heart disease is the number one killer of Americans. Because less heart disease is generally seen in people who eat diets high in fruits and vegetables and because β-carotene is a component of these foods, some speculate that β-carotene supplements might reduce the risk of heart disease. Unfortunately, this does not appear to be so. When β-carotene was given to healthy men and women for years, their rate of getting heart disease is no different than other men and women who didn't use β-carotene supplements.[285,299,300,301] When given to people who already have significant amounts of heart disease, β-carotene likewise is ineffective at slowing its progression.[302] Furthermore, if you smoke and have had a heart attack, there is worse news—β-carotene supplements (20mg per day) appear to increase your risk of having another heart attack by as much as 43%.[303]

The bottom line of all of this is simple: if you want to reduce your risk of heart disease, don't smoke (or quit if you do smoke), eat healthy (plenty of fruits and vegetables), drink moderately, reduce stress and exercise 20 to 60 minutes at least 4 times per week.

β-Carotene and Cancer

Beta carotene is an antioxidant, a substance which neutralizes the formation of free radicals. Hundreds of studies over the years have found that people who eat a wide variety of fruits and vegetables get less cancer, heart disease and other degenerative conditions.[285,294,295] Since β-carotene is contained in many fruits and vegetables, it was assumed that β-carotene might be the protective force behind these foods. To test this theory, studies were conducted in the 1990s to see if β-carotene could protect against cancer. Large numbers of people were given both β-carotene supplements (20mg per day) and vitamin E supplements (50mg per day) for several years and told to go about their normal daily lives.[296,297] In the end, β-carotene did not reduce the risk of getting uterine cancer, skin cancer, bladder cancer, pancreatic cancer, thyroid cancer, brain cancer, colon cancer or lung cancer. One very interesting outcome of these studies, however, was that smokers who used β-carotene supplements had almost a 30% *higher* rate of lung cancer than those not receiving β-carotene supplements.[285] For this reason, smokers are highly discouraged from using β-carotene supplements. In contrast, eating foods that contain β-carotene, does not increase the risk of lung cancer in smokers. If you are not consuming a healthy diet, preliminary evidence hints that β-carotene (when combined with vitamin E and selenium) may reduce the risk of stomach cancer in malnourished Chinese individuals.[298] This most likely would not apply to most Americans. In other words, if you have the money to buy β-carotene, vitamin E and selenium supplements, you also have the money to buy food and are most likely not malnourished.

Side Effects and Concerns

Aside from turning your skin orange if you use too much of it, for the most part β-carotene seems pretty safe in healthy, nonsmokers.

In smokers, β-carotene appears to increase the risk of lung cancer when used long-term in supplements containing 20 milligrams. Whether or not less than 20 mg also has this effect needs more study. Smokers are highly advised to consult with their physician before using β-carotene supplements. Fortunately, obtaining β-carotene naturally from food does not increase lung cancer risk in smokers.[304]

My Thoughts

Honestly, I've never been a fan of using individual nutrients like β-carotene as cure-alls to promote health or reduce disease risk. β-carotene is a prime example why I feel this way. People thought β-carotene would stop them from getting cancer. Studies find not only does β-carotene not reduce cancer risk but actually raises the risk of lung cancer if you smoke! Beta is the second letter of the Greek alphabet. Nutrients are sometimes labeled in order of their discovery with alpha being first, beta being second and so on. Whenever you see a nutrient listed as alpha, beta, gamma etc. this is usually a tip off that many different types of the nutrient exist. In fact, there are hundreds of carotenoid molecules of which β-carotene is only one. Studies find that people who eat fruits and vegetables get less cancer, heart disease, etc. It appears that it is the unique interaction of β-carotene, with all of the other known (and unknown) nutrients in food, in addition to other healthy lifestyle habits that are responsible for these effects. If you're a smoker and looking to reduce your cancer risk, quitting smoking will do this better than any supplement.

Beta Glucans

Beta glucans are essentially fancy sugar molecules that act as parts of the cell walls of bacteria and yeasts. These compounds are sometimes used to address issues of high cholesterol while others may use them to treat more serious problems like cancer. Other names which also refer to beta glucans include *beta-1,3-D-glucan*, *Gifolan* (GRN), *Lentinan*, *Schizophyllan* (SPG), and *PGG-Glucan*.

Beta Glucans and the Immune System

Some research suggests that beta glucans appear to have antiviral and antibiotic properties. When injected, beta glucans seem to stimulate the immune system by promoting the release of immune chemicals and enhancing the number of different types of immune cells.[280,281] Beta glucans might also reduce the risk of infections following surgery.[284] It seems that beta glucans don't directly attack microorganisms but rather kick the body's defenses in the butt to help them battle the attacking invaders better. Whether oral beta glucan supplements have the same effects on the immune system needs more study.

Beta Glucans and Cholesterol

Beta glucans contain both soluble and insoluble fiber.[279] It is thought by some that the soluble fiber components of beta glucans are responsible for the cholesterol-lowering effects of oats.[283] Since oat fiber has been shown to lower cholesterol levels, would beta glucan supplements also show this effect? Some investigations have found that the answer is yes.[279,282]

In one study, the use of 15 grams of yeast-derived beta glucans per day was found to modestly reduce cholesterol in men who had high cholesterol levels.[279] With respect to oat-derived beta glucans, the FDA now allows oat-containing products to make the claim that they are heart healthy if they contain 0.75g of soluble fiber per serving.[283] Three grams of oat fiber per day, combined with a low cholesterol, low saturated fat diet, is thought to be the least amount needed for the cholesterol-lowering effect to occur.[283]

Beta Glucans and Cancer

Some research finds that when used alongside conventional cancer treatment, beta glucans may prolong survival time of people with some forms of cancer.[272,273] The beta glucans called *lentinan* and *schizophyllan* are two of the most studied types for this purpose.[275,276] The types of cancer which seem to respond most include head and neck cancer and cervical cancer.[275,276] Because of evidence like this, beta glucans are sometimes used by people with cancer. A problem however arises when it becomes known that most of the research stems from beta glucans that were *injected* into the body.[272] The evidence for orally-taken beta glucan supplements is scant at best. Another issue complicating the use of beta glucan supplements for cancer is the fact that they do not seem to be absorbed very well when taken orally.[274]

Beta Glucans and HIV

Preliminary evidence hints that beta glucans may enhance various facets of immunity in people who have HIV.[277,278] As with cancer mentioned previously, most of the research is on intravenously administered beta glucans. Oral supplements of beta glucans have little evidence as to their efficacy for HIV. Those with HIV should see their physician for the most up to date information on this topic.

Side Effects and Concerns

Orally used beta glucan supplements appear to have relatively few negative side effects in healthy people. Intravenous injections of beta glucans may be accompanied by fever, joint and lower back pain, and hypertension (or hypotension), to name a few.[277]

People who receive new organs often must use anti-tissue rejection medications to suppress their immune systems. If they did not take these medications, the person's immune system would attack the new organ, as it normally would a bacteria or virus! In theory, beta glucan supplements might be inappropriate for people who have received new organs because they might cause organ rejection. Currently, there are no reports of this scenario occurring but caution should be exercised because of the seriousness of this situation.

My Thoughts

The evidence seems clear that injections of various beta glucans may be effective at stimulating the immune systems of some individuals. As for oral beta glucan supplements, those that are well made are unlikely to cause any serious side effects in healthy people. One problem with supplements though is that they may not be absorbed very well. If you are con-sidering using beta glucan supplements, ask the maker of the product to produce published peer reviewed studies attesting to absorbability and effectiveness.

Bitter Orange

Bitter orange is the extract from the bitter-tasting Seville orange, a citrus fruit that contains a substance called *synephrine*. Chemically, synephrine *looks* like the active ingredient in ephedra—ephedrine.[11] So, synephrine and ephedrine are almost like *kissing cousins!* Bitter orange is one of the ingredients that is often included in "ephedra-free" weight loss supplements.[16] Those who eat oranges usually get some bitter orange in their diet but this is probably much less than is in supplements containing this compound. Other names that refer to bitter orange include *Citrus aurantium, Aurantii Pericarpium, Seville Orange, Sour Orange,* and *Green Orange.*

Bitter Orange and Weight Loss

Previous studies have noted that the herb ephedra is moderately effective for short-term weight loss.[17] Ephedra, though is a controversial herb that some companies may shy away from because of possible negative side effects. Because synephrine (which is in bitter orange) is chemically similar to ephedrine—the active ingredient in ephedra—it makes sense that it would be used as an alternative in weight loss supplements. The science on this issue though is limited, so for the moment, it's difficult to say whether bitter orange is effective for weight loss or not.

One issue that is not often talked about is that at least six different types of bitter orange are known to exist. They are called *ortho bitter orange, meta bitter orange* and *para bitter orange.* Each version has both a right-handed and left-handed form (technically called D or L), which brings the total to six. All versions differ slightly in their chemical structure and most likely have different properties, side effects, etc. Some bitter orange supplements indicate the version they contain but others may not. Supplements may contain any of these types as well as various combinations of each. Studies of the effects of bitter orange may also not specifically state which type they are using. This is a problem because side effects as well as beneficial effects attributed to one type may not necessarily be the same for the other types. Because little is known about each version, it's difficult to say which would be most effective for weight loss or for that matter, whether any of them would.

Side Effects and Concerns

Many experts agree that bitter orange can elevate both blood pressure and heart rate.[13] These responses are most likely increased when bitter orange is combined with other stimulants like caffeine. For this reason, bitter orange is not appropriate for those with blood pressure, heart or kidney problems.

In children, there is some evidence that convulsions and death may occur after bitter orange use.[12] Pregnant women should avoid bitter orange during pregnancy. Pregnant women should not be attempting to lose weight unless directed to by their physician.

People with glaucoma should avoid bitter orange supplements because it may worsen symptoms.

Bitter orange extracts may also contain another chemical called *octopamine* which is similar in chemical structure to adrenaline. Octopamine can constrict blood vessels and increase heart rate and probably acts synergistically with synephrine.

Fair-skinned individuals may experience an over-sensitivity to sunlight.[14]

Some evidence finds that bitter orange may inactivate enzymes that are responsible for the elimination of toxic substances.[15] In theory, this means bitter orange may result in the build-up of toxins that are normally flushed from the body. Bitter orange might also inhibit the normal metabolism and breakdown of some medications, causing them to build up in the body to dangerous levels.[15]   Individuals who are taking medications for depression, such as *MAO inhibitors* should exercise caution when using bitter orange because of the possibility that they may add together and spike blood pressure to dangerous levels.[13]

My Thoughts

Bitter orange is found in many "ephedra free" weight loss supplements because it kind of looks like ephedra. While that may be, because of the lack of good human research, its difficult to tell how effective it might be. Weight loss is a complex problem and that's one of the reasons people have trouble in this area. Regardless of its effect on weight loss, its chemical similarity to ephedrine means that bitter orange probably has many of the same negative side effects associated with ephedra. This possibility is highlighted on bitter orange-containing supplements themselves when you read the cautions listed on their labels.

Black Cohosh

Black cohosh is an herb which grows in North America and was first introduced to early European settlers by the American Indians. These days the main reason people use black cohosh is to relieve menopause symptoms; the herb, is also sometimes rumored to treat sore throats, arthritis and even used by some as an insect repellent! The scientific names for black cohosh are *Actaea racemosa* and *Cimicifuga racemosa*. Other names that also refer to black cohosh include, *Black Snakeroot*, *Bugwort*, and *Baneberry*, to name a few.

Black Cohosh and Menopause

Some studies have found that black cohosh may be of modest help at reducing hot flashes and other symptoms associated with menopause and premenstrual syndrome (PMS).[333] However, not all research shows positive results. In addition, most studies agree that at least a few weeks of continued use is needed before any reduction in symptoms is noticed.[334] Because of its apparent ability to reduce some symptoms of menopause, it has been generally believed that black cohosh has estrogen-like activity in the body. This theory is still being investigated and debate continues as to how black cohosh works. A good amount of research on black cohosh has been on a specific formula called *Remifemin®*, which is marketed by GlaxoSmithKline.[335] Other products might work similarly.

Black Cohosh and Osteoporosis

Osteoporosis is a disease where bones become brittle and break easily. Estrogen is needed to help keep bones strong. Because black cohosh is thought to possess estrogen-like qualities, some feel this herb may help osteoporosis. Currently, this is a controversial issue and the impact of black cohosh for this purpose is unknown.

Side Effects and Concerns

While black cohosh is generally well-tolerated in healthy adults, there are a few issues that should be remembered when using this herb.

Black cohosh should not be used by pregnant women because of concern that it may stimulate contractions of the uterus.[336] In theory, this might result in miscarriage. Likewise, black cohosh should not be used by lactating women because of its unknown effects on the baby.

There is some evidence that black cohosh may cause hepatitis, a liver condition.[337] The probability of hepatitis occurring seems small when compared with the millions of women who have used black cohosh. Until more is known, it may be wise to have periodic liver function checkups while using this herb. In theory, black cohosh might interact with other supplements like Kava and niacin which also may affect liver function.

Some evidence suggests that black cohosh may increase the toxicity of some chemotherapy drugs.[339] People with cancer should inform their physicians and oncologists about black cohosh as well as other supplements they may be using.

What is Blue Cohosh?

Blue cohosh (also called *Caulophyllum thalictroides*) is an herb that stimulates contractions of the uterus and may be used by some midwives to induce labor. While controversial, some evidence suggests that this practice may cause heart failure to occur in the baby who is about to be delivered.[340] Blue cohosh can also interact with a variety of medications such as those to treat hypertension and diabetes.[10] Don't confuse blue cohosh with black cohosh; they are not the same.

My Thoughts

Evidence suggests that black cohosh holds promise for many women suffering from menopausal and possibly PMS symptoms. The active ingredients seem to be in the root of the plant, so the roots should be the main constituents of black cohosh supplements. As for black cohosh causing liver problems, this is a contro-versial topic.[338] It is not yet known if black cohosh alone is the culprit or if it is the interaction of black cohosh with other supplements taken by the individual.

With respect to black cohosh helping osteo-porosis, the evidence is weak. Because bone loss starts around the age of 35, many medical professionals are viewing osteoporosis as a syndrome that starts in youth and not old age. Thus, building strong bones when we are young is probably the best defense against osteoporosis. Those who are now experiencing osteoporosis and want an alternative solution for this condition are better served by performing weight-bearing and strength training activities on a regular basis and consuming adequate amounts of calcium and vitamin D.

Blue-Green Algae

Blue-green algae is a general term that refers to a variety of microscopic sea-dwelling plants. One of the most popular types of blue-green algae is *spirulina*. Other names for this supplement can include *Spirulina platensis*, *dihe*, *BGA* and *tecuitlatl*.

Blue Green Algae and Weight Loss

While rumors that blue-green algae might help people shed excess pounds date back to the 1980s, it is surprising that there is little peer-reviewed research showing that it works. At least one study from the mid-1980s failed to find that spirulina promoted weight loss in humans.[22] Blue-green algae does contain the essential amino acid *phenylalanine*, which some have speculated may play a role in appetite suppression.[9] While intriguing, it is not universally accepted that phenylalanine supplementation suppresses appetite—or even if it did, what the optimal dosage might be. Blue green algae is a good source of protein with spirulina containing about 65% protein.[16] However, it can be more expensive than more traditional foods like tuna, chicken, turkey, etc., making it not a wise choice for those on a budget.

Side Effects and Concerns

Side effects from blue-green algae are relatively minor; that being said, it is important to deal only with reputable manufacturers in light of evidence that some products may contain pollutants like mercury, lead and arsenic.[10]

Another source of concern is the possible contamination with blue-green-algae-derived toxins. One such toxin, *microcystin*, can cause liver damage.[19] One study investigating microcystin contamination in blue green algae supplements found that 85 out of 87 products tested were found to contain microcystin with 72% of these products containing levels that were higher than that deemed safe for long-term human consumption.[20] Blue-green algae is not recommend for those with kidney or liver disorders. Theoretically, children may be at greater risk of microcystin toxicity because of their lower body weight.[21]

Currently, there are no known drug interactions with blue-green algae and it appears relatively nontoxic when not contaminated by harmful substances like mercury, arsenic, lead or microcystin. Because blue-green algae contains the amino acid phenylalanine, it should not be used by persons who have a genetic syndrome called *PKU*, where individuals are unable to break down phenylalanine.

My Thoughts

Blue-green algae is a good—albeit relatively expensive—source of protein that contains all essential amino acids that the body needs. Little testing has been done on any effect blue-green algae may have with respect weight loss in humans. Combining blue-green algae with a low calorie eating program theoretically might help weight loss. Whether adding blue-green algae to a low calorie diet would promote greater weight loss than consuming a low calorie diet alone is not currently known. Because of impurity issues, consumers should deal only with reputable manufacturers. Those with existing medical concerns such as PKU should consult their physician before using blue-green algae supplements.

Boron

Boron is a trace mineral that is required in small amounts in the body. Food sources of boron include broccoli, grape juice, peanuts, apples, potatoes, wine and milk to name a few. Currently, there is no recommended dietary allowance (RDA) for boron and its main function in the body remains a mystery. Boron supplements at one time were popular among people who exercise and others may use it for additional reasons as well. Other names that might also refer to this mineral include *boric anhydride* and *borate*.

Boron and Exercise

Boron was popular among bodybuilders and strength trainers in the early 1990s because of research finding that boron supplements raised levels of testosterone. Higher testosterone levels might lead to bigger, stronger muscles. The problem with this becomes obvious when one discovers that this research investigated how boron supplements affected older, postmenopausal women who were eating a boron-deficient diet.[237,244] The last time I checked, there were major differences between bodybuilders and other athletes (male or female) and postmenopausal women, consuming a diet low in boron. All kidding aside, the majority of studies conducted since the 1990s *do not* find that boron elevates testosterone levels in men or women who consume a nutritionally sound diet and who exercise regularly. In fact, boron supplements have even been tested on male bodybuilders with no effect.[238,239,240] One possible negative outcome of using boron supplements may be the elevation of estrogen levels in men.[242] The dosage used in this study was 10 milligrams per day, which is much more than most Americans get from a healthy diet. It has not been determined how this possible rise in estrogen affects muscle mass or exercise performance. So, for the bodybuilders and other fitness enthusiasts reading these words who have used boron in the past, I wouldn't lose any sleep over this. The main thing to remember is that boron is highly unlikely to improve testosterone levels in men and even more unlikely to improve strength or exercise performance. As long as you are eating a healthy diet, your boron levels are most likely fine and boron supplements are not needed.

Boron and Seniors

Preliminary evidence finds that boron may improve some aspects of brain function in seniors as well as improve their ability to perform tasks requiring manual dexterity.[243]

At least one study also finds that boron may increase bone density, making it a possible effective co-treatment for osteoporosis when used alongside other more traditional therapies.[245] While this particular study looked at athletic females and not seniors, in theory, one might speculate that it may act similarly in older adults. Currently though, there is little research on how boron affects osteoporosis. Still, for these reasons boron may be an ingredient in some supplements geared toward improving osteoporosis.

Boron and Arthritis

Osteoarthritis is a form of arthritis in which the cartilage between bones wears away. This results in pain as bone grinds against bone. Some research has found favorable results on osteoarthritis-related pain following boron supplementation.[241] This investigation used 6 milligrams of boron, which is far more than the 1.5 to 3 milligrams a day typically consumed by Americans.[137] Thus, based on these preliminary results, boron may be included in some supplements touted to reduce osteoarthritis pain. So far, there is no evidence that boron helps rheumatoid arthritis.

Side Effects and Concerns

Boron appears to be relatively safe for healthy adults especially when consumed in amounts normally found in food. Because boron may elevate estrogen levels,[242] women who have cancers (such as breast cancer or ovary cancer) that are sensitive to estrogen levels should not use boron supplements unless approved by their physician. Women who are undergoing hormone replacement therapy should likewise also use caution when using boron supplements.[242]

In theory, boron might also be inappropriate for men with prostate cancer; this is controversial however in light of research noting that boron is associated with a reduced risk of prostate cancer.[246]

The maximum upper tolerable intake (UL) for boron is 20 mg per day. Keeping daily boron intake below this level will reduce the chance of problems arising.

My Thoughts

Most of the research on boron that finds positive effects is several years old. I'd feel better if I saw some newer studies published on this stuff. Boron is almost certainly a nutrient that plays roles in many valuable functions in the body. Currently though, nobody is sure what those roles are. I am admittedly not a fan of loading up on any one mineral or vitamin, because of the possibility that it might crowd out other important nutrients. Until newer studies are published on boron, it's probably wiser if you get this nutrient from apples and other boron-containing foods and leave the supplements alone for now.

Branch Chain Amino Acids

Amino acids are often called the building blocks of proteins because proteins are made of amino acids. The branch chain amino acids (BCAAs) are *leucine*, *isoleucine* and *valine*. They are called *branch chain* because these amino acids have *branches* in their molecular structure, that sprout out from the side, kind of like branches of a tree. This makes BCAAs look slightly different from other amino acids. While BCAAs have been typically promoted for improving exercise ability, they may be used for other reasons as well.

BCAAs and Exercise

Among people who work out very intensely, fatigue is an almost inevitable part of their exercise routine. Over the past several years, the idea of supplementing with the branched chain amino acids has become a recognized practice among some fitness enthusiasts as a way of warding off the mental fatigue that occurs during long duration exercise. The theory behind using branch chain amino acids is based on the fact that they compete with the amino acid tryptophan for entry into the brain.[55] Since tryptophan is needed for the production of serotonin, a brain chemical that causes fatigue, high levels of BCAAs might prevent tryptophan from gaining entry into the brain and thus may limit the production of serotonin. This in turn might decrease mental fatigue and improve exercise performance. The theory sounds plausible; but, research is mixed. Some investigations find that BCAAs may improve performance[215,216] while other studies show no effect.[213,214] Most of the research on BCAAs has involved aerobic exercise such as long distance running. Very little research examining how BCAAs might affect those involved in weight lifting has been conducted.

Some have speculated that BCAAs may impair exercise performance by decreasing coordination due to high levels of ammonia that are created when BCAAs are broken down.[219,220] To date, little research has looked at BCAAs for impairment of athletic coordination. For athletes whose sport requires balance, agility or coordination this may be something to consider until more is known.

BCAAs may also decrease the breakdown of muscle proteins during exercise.[220] While this may be true, so, too, will eating carbohydrates. Obtaining BCAAs from food is relatively easy. Three ounces of tuna fish appear to supply all of the BCAAs needed to prevent muscle breakdown during exercise.[229]

Tyrosine

The amino acid, tyrosine also appears to inhibit the entry of tryptophan into the brain and as such may also be used by athletes to help reduce exercise-induced fatigue. Some research does hint that tyrosine may help mental alertness. This might help improve exercise performance for those participating in marathons and other grueling types of physical activity. The effect of tyrosine on exercise is still under study. For the moment, tyrosine has not been adequately field-tested in athletes to see whether theory holds up to reality.

BCAA and Appetite

Some research suggests that diets that are deficient in BCAAs may somehow dull the sensation of taste. Replacing BCAAs (particularly leucine) in the diet seems to reverse this situation and stimulate appetite. Indeed, there appears to be some support for this. Emerging research finds that BCAAs may improve appetite in malnourished elderly individuals. In one study, the addition of 12 grams of BCAAs per day stimulated appetite after only one month and resulted in greater amounts of calories and protein being consumed.[217] Other research finds similar results when BCAAs are consumed by cancer patients.[218] If this holds true for all people, in theory, BCAAs might also be of benefit to those with eating disorders like anorexia nervosa.

BCAAs and the Brain

Tardive dyskinesia is an uncontrollable movement disorder that sometimes results in individuals who use certain psychiatric drugs. Several studies exist showing that BCAAs can improve the symptoms of tardive dyskinesia.[221,222,223] It is believed that BCAAs better stabilize various brain chemicals which cause the uncontrollable movements that are characteristic of tardive dyskinesia. Studies finding positive results generally use about 200 mg taken three times per day for several weeks. People using prescription medications for Parkinson's disease should not use BCAAs without the OK from their doctor. Theoretically, BCAAs might reduce the effectiveness of Parkinson's medications.[224]

Mania is a mental disorder where individuals experience high levels of energy and restlessness.

Other criteria that may accompany manic episodes include difficulty concentrating, impairment of judgment and rational thinking as well as having unrealistic beliefs about one's skills, abilities or status. Some evidence hints that a beverage containing 60 grams of BCAAs may be an effective short-term way to reduce mania in some individuals.[226] BCAAs do not seem to be a cure for mania and further investigation is needed to verify these conclusions before concrete conclusions can be drawn.

BCAAs and Diabetes

Research finds that leucine (which is a BCAA), when taken with carbohydrates, may promote the release of insulin.[225] If this is true, then using leucine with insulin or other anti-diabetes drugs might theoretically lower blood sugar levels. This might negatively affect exercise performance. Until more is known, diabetics and those prone to hypoglycemia should consult their physician before using BCAAs. It should be stressed that leucine is not a cure for diabetes and should not be used in place of traditional diabetes therapies.

BCAAs and ALS

Amyotrophic lateral sclerosis (ALS), also known as Lou Gehrig's disease, after the famous baseball player who was afflicted with the syndrome, is a neurological disorder marked by progressive destruction of brain areas responsible for voluntary movement. While no cure for ALS exists, some with this condition may be tempted to experiment with BCAAs because of research finding that BCAAs may improve ALS symptoms.[227] Other research however finds that long term use of BCAAs do not improve ALS symptoms and may actually make the condition worse by interfering with lung functioning.[228] People with ALS should consult with their physician before experimenting with BCAAs in amounts greater than that found in food.

Side Effects and Concerns

BCAA supplements appear to be safe for the majority of healthy people, with nausea being one of the most commonly noted side effects.

Because high intakes of BCAAs might lead to an increase in ammonia production, this might theoretically increase fatigue levels felt during exercise or at rest.[220]

Diabetics should monitor blood sugar levels during BCAA use to minimize the possibility of hypoglycemia.[225] In theory, the use of high potency BCAA supplements might be inappropriate for persons with liver or kidney disorders because the elevation of ammonia from BCAA metabolism might overstress these organs.

My Thoughts

Currently, the debate continues as to whether BCAAs result in significant improvement in aerobic exercise performance. While exercisers continue to be large purchasers of BCAAs, the finding that these amino acids may stimulate appetite is very interesting and deserving of more research. If corroborated, BCAAs may benefit people with eating disorders as well as seniors, who sometimes don't eat as much as they should, and those with various diseases where muscle wasting and weakness are of concern.

Caffeine

Caffeine, a stimulant found in coffee, teas, soft drinks and even some medications has been around for centuries. Aside from being a morning pick-me-up for millions of coffee drinkers, caffeine is also used for a variety of purposes including weight loss and to boost exercise capacity.

Caffeine and Weight Loss

When consumed, caffeine stimulates the central nervous system, which in turn causes the release of the hormone *adrenalin*. Adrenalin, in addition to making people more alert, also increases the release of fat from fat cells where it can be burned for energy. Because of this, caffeine is sometimes incorporated into nutritional supplements touted for weight loss. That being said, caffeine's ability to move fat from fat cells to be burned for energy is probably mild at best. Thus, caffeine is often combined with other supplements to produce a greater effect.[24] In addition, because of caffeine's ability to enhance alertness, it is probably also used in weight loss supplements because of the assumption that a more alert person is more likely to perform more exercise. Greater amounts of exercise performed equal more calories burned, which, in turn, theoretically means, more weight loss. The optimal amount of caffeine for weight loss is not well known. Caffeine seems to have no direct effect on appetite so it is unlikely to decrease your desire to pig-out Saturday nights at your favorite restaurant.

Caffeine and Grapefruit

Some research suggests that grapefruit can enhance the stimulatory effects of caffeine in the body. Because of this you may notice grapefruit incorporated into some caffeine-containing weight loss supplements. When considering supplements containing grapefruit, you should remember that not all evidence shows grapefruit increases caffeine's effects.[31] In addition, other research finds no increase in resting metabolism occurs when grapefruit is combined with caffeine.[32] Those who are using medications should consult their physician before consuming grapefruit or grapefruit-containing supplements because negative interactions between grapefruit and various medications are well known.

Caffeine and Exercise

A number of studies have noted that caffeine can extend the time it takes to totally exhaust oneself during exercise lasting 30 minutes or less in duration.[419,420,421,422] Caffeine may also improve reaction time. Thus, a cup of coffee, diet soda or a caffeine supplement may be part of an athlete's pre-race preparation.

It is currently unknown how caffeine impacts those who take part in strength training-type activities, with some studies finding that it helps while others showing no effect.

While the optimal amount of caffeine needed to improve performance is open to debate, some experts have advocated that caffeine be consumed about one hour prior to exercise at a dosage equal to 5 milligrams per kilogram of body weight.[55] Since there are 2.2 pounds in a kilogram, this would equal 340 mg for a 150-pound athlete. People who are not accustomed to caffeine (and thus more sensitive to its effects) may be able to get by with less.

How caffeine works is not well understood but it is thought that it functions through multiple avenues including stimulating the nervous system and promoting the release of calcium, which helps muscles contract more forcefully.

One criticism of the use of caffeine for exercise improvement is that most of the research has been conducted under strict laboratory settings. In other words, just because something works in the lab doesn't automatically mean it will work in the "real world".[55,418]

Caffeine Content of Common Beverages[423]	
Beverage	Average Caffeine Content (mg)
Coffee, brewed, 8 oz	135
Coffee, instant, 8 oz	95
Coffee, decaf, 8oz	5
Tea, 8 oz	50
Snapple iced tea, 16 oz	42
Green tea, 8 oz	30
Mountain Dew, 12 oz	55
Diet Coke, 12 oz	46
Coca-Cola 12 oz	35
7 UP and Diet 7 UP	0
Sprite	0

Caffeine and Headaches

Caffeine is an ingredient in some over-the-counter pain medications to treat headaches because it helps speed the absorption of the medication into the body as well as boost the effectiveness of the medication.[415] Food for thought; caffeine can be addicting and cutting back may also cause headaches.

Taurine

Taurine is an amino acid that is sometimes found alongside caffeine in some energy drinks and supplements. Some research suggests that taurine and caffeine may improve reaction time, as well as aerobic exercise performance.[832] Optimal amounts that might improve these issues require more study and those who experiment with taurine should start out with less than the recommended dose to see how they respond. Because of its effects on the heart, people with medical conditions—especially disorders of the heart, kidneys or blood pressure—should consult their physician before using taurine.

Side Effects and Concerns

Caffeine is relatively safe to use in healthy adults with usual side effects ranging from insomnia, anxiety and jittery feelings. Other side effects can include rapid heart beat (tachycardia), tremors and an increased desire to urinate. Thus, caffeine is not something that should be consumed before sleeping.

Very high intakes of between 3 and 10 grams of caffeine per day have been associated with death.[27] Fortunately, for the millions of us who begin our day with a caffeinated beverage, it would be difficult to obtain such high amounts normally and this shouldn't be a concern.

Because caffeine can promote the loss of calcium from the body, some have speculated that caffeine may be a risk factor in the development of osteoporosis.[416] So far, this is a debatable issue with no solid evidence one way or the other.[417] What can be said is that one or two cups of coffee or bottles of soda a day is unlikely to cause osteoporosis. Also, getting adequate calcium either from food or calcium supplements (along with exercise, of course) seems to offset any loss of calcium caused by caffeine.[417]

Since caffeine can elevate heart rate and blood pressure, people with heart, kidney or blood pressure issues should use caffeine sparingly, if at all.

My Thoughts

For many people, caffeine may be the real deal with multiple studies finding that it helps people exercise longer before total exhaustion sets in. This might be especially true for those who are unaccustomed to the effects of caffeine and who perform aerobic-type activities. Athletes training for the Olympics should check with their coach before using caffeine because high intakes are prohibited by the International Olympic Committee. With respect to weight reduction, caffeine seems to provide modest weight loss in the short run, especially in those who are not accustomed to its effects. This is one of the reasons why caffeine shows up so frequently in weight loss supplements.

Calcium

The mineral calcium is one of the most popular supplements in the US and is used by tens of millions of women every day because of substantial evidence that it can help off-set the ravages of osteoporosis. Milk and other dairy products are good natural sources of calcium. While osteoporosis is the main reason people use calcium, research is beginning to hint that this mineral may do more than help keep our bones strong.

Types of Calcium

There are several types of calcium available for those interested in increasing their calcium intake. When deciding which type of calcium supplement is best, consumers should be looking for *elemental calcium*. Elemental calcium is the form of calcium that is used by the body. The different types of calcium supplements each contain different amounts of elemental calcium. The table below lists the amounts of elemental calcium contained in some of the most well-known types of calcium found in supplements.

Elemental Calcium in Calcium Supplements

Calcium Type	Percent Elemental Calcium
Calcium Carbonate	40%
Calcium Citrate	21%
Calcium Lactate	13%
Calcium Gluconate	9%

As you can see from the table, calcium carbonate has the most elemental calcium with 40%. This means that 40% of the calcium in the supplement can be used by the body to help build bones and do other things that require calcium. This is why calcium carbonate is usually the most recommended form to use. As an added bonus, calcium carbonate also tends to be less expensive than its counterparts. Calcium citrate is the next highest, containing 21% elemental calcium followed by calcium lactate with 13% and finally by calcium gluconate which has only 9% elemental calcium. The greater the amount of elemental calcium in a supplement means you can take less to reach the recommended 1200-1500 milligrams per day.

How Much Elemental Calcium is in *Your* Supplement?

Some calcium supplements list the amount of elemental calcium that the supplement contains. Others may not. Figuring out the amount of elemental calcium your supplement has is pretty easy though. All you need to know is the total milligrams of calcium in the supplement, the type of calcium (calcium carbonate, etc.) and the percentage of elemental calcium that it contains. For example, suppose you had a calcium carbonate supplement that contained 600 mg per tablet. All you have to do is multiply the total milligrams of calcium (600 mg) by the percentage of elemental calcium, which in this case is 40%. In other words, 600 mg X .40 = 240 mg. So, there is 240 mg of elemental calcium in each 600 mg calcium carbonate tablet.

Calcium and Caffeine

Some research finds that caffeine intake of greater than 300 mg per day may be linked to greater bone loss.[104] This would be equal to consuming about 6 cans of caffeinated soda per day. Whether this means caffeine is linked to osteoporosis for everybody needs more study. Studies do link increased caffeine intake to more fractures in the elderly. More research is needed to determine if this effect also holds true in those who exercise and eat well. Also, not all studies find that caffeine intake results in bone loss. Those who consume caffeine should make sure they obtain enough calcium from foods and supplements as well as participate in regular physical activity to maintain bone mass.

What About Phosphorus?

Phosphorus is another mineral, which along with calcium helps keep bones strong. For this reason some calcium supplements may be fortified with phosphorus. Besides helping bones, phosphorus plays key roles in many other crucial processes needed to keep us healthy. However, phosphorus is found in a wide range of foods such as meat, chicken, eggs, milk, nuts, grains and even chocolate. Thus, a deficiency in this mineral is unlikely.

Calcium and Weight Loss

Calcium has found its way into the weight loss arena with published scientific studies showing that as calcium intake increases, weight loss also increases.[34] The research, while limited, so far indicates that only *dairy calcium*, such as from milk and yogurt, seems to promote weight and fat loss. Studies generally use 800-1000 mg of dairy calcium and combine this with a low calorie diet. Keep in mind that not all research shows that calcium helps, so this is not a magic bullet and individual weight loss results are likely to vary.[35]

Got Coral?

Coral calcium is a type of calcium that's derived from coral reefs. Currently very little published research exists to substantiate the claims of coral calcium supplements and it has not been adequately tested for its role in disease treatment or prevention. One study did note that coral calcium was a little better absorbed than calcium carbonate[37] but that doesn't mean it's going to help you live to be 140, ward off disease or make anybody a *skinny minny*. In addition, at least one test of coral calcium supplements noted the presence of low levels of lead in some brands.[41] Until more research is conducted, stick to calcium carbonate, calcium citrate and other more well accepted brands.

Side Effects and Concerns

Calcium is safe when consumed in foods that contain this mineral and when used in supplement form. A few things to consider when using calcium supplements are listed below.

Fiber tends to decrease the absorption of calcium. To lower the chance of this occurring, separate calcium supplements from high fiber meals by several hours.

Vitamin D enhances calcium absorption. See the section on vitamin D for more information on this vitamin.

Some steroid hormones, like prednisone, used for medical reasons, can cause bone loss and contribute to osteoporosis. Using these medications short term is unlikely to be a problem but long term use may be.

Some antibiotics may reduce the absorption of calcium. This shouldn't be a problem for short term use. Those concerned about this issue should first check with their doctor or pharmacist to see if their antibiotics interact with calcium and if yes, separate antibiotics and calcium supplements by a few hours to improve calcium absorption.

People who have under-active thyroid glands may use a drug called synthroid to help maintain their metabolism. When taken together, calcium carbonate may decrease the absorption of synthroid. This might result in people feeling tired. Separating their use by about 4 hours should avoid this possible interaction.

Besides causing cancer and many other diseases, smoking also increases the loss of calcium from the body, making it a risk factor for osteoporosis.

Sodium can increase calcium loss. New guidelines call for no more than 2300 mg of sodium be consumed per day. Those with high blood pressure, heart disease and other conditions should consume less sodium.

My Thoughts

When you start reading about all of the different uses calcium has in the body, it almost seems as though this mineral does everything! Calcium (along with exercise) is definitely a major player in the fight against osteoporosis. Of the different types of calcium available, calcium carbonate is the cheapest, making it an attractive option for those on a budget. Calcium citrate, while containing less elemental calcium, tends to be better absorbed.[105] Calcium is absorbed best in 500 mg doses or less. Thus, it's probably better to consume smaller amounts over the course of the day rather than one big dose. With respect to calcium and weight loss, remember, obesity and weight loss are complex issues that almost certainly involve multiple factors. If you are going to experiment with calcium to help shed a few pounds, I suggest adding a low-calorie diet and exercise program to your regimen to enhance any effects calcium may have.

Carbohydrate Blockers

Carbohydrate blockers (also called carb blockers or starch blockers) refer to supplements reputed to block the absorption of carbohydrates. The theory behind these supplements is that if the absorption of carbohydrates can be blocked or reduced, weight loss would occur. Carbohydrate blockers were a natural evolution of the fat blocker supplements which seemed all the rage during the late 1980s. Carb blockers are sometimes popular among people who subscribe to low carb diet philosophies as well as those who want to have their cake and eat it too—literally and figuratively!

Carb Blockers and Weight Loss

Carb blockers are usually reported to work by blocking or inhibiting an enzyme called *alpha amylase*, which breaks down sugar in the body. The theory goes like this: if you can block the enzyme that breaks down sugar, you prevent sugar from turning into fat. Nutritional supplements that are touted to block the alpha amylase enzyme usually contain an extract from kidney beans called *phaseolamin*. They may also contain other reputed fat burner supplements such as chromium.

Thus far, the evidence for carb blocker supplements is less than inspiring. Carb blockers received attention from the scientific community in the early 1980s. In one study published in the *New England Journal of Medicine*, carb blockers were found to be ineffective at preventing the absorption of carbohydrates in humans.[38] Another human study, from the early 1980s, also found carb blockers ineffective.[39] Carb blockers were also investigated during the early 1990s—again with less than spectacular results.[40] Thus far, the majority of research on these supplements finds the same thing–they don't work.

Side Effects and Concerns

Currently, little is known about carbohydrate blocker supplement side effects or how they interact with medications. In theory, people with intestinal or digestion problems should exercise caution until more is known.

My Thoughts

It's ironic that the most popular substance found in most carb blockers—phaseolamin—is itself derived from kidney beans, which contain carbohydrates. Regardless, most research finds that carbohydrate blockers would probably not make a significant dent in our waistlines. Many of the studies investigating carb blockers are several years old. It is possible that the preparations being marketed today are more advanced than their counterparts from the 1980s and 90s; however, with little research on them available, it is difficult to draw conclusions. My gut instinct is to keep working out, eat fewer calories and wait for more research.

Carnitine

Carnitine or *L-carnitine*, as it is also called, is an amino acid. Made in the liver and kidneys from the amino acids *lysine* and *methionine*, carnitine has a reputation as a fat burner because of its role in moving fat from fat cells to the mitochondria—the area of our cells where fat is broken down for energy. Essentially, carnitine is a fancy *taxi-cab* molecule. In other words, it takes fat to where it needs to go to be broken down. Thus, the theory behind carnitine as a fat burner is that if you had more carnitine, you'd have more taxicabs available to help with the fat burning process. Sounds interesting enough. So, is there any evidence that carnitine might help burn fat and promote weight loss?

Carnitine and Weight Loss

It appears that the reputation of carnitine as a fat burner stems from studies where carnitine was given to low-birth- weight babies who, as a rule, don't do a good job at making carnitine to begin with. Studies show that when given to low-birth-weight babies, carnitine enhances the breakdown of fat for energy.[42] With respect to adults looking to shed a few pounds, studies have generally been less than encouraging. One study investigated the effects of eight weeks of the combined effects of carnitine supplementation (4 grams per day) and aerobic exercise in 36 overweight women.[43] The results of this study showed no greater change in weight or fat loss compared to women who only exercised.

Another study looked at how the combination of carnitine and a low-calorie diet might impact weight loss.[44] This study also found no greater reduction in weight as compared to dieting alone.

Yet another investigation concluded that carnitine promoted fat loss in lab rats as well as aerobic exercise did when the carnitine was combined with choline and caffeine.[45] These results are opposite of another rat study that found that aerobic exercise was superior to carnitine.[424]

What Does the "L" in L Carnitine Mean?

Those who have used carnitine may have wondered what the letter "L" in the name of the supplement means. The letter L essentially means the molecule is *left-handed.* Yes that's right—just as there are left-handed and right-handed people in the world, so, too, are there left-handed and right-handed molecules! The letter L stands for the word *levorotory,* which is science-talk for "left-handed". You see, molecules can exist in two different forms—either right-handed or left-handed. These different forms are identical to each other with the exception that one molecule rotates light that is shined on it counterclockwise (to the left). The other form of the molecule, which is right-handed, rotates light clockwise—or to the *right.* The right-handed version of molecules is referred to as "d" or dextrorotary.

Carnitine and Exercise

Because of some evidence that carnitine supplementation may improve walking ability in those with heart disease,[110] some fitness enthusiasts use this nutrient to improve their exercise ability. So far the verdict on carnitine for this purpose is debatable. Some research shows that carnitine may delay fatigue and improve aerobic ability during exercise.[111,112] Conversely, other research shows no improvement following carnitine use.[113] Thus, it is not known if carnitine can improve exercise ability in healthy individuals. For those who wish to experiment with carnitine, exercise studies generally have used 2-4 grams per day with mixed results.

What is Acetyl L Carnitine?

Acetyl L carnitine refers to a supplement that has a slightly different chemical structure than the more traditional carnitine that most people may be familiar with. Acetyl L carnitine has been studied mostly to improve memory and help people with Alzheimer's disease. Research to date however is not encouraging. One study followed over 400 people with Alzheimer's disease for a year to see if acetyl L carnitine helped.[116] It didn't. This lack of effect was corroborated by the results of another year-long study which followed 229 people with Alzheimer's.[117] Likewise, little evidence exists to support the use for acetyl L carnitine for weight loss or improving exercise ability in humans.

Other Uses of Carnitine?

There is preliminary evidence that carnitine may help some medical conditions but it is too early to know for sure. For example, some research hints that carnitine may help some people with heart failure.[106,107] carnitine supplementation has also been shown to improve the walking ability of some individuals with heart disease.[110] Carnitine may also increase the amount of red blood cells in those who are experiencing kidney failure.[108] Preliminary research also hints that carnitine may help some children with attention deficient hyperactivity disorder (ADHD).[114] This research is ongoing. These are all serious conditions and self experimentation with carnitine for these reasons is not recommended.

Side Effects and Concerns

Carnitine is usually considered safe in healthy adults. Side effects from carnitine may include nausea, vomiting, abdominal cramps and diarrhea. Body odor has also been reported following carnitine use.

People with liver disease should avoid carnitine because of speculation that it may overtax the liver, resulting in a buildup of carnitine in the body.[115]

People who have hypothyroidism or those who are using synthetic thyroid hormone medications should consult their physician before using carnitine supplements. There is some evidence that carnitine may inhibit the action of thyroid hormone.[118]

One often-reported warning regarding carnitine is to avoid both the "D" and "DL" versions of this supplement. These refer to the *right-handed* version and mixture of the left and right-handed molecules, respectively. Using either the D or the DL version of carnitine has been associated with muscle wasting, weakness and fatigue as well as carnitine deficiency. To reduce any small chance of this occurring, deal only with established companies that you trust.

My Thoughts

In my book—literally and figuratively—carnitine just doesn't live up to its reputation as a major league fat burner. Taken as a whole, the majority of evidence appears to show that for adults looking to drop a few pounds (or several pounds for that matter) carnitine alone is unlikely to have much of an effect. As for carnitine improving exercise performance, based on the research available to date, one might speculate that if it works, its effects might be minimal and not noticed by most people. For those who want to try carnitine, you should know after a few months whether it is working or not.

Chitosan

Chitosan, also called *chitin*, is a carbohydrate-like fiber that forms the hard, exterior shells of crabs, lobsters and shrimp. Chitosan also forms the exterior skeletons of insects and is the reason that bugs make that "crunch" sound when you step on them. In America, people are usually attracted to chitosan because of the claim that it will promote weight loss. Supplements that contain chitosan are easily spotted because they usually contain the word *chito* somewhere in their name.

Chitosan and Weight Loss

The general theory of chitosan's apparent role as a fat burner goes this way: chitosan contains positive electrical charges that attract fat, which is negatively charged. This allows chitosan to bind up fat so it can be excreted from the body.[428] While some studies have found that chitosan may enhance fat excretion, most research to date seems to show no effect.[47,48,49,50] In fact, a recent review of the most well-done chitosan studies found that it did not significantly effect weight loss in humans.[425] One study did observe that chitosan may work better at promoting fat excretion when combined with vitamin C, but these outcomes were obtained from a study of people with Crohn's disease and may not be applicable to healthy individuals.[52]

Chitosan and Cholesterol

Some research finds that chitosan can lower cholesterol levels.[426] The effect of chitosan on cholesterol appears to be modest at best.[119] For the time being the use of chitosan for lowering cholesterol is controversial because not all studies find that it works.[120] People attracted to chitosan because of its cholesterol-lowering properties should keep in mind that other supplements have a stronger track record. For example, there is far more research for soy improving cholesterol levels than chitosan.

Side Effects and Concerns

Chitosan is usually considered safe in healthy adults with occasional diarrhea sometimes reported. In theory, because chitosan is derived from shellfish, there is some concern of allergic reactions following consumption of chitosan-containing products.[428]

Because of research showing chitosan can bind fat, another possible issue is that it may also hinder the absorption of the fat-soluble vitamins—vitamins A, E, D and K. In theory, chitosan might also block essential fatty acids from being absorbed.

Chitosan has been shown to increase the loss of calcium from the body.[121,122] This hints that long-term use of chitosan-containing products may increase the risk of osteoporosis. Currently though, this is speculation. Those using chitosan should consume adequate amounts of calcium and participate in regular physical activity to minimize any possible effects on bone loss that might occur.

Preliminary evidence also suggests that long-term use of chitosan may lead to arsenic poisoning.[123] This case report stems from one person and should be viewed with skepticism until more research is conducted.

My Thoughts

Personally, I am not impressed with chitosan for weight loss. It's important to remember that whether or not chitosan increases fat excretion from the body does not automatically mean it promotes weight loss. Remember, weight loss (and weight gain, for that matter) has much more to do with how many calories are eaten than how much fat is consumed. Americans are heavier than ever today in spite of the availability of hundreds of low-fat foods. Taken as a whole, the studies conducted to date show a trend that chitosan does not promote weight loss in healthy people.

The effect of chitosan on cholesterol levels is also debatable. Food for thought: there is much more evidence for exercise as a cholesterol-lowering agent than chitosan. For the healthy individual, chitosan seems relatively harmless for short-term use. At best, one might see modest weight loss if chitosan is combined with a reduced-calorie eating plan and exercise. At worst, it may cause you to spend more time sitting on the toilet while chitosan sucks some of the fat out of the food that you eat.

Chromium Picolinate

Chromium is a mineral that is involved in the utilization of sugars for energy through its actions on the hormone, insulin.[54] Chromium helps lower blood sugar because it functions as part of a molecule called *glucose tolerance factor* (or GTF). Basically what GTF does is *sandwich* itself between insulin and the insulin receptors on the surface of the cells in your body. It is in this way that chromium—as part of GTF—allows insulin to work better.[55] Occasionally chromium is called GTF but in reality the two are not the same. Chromium is a very important part of GTF, though.

Another name occasionally used is trivalent chromium (chromium III). This is to separate it from other, more toxic forms like *hexavalent* chromium (chromium VI)—made popular in the movie *Erin Brockovich*. Hexavalent chromium is employed in some industrial settings and not used in supplements because it can cause cancer and heart failure.[71]

Types of Chromium

Chromium Type	Description
• Trivalent chromium (chromium III)	Natural form. Used in supplements
• Hexavalent chromium (chromium VI)	Toxic. Causes liver, kidney and heart failure. Not normally found in supplements

Because chromium is not well absorbed by the body, some manufacturers combine this mineral with a compound which will enhance its absorption. For example, chromium picolinate is formed by attaching chromium to picolinate acid, a natural breakdown product of the amino acid tryptophan. Natural sources of chromium include beef, chicken, spinach and apples to name a few.

Chromium and Weight Loss

Since the late 1980s, chromium—especially its most popular dietary form, chromium picolinate—has enjoyed a success which has been almost unparalleled in the nutritional supplement industry, stemming from early research finding that in young animals, chromium might burn fat and build muscle.[55] Clinical studies do indeed exist showing that chromium supplements may do this; however, many of these studies have been criticized by researchers for various reasons. For example, some research showing that chromium burns fat and builds muscle arrived at these conclusions based upon less than accurate measures of body composition.[56] One of the most accurate tests to determine how much fat and muscle a person has is *underwater weighing*—a technique that involves weighing a person who is completely submerged under the water. Studies determining body composition by other methods have the possibility for greater levels of error. This may be what is happening with chromium because, taken as a whole, there are far more studies showing that chromium picolinate does not burn fat or build muscle in healthy adults.[57,58,59,60,61,62]

Chromium and Diabetes

Diabetics sometimes appear to have low levels of chromium and this may impact how well they deal with blood sugar. There is evidence that chromium picolinate supplements can reduce blood sugar and cholesterol levels in some people with type II diabetes.[61,63] Studies examining this issue generally use between 200 micrograms (mcg) to as much as 1000 micrograms divided up into several equal doses throughout the day. The effect of chromium on blood sugar is highly variable and doesn't appear to work for everybody. Also, when it does work, chromium may take a few months before results are noticed. Diabetics considering chromium should be reminded that this mineral is not a cure for diabetes. Some speculate that chromium may only work in those who have low chromium levels to begin with.[74] Diabetics should talk to their physician before experimenting with chromium to minimize any side effects which might occur.

Can Chromium Cause Weight *Gain*?

It is sometimes reported that chromium may not be appropriate for some individuals because of the possibility that it may promote not weight loss but rather, a *gain* in weight.[64] This caveat stems from an investigation of young, overweight women who were given chromium picolinate supplements. The dosage used was 400 micrograms—a level found in many chromium products. Some of the women in the study exercised while others did not. Following the study, it was found that chromium picolinate caused *weight gain* in the women who did not exercise. Those who combined chromium with exercise lost weight. The big questions are how significant is this effect and does it really occur? Unfortunately, little research exists to answer these questions or to substantiate these conclusions. If chromium does cause weight gain (and that's debatable), the effect is probably small. Regardless, until more is known, the take home message is that if you are going to use chromium supplements to aid weight loss, make sure you also exercise—just to be on the safe side.

Side Effects and Concerns

Chromium is safe when consumed at levels found in food. In healthy adults, chromium supplements are probably also safe when used short term.

Because chromium may lower blood sugar, diabetics should not experiment with chromium without first consulting with their physician. The use of both chromium supplements and insulin might cause blood sugar levels to decrease too much, producing a condition called *hypoglycemia*. Diabetics using chromium supplements should monitor blood sugar closely.

Chromium supplements should be avoided by persons with kidney disease. There is some evidence that chromium supplements may aggravate some forms of kidney disorders.[65]

There is conflicting evidence on the role of chromium and those who suffer from depression. Some research hints chromium may make symptoms of depression worse while other studies suggests it may help.[72,73] Those who suffer from depression or other mental illnesses should consult their physician and mental health professional first.

Since the 1990s there has been some concern that chromium picolinate might cause alterations (mutations) in the genetic material (DNA) of humans, which, in theory, might lead to diseases like cancer.[66] Since the initial reports, other research has also been published which hints that long-term exposure to chromium picolinate may not be healthy.[67,68,69,70] It is theorized that chromium picolinate acts negatively in the body by producing free radicals.[70] So far, the bulk of the evidence showing that chromium picolinate can be dangerous to DNA stems mostly from studies of isolated cells taken from animals and insects. To date, no strong evidence links chromium picolinate to cancer in humans. It is worth noting that it appears to be the picolinate acid in chromium picolinate that seems to be detrimental. Chromium by itself appears perfectly fine to use.

One disturbing outcome from an independent assay of the quality of chromium supplements was the discovery of small amounts of toxic, cancer causing *chromium VI* in one of the products tested.[76] This finding highlights the need to only do business with companies that you have investigated and trust.

Chromium Nicotinate

Chromium nicotinate is another form of chromium that is different from the more familiar chromium picolinate. Unlike chromium picolinate which is formed by the combination of chromium and picolinate acid, chromium nicotinate is made by combining chromium with the B vitamin, niacin. Another name for chromium nicotinate is *niacin-bound chromium*.

Chromium nicotinate, like other forms of this mineral, is usually marketed for weight loss. In the study mentioned above, where chromium picolinate was found to facilitate weight gain in young women, chromium nicotinate was observed to promote weight loss.[64] This effect appears to have been reinforced by the findings of at least one other study also observing that chromium nicotinate promotes weight loss in humans.[75] While these results are encouraging, more research should be performed before they are taken as gospel.

My Thoughts

According to the research at hand, chromium may aid in stabilizing blood sugar in some people with type II diabetes. In contrast, the studies to date appear to be overwhelming that chromium does not significantly burn fat or build muscle. For those who want to try chromium to help them lose weight, remember that downing a chromium supplement with a milkshake is unlikely to produce the results you seek. The effect of all supplements is of course enhanced when they are accompanied by a healthy lifestyle. In the case of weight loss, this means eating fewer calories and getting more regular exercise.

Coenzyme Q_{10}

A coenzyme is a substance that helps enzymes work better. Coenzyme Q_{10}—also referred to as "CoQ_{10}"— is actually a molecule that is found in every cell of the body. Because it is so abundant, this nutrient also goes by the name *ubiquinone* because it is said to be *ubiquitous,* or everywhere in the body.[146] Coenzyme Q_{10} plays a very important role in our ability to generate energy aerobically. In fact, some studies show that coenzyme Q_{10} can enhance the aerobic exercise ability in people with congestive heart failure.[147] Because of this, athletes may also use this compound because of a belief that it will help improve their exercise ability as well. Today, millions of people in Japan use coenzyme Q_{10} as part of their daily medical regimen to help treat symptoms of heart disease.

CoQ_{10} and Congestive Heart Failure

Congestive heart failure results when the heart becomes so weak that it can no longer pump enough blood to sustain normal activities. Evidence suggests that when used alongside conventional therapies, CoQ_{10} may help assuage some of the symptoms of this condition.[435,436,438] It is noteworthy however that not all investigations find that this nutrient works.[437,439] Studies generally use about 60 mg a day but because the degree of heart disease can vary from person to person, the wisest choice of action on this matter is for people to talk to their cardiologist—who is most likely very familiar with all of the research on CoQ_{10} and how applicable it might be to their specific condition.

CoQ$_{10}$ and Exercise

Because of the positive research on heart patients, coenzyme Q$_{10}$ is sometimes advertised to enhance aerobic exercise performance in healthy individuals. Little clinical evidence however supports the idea that coenzyme Q$_{10}$ produces the same beneficial effects in healthy people as it appears to in those with heart disease. For example, one investigation found no improvement in aerobic exercise ability in either younger or older men following six weeks of CoQ$_{10}$ supplementation at 120 mg per day.[148] Those involved this study were regular exercisers—the very people who are sometimes attracted to CoQ$_{10}$ supplements. Most studies of coenzyme CoQ$_{10}$ essentially find the same thing—that supplementation does not noticeably improve aerobic exercise performance in healthy people. In theory, coenzyme Q$_{10}$ may help healthy people in other ways that is not being measured by researchers, but that is speculation.

Studies investigating how coenzyme Q$_{10}$ affects people engaged in strength training are less numerous. This makes it difficult to determine if it helps these individuals or not. One study found that 150 mg of CoQ$_{10}$ per day for two months had no effect on the ability of middle-aged men to exert force using a *dynamometer*, a device that determines grip strength in the hands.[149] So, from this study, one might conclude that coenzyme Q$_{10}$ would have minimal effect on strength training performance. However, squeezing something as hard as you can with your hand is not the same as performing traditional strength training exercises.

Does Coenzyme Q_{10} Have Other Uses?

Besides its more traditional uses mentioned previously, people may supplement with this nutrient for a number of other reasons. These other situations are summarized below.

Cancer. For many years it has been known that people with a variety of cancers tend to have low levels of CoQ_{10} in their blood.[433] Preliminary research suggests that CoQ_{10}, when used alongside conventional cancer therapies and when combined with other supplements, may be effective against breast cancer.[434] Currently, there is no evidence that CoQ_{10} prevents cancer or that it is effective alone against cancer. Persons with cancer should consult their oncologist for the most up-to-date information on this aspect of CoQ_{10} research.

HIV Infection. Some studies suggest that 200 mg per day of coenzyme Q_{10} may be effective at improving the immune systems of those infected with HIV.[46,150] Unfortunately, few studies seem to exist, so it is difficult to determine how big of an impact, if any, CoQ_{10} has on the progression and symptoms of HIV infection. Individuals should consult their physician for the most current information on how CoQ_{10} impacts HIV.

High Blood Pressure. Preliminary evidences hints that CoQ_{10} may lower blood pressure in people with hypertension.[151,429] So far, studies have used between 120-200 mg spread out over the day.[151,429] In addition, it may take up to three months of continued use before blood pressure is lowered.[152]

Heart Attacks. Preliminary studies suggests that 120 mg of coenzyme Q_{10} may help prevent future heart attacks in some people who have already had a heart attack.[153] This may have something to do with the ability of this nutrient to elevate good cholesterol (HDL) levels while decreasing both total cholesterol and bad cholesterol (LDL).[46] Because, in theory, coenzyme Q_{10} may interact with a number of medications, persons who have had a heart attack should consult their physician before using this supplement.

Angina Pain. Angina refers to chest pain that is sometimes associated with heart disease. There is some evidence suggesting that 50 mg of coenzyme Q_{10} per day may reduce angina pain.[161] Most of the good research in this area is rather old which makes gauging its effectiveness difficult. Those interested in coenzyme Q_{10} for this purpose are encouraged to speak to their physician for the most up to date information.

Parkinson's Disease. Parkinson's disease is a brain syndrome that can effect movement. Some research suggests that coenzyme Q_{10} may slow the progression of this condition.[157] The optimal amount of coenzyme Q_{10} needed to improve Parkinson's symptoms is not clear but research hints it may be somewhere between 300-1200 mg per day.[157] Those with Parkinson's should see their physician for the most up-to-date information on this topic.

Diabetes. The results on how CoQ_{10} impacts diabetes are conflicting. Some studies find that coenzyme Q_{10} may help regulate blood sugar in those who have diabetes.[154] Other research, though, does not find any effect on blood sugar.[432] Studies finding positive effects have generally used about 150 mg of coenzyme Q_{10}.[155]

Fibromyalgia. Fibromyalgia is an arthritis-type syndrome where people essentially feel tired and achy most or all of the time. Some research hints that a daily dose of a combination of 200 mg of coenzyme Q_{10} and 200 mg of ginkgo may be of some benefit to those with fibromyalgia.[159] Currently, there is little research supporting the use of coenzyme Q_{10} alone for fibromyalgia. See the section on ginkgo for a review of this supplement.

Gum Disease. Some research hints that coenzyme Q_{10} may alleviate gum disease. Most of the research on this topic dates back to the 1970s and there is not total agreement that coenzyme Q_{10} works for this purpose.[158]

Wrinkles. CoQ_{10} is sometimes found in cosmetics. The reason for this is that CoQ_{10} is an antioxidant and antioxidants neutralize free radicals. Free radicals, aside from their implication in diseases like cancer and heart disease, also contribute to wrinkles. So, the thought is that by neutralizing free radical damage to the skin, coenzyme Q_{10} might help reduce wrinkles. Some research does hint that exposure to ultraviolet light reduces the levels of coenzyme Q_{10} and vitamin E in the skin.[160] Might this reduction in CoQ_{10} contribute to wrinkles? Maybe. Aside from being more expensive, cosmetics containing CoQ_{10} couldn't hurt and might help.

> ## Coenzyme Q_{10} and Statin Drugs
>
> Statins are a class of drugs that lower cholesterol levels and are used in the treatment of heart disease. Statins work by interfering with the production of cholesterol. It turns out that statin drugs also lower CoQ_{10} levels.[621] Giving CoQ_{10} supplements to people using statins has been shown to maintain CoQ_{10} levels.[622] That being said, does this mean that people who use statin drugs should supplement with CoQ_{10}? Maybe, but the answer to this question is not fully known. Because research is ongoing, this is something to discuss with a physician.

Side Effects and Concerns

Coenzyme Q_{10} appears to be generally safe with multiple studies reporting no harmful side effects in adults. Regardless, there are some things to consider before using this supplement. Because of lack of evidence one way or the other, some of the areas listed here are either speculation or are extrapolations based on what we currently know about this supplement.

Because there is some evidence suggesting that coenzyme Q_{10} can lower blood pressure, individuals who are using medications to treat high blood pressure should consult their doctor before using coenzyme Q_{10}. Theoretically, the combination of coenzyme Q_{10} with high blood pressure medications could lower blood pressure too much.[431]

People who are undergoing radiation or chemotherapy should talk to their physician before using coenzyme Q_{10}. There is some evidence that CoQ_{10}—as well as any antioxidant for that matter—may make it harder for radiation or chemotherapy to destroy cancer cells.[430] This makes sense when you consider that both of these therapies destroy cancer by creating free radicals. Antioxidants—including CoQ_{10}—neutralize free radicals. So a worst possible scenario could be that the use of antioxidants might decrease the effectiveness of these therapies.

Those using blood thinner medications should exercise caution when using coenzyme Q_{10}. Chemically, coenzyme Q_{10} *looks* like vitamin K—a vitamin which plays a crucial role in the blood clotting process. Theoretically, the use of coenzyme Q_{10} might work against blood thinner medications.[162] Research thus far has not shown that coenzyme Q_{10} interferes with Coumadin, a blood thinner medication.[163] To be safe, consult with a physician first if using blood thinners.

Diabetics should monitor their blood sugar levels closely if they use coenzyme Q_{10}, in light of some evidence suggesting that this supplement may lower blood sugar levels. The use of coenzyme Q_{10} along with insulin or oral diabetic medications might have an additive effect and lower blood sugar more than is desired.

My Thoughts

Coenzyme Q_{10} has been known to exist since the 1950s and is now used for a variety of reasons. The strongest evidence seems to be for those suffering from congestive heart failure. Other claims for CoQ_{10} probably have simpler, less expensive, solutions. For example, take gum disease. If you're looking to keep your gums healthy, don't smoke, brush and floss daily, and see your dentist regularly. While undoubtedly essential for life, the usefulness of CoQ_{10} supplements by healthy people needs more study before anybody can say for certain whether it's needed or not.

Colostrum

If you are a guy—especially an unmarried guy—you probably have never heard of colostrum. Colostrum is a milky fluid that is made in the breasts of women shortly after they give birth. Because colostrum is full of antibodies, proteins, fats, carbohydrates and other growth factors, it makes a great "first meal" for newborns and helps their tiny bodies get a head start in the world. Because colostrum contains antibodies, some may also use colostrum supplements as an immune stimulator. The theory is that the immune factors in the colostrum are transferred to the person using the supplement. The colostrum in nutritional supplements usually does not come from humans, but rather, cows. Because of this, another name for colostrum is *bovine colostrum*.

Colostrum and Immunity

Because colostrum contains antibodies, some people use bovine colostrum supplements to boost their immune system and help fight disease. One criticism of this position is that colostrum contains antibodies against diseases that affect *cows*—not humans. The extent to which cow antibodies can impact disease in humans needs more study and is controversial. Also, some speculate that the concentration of antibodies in bovine colostrum is too low to significantly prevent disease in humans. There is also the often-mentioned criticism that antibodies are made of protein and as such would be largely, if not entirely, digested in the stomach before they could be assimilated. While it is possible that something from the colostrum of cows may positively impact health in humans, the lack of good research in this area makes this issue open to speculation.

Much of the research on the immune-stimulating aspects of bovine colostrum involves a form of colostrum that is not available to consumers. It is called *hyper-immune colostrum*. Hyper-immune colostrum is created when pregnant cows are inoculated with microorganisms that cause disease in *humans*. This causes the cows to make antibodies to those human diseases. The antibodies in turn are excreted in the colostrum. Hyper-immune colostrum is classified by the FDA as a drug to treat various conditions and is not the type used in supplements.[137] Whether hyper-immune colostrum and bovine colostrum supplements work the same way is controversial.

Colostrum and Exercise

Bovine colostrum is rich in protein which is very popular among weightlifters and other fitness enthusiasts. This, combined with other possible muscle-enhancing compounds, makes bovine colostrum attractive to those looking to gain an edge during exercise. The concept of bovine colostrum improving exercise performance is actually a fairly popular area of research that has some support. For example, one study found that cyclists who used 20 grams and 60 grams of bovine colostrum a day were able to pedal faster during a 2-hour ride, compared to cyclists who consumed 60 grams of whey protein.[164] Another study noted that 8 weeks of colostrum at 20 grams per day along with a strength training program seemed to result in an increase in muscle mass, although strength did not appear to increase.[165] Another investigation noted increases in power, measured by how high people could jump, following bovine colostrum use.[440]

During exercise, metabolites such as lactic acid build up in the blood. These metabolites must be kept in check (buffered) if exercise is to continue. At least one investigation has observed that bovine colostrum improved the buffering capacity of blood in world-class female rowers.[166] Interestingly, the authors of this study were unable to reproduce their findings in a similar investigation.[167]

Currently, most of the studies showing positive effects have used about 60 grams of colostrum per day. Also, any improvements that might occur won't happen over night. It might take eight weeks before any performance enhancements take effect.

Side Effects and Concerns

Bovine colostrum supplements seem relatively safe for healthy adults. There are no known drug interactions of significant side effects.

Consumers may want to exercise caution when dealing with colostrum that is derived from cows in countries where mad cow disease has been found. Thus far, there have been no cases of mad cow disease in humans that have been attributed to bovine colostrum or any nutritional supplement. The FDA and supplement companies both work to restrict various cow-derived products from being incorporated into supplements so as to decrease even further any possible transmission of mad cow disease to humans.[171]

My Thoughts

I'm not yet convinced that colostrum supplements improve resistance to infection in people. Those looking to lower their risk of getting sick are probably better served by washing their hands regularly and getting some exercise. The evidence for exercise enhancing immunity is overwhelming and far surpasses that of colostrum supplements. As for colostrum improving exercise performance, the studies to date are very interesting and this may be something worth looking at if you are a competitive athlete, like a rower or cyclist. Since not all studies find that it helps, I still want to see more research performed before I give it two thumbs up.

Conjugated Linoleic Acid

Conjugated linoleic acid, also called *CLA*, is a type of fatty acid that is based on the essential fatty acid, linoleic acid. Found mostly in beef and dairy products, linoleic acid is one of the omega-6 fatty acids which have generated much public and scientific interest over the past few years. Contrary to popular opinion, CLA actually represents a group of linoleic acid types, with each form differing slightly from the others and having different properties. The forms of CLA which have received the most attention are as follows:

- cis-9, trans-11 linoleic acid
- trans-10, cis-12 linoleic acid

These are some pretty strange names to be sure. The names "cis" and "trans" refer to the arrangement of the atoms that make up the fat. If, when you saw the word *trans*, you thought "trans fatty acid" pat yourself on the back because CLA is an example of a trans fatty acid—the type of fats that are traditionally thought to be harmful to the body. More about that later...

CLA and Weight Loss

There is evidence that CLA may promote fat loss but not weight loss.[78,82,86] How CLA affects body composition change is not well known, but some speculate that CLA causes fat cells to die off.[448] At least one study has found that CLA may be more effective when combined with regular exercise.[83] Since fat takes up more space than muscle, losing fat from the body could make people look thinner—which is the reason people gravitate toward weight loss supplements to begin with. Related to this, at least one study has found that CLA may reduce appetite in humans.[442] It should be mentioned that most of the evidence to date for CLA stems from animal studies.[80] In addition, not all human studies find that CLA works.[80,81,84] Most weight loss studies finding favorable results have used between 2-7 grams of CLA per day. Some research hints that the optimal dose for weight loss may be somewhere around 3.5 grams.[78]

Of the different types of CLA, the evidence for fat loss seems strongest for the *trans-10, cis-12* form.[85] Thus, consumers interested in fat loss should look for *trans-10-, cis-12 linoleic acid* since it has the most evidence to date. Diabetics who are considering CLA should consult their physician first. Some evidence shows that the same type of CLA that may promote fat loss may also make the body less responsive to insulin.[86]

CLA: The Trans Fatty Acid Connection

Trans fatty acids are typically vilified by the media because of evidence that high intakes may increase the risk of heart disease. However, some speculate that all trans fatty acids may *not* be created equal. CLA is an example of a trans fat that may have positive qualities. In addition to possibly helping some people lose fat, another type of CLA—*cis-9, trans-11 linoleic acid*—may have potential anti-cancer properties. Thus, while, more research is needed, CLA may be an example of a trans fat which has health benefits.[87]

CLA and Cholesterol

Some research finds that CLA may lower both total cholesterol and low-density lipoprotein (LDL)—the so-called "bad" cholesterol.[77,78] But, not all human studies show these effects.[79] Food for thought: there are more studies documenting the cholesterol-lowering effects of regular exercise than CLA.

CLA and Cancer

Some research suggests that CLA may have anti-cancer properties.[446] This comes from the observation that older women who have the greatest intake of CLA from foods have a lower risk of breast cancer.[443] Unfortunately, other research shows no connection between breast cancer and CLA intake.[444,445] This does not mean CLA is useless against cancer but rather that a lot of questions need to be answered before CLA can be universally recommended. For example, it's not known if CLA can prevent cancer.

Side Effects and Concerns

CLA seems to be pretty well tolerated in healthy people, with the most usual side effects being occasional diarrhea and GI problems.

One group of people who might want to steer clear of CLA are nursing mothers. CLA has been shown to reduce fat from breast milk.[447] Given that fat is a valuable source of calories for growing babies, the use of CLA might affect the baby's development.

Because the trans-10, cis-12 form of CLA may reduce blood glucose levels, diabetics should monitor blood sugar while using CLA.

My Thoughts

While controversial, several studies have found that CLA (especially, the trans-10, cis-12 form) may be moderately effective for some people looking to drop excess body fat. We typically get very little CLA in our diets with meat and dairy products being the main contributors. So, those who want to increase their consumption of CLA should probably look for a quality supplement because obtaining high levels of CLA in the diet means consuming a lot of fat and calories—which does nothing for the waistline.

Cordyceps

Cordyceps refers to a supplement that has the unique distinction of being traditionally derived from a fungus that grew on the bodies of dead caterpillars.[345] Cordyceps may be used for a number of reasons but the most popular include improving energy levels, enhancing exercise performance and fat loss. Other names which also refer to cordyceps include *Cordyceps sinensis*, *caterpillar fungus*, and *Dong Chung*.

Cordyceps and Exercise

The published research on cordyceps improving exercise performance in humans is not plentiful, so it is difficult to draw conclusions one way or another. One published study found that cordyceps was ineffective at improving aerobic exercise performance in male cyclists who used 3 grams of cordyceps a day for five weeks.[346] It is possible that cordyceps may help those who are less exercise-conditioned; however, more research should be conducted before anyone can say for certain. Some older animal research originating in China indicates that cordyceps may increase red blood cell production.[352] Red blood cells carry oxygen. Theoretically, an increase in red blood cells could translate into greater oxygen delivery to the muscles and thus enhance the ability to perform aerobic exercise such as cycling and jogging. While that sounds feasible, because of the lack of consistent proof that it works in humans, the effects of cordyceps as an exercise booster might be expected to be minimal and would probably vary from person to person.

Cordyceps and Cancer

Emerging research indicates that cordyceps may increase cancer-fighting natural killer cells as well as other immune system defenses.[348,349,350] Some animal research finds that cordyceps may also improve cancer survival rates.[351] While these are interesting results, most of the research on this aspect of cordyceps currently stems from animal research.

Side Effects and Concerns

Cordyceps is probably safe for most healthy adults. So far there have been no significant side effects or drug from the use of cordyceps. The typical amount used by people is 3 grams per day.[353]

My Thoughts

Most of the published evidence in America showing positive effects from cordyceps stems from studies of mice and other lab animals. This is much different than research in humans. While its effects on cancer is interesting, the types of human cancer upon which it might work and the amounts which might help are not known. With respect to cordyceps improving exercise capacity, I think that if it works, any improvement would be small at best. This is supported by research finding that cordyceps might improve aerobic capacity by about 5 percent in people age 40-70.[347] While more research is needed, if this holds true, then cordyceps might be something worth checking out if you are an elite athlete. For those who are not at the top of their athletic game, the effects of cordyceps might be less pronounced.

Creatine

Creatine, a natural product that is made in the body as well as found in meat and fish, is arguably one of the most highly researched dietary supplements in history. Creatine is very popular among those who exercise although research hints that it may have other uses as well. The strongest research is on exercise though. Over the last several years creatine has enjoyed unprecedented popularity in the fitness community because research finds that it tends to make people stronger and more powerful.

How Creatine Works

Let's talk chemistry for a moment. The main energy-producing molecule in our bodies is called *adenosine triphosphate* or ATP for short. In a nutshell, ATP, basically breaks apart, and in doing so, releases energy that allows us to continue to do all of our activities. Because the body has only a limited supply of ATP at any given moment, it must constantly be made. One of the methods the body uses to regenerate ATP is by using another molecule called *creatine phosphate* (or CP for short). Creatine (as creatine phosphate) is the main way our bodies replenish ATP during bouts of very intense, short-lasting exercise like sprinting or lifting a very heavy weight. Basically, what CP does is *donate* its energy to reenergize ATP very quickly, so ATP can once again break apart and release its energy so you can continue exercising. You can think of creatine as a *supercharger* because it helps make ATP when it must be made super-duper fast. Normally, we make about 2 grams of creatine a day and obtain between 0.25 and 1 gram of creatine per day from the foods we eat.[357] Creatine supplements typically contain more than this amount.

Creatine and Exercise

As was mentioned before, creatine is a supplement that some people use to help make them stronger and more powerful. This effect has been validated by a large number of published, clinical studies.[354,355,356,357] Most investigations find that creatine helps when combined with high intensity exercise, lasting less than 30 seconds.[357,358] What constitutes high intensity is best explained by the following scenario. Suppose you are out driving one day and you find a car along the side of the road that is turned upside down. To make matters worse, the occupants of the overturned car are *nuns and kittens!* Your job is to lift the car up and save the nuns and kittens from certain doom. Obviously, this task requires a lot of strength and power and this is where creatine comes in to play. It can't be restated enough that the creatine energy system is only used during activities that require explosive bursts of strength which are also short-lasting. While you are unlikely to ever encounter a car that's filled with nuns and kittens, other, more down-to-earth activities such as heavy strength training and sprinting also utilize the creatine energy source. Below is a list of activities which might benefit from creatine supplementation.

Sports Which May Benefit from Creatine	
• Powerlifting	• Bodybuilding
• Football	• Shot putting
• Javelin throwing	• Sprinting
• Boxing	• Martial arts

Now that we have established where creatine might be effective, let's talk about where it probably wouldn't work. Creatine does not seem to offer any competitive benefit in athletic events that are not high intensity. Activities like jogging, walking or other similar aerobic-type exercise are examples of this. When you think about it, this makes perfect sense if you remember that creatine is only coming into play when ATP must be made very quickly. The energy needs of activities such as walking, jogging, cycling, etc. can be met very nicely by the breakdown of carbohydrates and fats. In fact, I would go so far as to speculate that some sports might even be impaired by creatine use. For example, marathon runners would probably be hindered by creatine supplements because its most common side effect is weight gain. The heavier the person is, the slower he or she might be. Thus, in general, I do not feel creatine is appropriate for any sport where how much one weighs is an issue.

Activities That May Not Benefit from Creatine	
• Triathlons	• Marathons
• Circuit weight training	• Group aerobics classes
• Horse racing	• Bicycling
• Jogging	• Hiking

It should be mentioned that not all of the research finds that creatine works.[357,359,360,361] Everybody is different and it seems that there are people who just don't respond to creatine. This is puzzling and more research is needed to further investigate this topic.

Types of Creatine

It seems like everybody is always trying to invent a better mousetrap and creatine is no different. Today, stores are full of all sorts of different types of creatine. The type of creatine, that has the most scientific research backing up its claims is *creatine monohydrate*.[357] Other formulations may also work well but until more research is conducted on them, creatine monohydrate is probably the best to use.

Types of Creatine Available to Consumers	
• Creatine monohydrate	• Magnesium creatine
• Creatine malate	• Creatine phosphate
• Creatine citrate	• Creatine tartrate
• Micronized creatine	• Anhydrous creatine
• Effervescent creatine	• Liquid creatine
• Chewable creatine	• Creatine titrate

An often mentioned claim for some of the various types of creatine is that they might be absorbed faster than creatine monohydrate and in turn promote faster enhancements of strength and power. It may be that combining creatine with another molecule might help it be absorbed faster. The question is does that automatically translate into more strength? This is a very good question and one that has not been adequately studied.

How Much Is Needed?

When creatine first became popular among fitness enthusiasts, many recommended that people consume approximately 20 grams of creatine for the first week, followed by using 2-5 grams per day thereafter. These were referred to as the *loading phase* and *maintenance phase*, respectively. Following this regimen will increase the amount of creatine in muscles and promote greater strength in many people. It is now known however that the loading phase is not necessarily needed, which is good news for people on a budget. It has been shown that using 3 grams of creatine per day for a month will increase muscle creatine levels as much as using 20 grams for a week.[364]

Combining creatine and carbohydrates will also increase the absorption of creatine. Specifically, some evidence suggests that combining 20 grams of creatine with 93 grams of carbohydrates may increase the absorption of creatine by as much as 60%.[368] Other research finds similar elevations in absorption when creatine is combined with 50 grams of protein and 50 grams of carbohydrate.[369] It is reasonable to assume that using lesser amounts of creatine, protein and carbohydrates would produce similar results.

Medical Uses for Creatine?

Emerging research is finding that creatine may hold value that goes beyond its popularity by those in the fitness community. Below is a list of conditions where creatine may be beneficial.

Gyrate atrophy is a rare genetic degenerative eye disorder that can result in near-sightedness, night blindness and cataracts. Some evidence suggests that using 1.5 grams of creatine per day may improve and delay the progression of gyrate atrophy.[370]

Congestive heart failure results when the heart can no longer pump enough blood to sustain normal activities. People with this condition usually become tired and short of breath during activity. Some studies have found that creatine may improve the way people with congestive heart failure deal with the stress of exercise.[371,372] Regardless, because of the seriousness of this, condition, those with heart disease are strongly urged to see their physician before experimenting with creatine or any other supplement.

Preliminary evidence from at least one study suggests that several weeks of creatine at 5 grams per day may help lower cholesterol, LDL and triglyceride levels in some individuals.[373]

Muscular dystrophy actually refers to a family of related syndromes characterized by a progressive degeneration and weakness of muscle. Some studies have found that creatine can mildly improve strength in people afflicted with some forms of this condition.[374,375]

Most of these other possible uses of creatine require more study before they are formally accepted and some, like reducing cholesterol, have simpler, more effective solutions, like exercise.

Side Effects and Concerns

Aside from complaints of nausea, abdominal cramping and diarrhea that are common among most supplements, studies to date have not found any serious negative side effects associated with creatine use.[357] Regardless, because everybody is different, it is possible that side effects not observed in research may be experienced by some people following creatine use.

Creatine does not appear to increase the risk of tendon or muscle injuries in most study participants. The most consistent side effect that has been observed is a gain in weight.[357] People can typically expect to gain between 1 to 3 pounds following the use of creatine.[365] This weight gain is generally thought to be the result of extra water being stored in the body and not due to extra muscle being formed.

Some have speculated that increased water retention may place some at increased risk of high blood pressure; however, so far this has not been observed in research.[449] Most studies to date have investigated creatine in people who do not have high blood pressure. While purely speculation, individuals with hypertension who use creatine should have their blood pressure monitored regularly.

Creatine supplements should be avoided by people with kidney disorders because creatine is broken down by the kidneys. In theory, creatine might worsen kidney function in those whose kidneys are already compromised by disease.[366] For those with healthy kidneys, creatine has not been shown to cause problems.

Creatine is broken down in the body to small amounts of formaldehyde, a toxic substance.[367] While no ill effects have yet been observed from this, more research is needed to ascertain what effect, if any, chronic exposure to heightened formaldehyde production might have in humans.

My Thoughts

There seems little doubt that for many people, creatine will increase strength and power during high intensity anaerobic exercise, like weight lifting or sprinting. While less is known about how creatine impacts various medical conditions, when it comes to exercise, creatine appears to be the real deal.

Devil's Claw

The name devil's claw is derived from the fact that the plant has little grappling hooks or claws sprouting from it. While in the past, devil's claw was used as an appetite stimulant and digestive aid, it is also thought to have anti-inflammatory properties. This hints that devil's claw may be effective for arthritis. Other names which also refer to devil's claw include *Harpagophytum procumbens*, *grapple plant* and *Uncaria procumbens*.

Devil's Claw and Arthritis

Several studies suggest that devil's claw may be effective at reducing the pain associated with *osteoarthritis*.[376,377,378,379] Because of this research, devil's claw may be found alongside other products like glucosamine, MSM and related supplements touted to improve osteoarthritis. The amount of devil's claw used in successful studies has ranged from 2 to 3 grams a day.

Most studies showing positive results have used specific brands of devil's claw extract (Harpadol and Doleteffin). Lesser evidence exists for devil's claw helping rheumatoid-arthritis-related pain. More research is also needed to validate claims that devil's claw helps other conditions as well.

Side Effects and Concerns

Even in high doses, devil's claw appears to be safe in healthy adults with few side effects. Side effects may vary in those with medical issues. Conditions where devil's claw may be inappropriate include the following:

Pregnancy. Some speculate that devil's claw may stimulate contraction of the uterus and theoretically cause a miscarriage.[10]

People using blood thinners. Theoretically, devil's claw may interact with some blood thinner medications and increase the risk of bleeding.[380]

People with ulcers. There is a possibility that devil's claw may increase the production of stomach acid. Thus, devil's claw may exacerbate ulcers or lessen the effectiveness of some ulcer medications.[10]

My Thoughts

The research for devil's claw helping osteoarthritis-related pain is interesting and may be something to consider. If you are going to experiment with devil's claw, keep in mind that its effects will probably vary from person to person. In addition, remember that the active ingredients are thought to reside in the roots of the plant. Also, like most supplements, if devil's claw is going to work, it may take several weeks before any effects are noticed. Lastly, if you're on the fence and trying to decide whether devil's claw or glucosamine might help your osteoarthritis, remember that of the two, glucosamine sulfate is generally more widely accepted.

DHEA

DHEA stands for a pretty big word—De-hydro-epi-andros-terone. Now you know why they call it DHEA for short! DHEA is actually a *hormone* that's made mostly in the adrenal glands which sit atop your kidneys.[88] Another name for DHEA is DHEA-S which stands for DHEA-sulfate. Both DHEA and DHEA-S are essentially the same thing. Because DHEA can also be made in some plants such as wild yams and soybeans, current US law allows this hormone to be sold over-the-counter as a supplement. The reasons people use DHEA are almost as numerous as the stars in the sky!

DHEA and Exercise

Before bodybuilders and other hardcore weightlifters discovered growth hormone, andro and pro-hormones, there was DHEA. Because DHEA is just *two* chemical steps from being converted to the male hormone testosterone, many strength trainers experimented with DHEA as a way to increase testosterone levels and thus muscle size and strength. In spite of its one-time popularity among bodybuilders, there is extremely little research on DHEA and its effects in strength trainers. One study found that a year of DHEA supplementation (50 mg/day), while effectively raising blood levels of DHEA, was ineffective at improving muscle strength or muscle mass in 280 elderly men 60-80 years of age.[125] Another study, investigating the effects of DHEA in young men (average age 24 years) found that DHEA (50 mg per day), when combined with a resistance training program did not elevate testosterone levels.[126] It's ironic that DHEA would be so popular among strength trainers when most of the research is conducted on people involved with aerobic exercise, like running and cycling.

DHEA and Obesity

The thought that DHEA might play a role in gaining weight dates back to the 1960s when researchers found that older, overweight diabetic people tended to make less DHEA than thinner, non-diabetic individuals.[89] This hints that using DHEA might cause weight loss. Other investigations however cast doubt on this.[90,91,92] Some research, in fact, even finds that overweight women have increased DHEA levels.[92] Other evidence finds that when DHEA is given to overweight people (as much as 1600 mg per day for 28 days), no change in body fat is observed.[93] Another study likewise found no change in body fat even after 6 months of DHEA treatment.[94] Thus, based on the evidence at hand, DHEA does not appear to be a major weapon in the battle against obesity.

DHEA and Sexual Function

Some research suggests that DHEA may be a possible therapy for men with erectile dysfunction.[131] However, it doesn't seem to work for everyone. This is probably due to the variety of reasons which might cause erectile dysfunction. In addition, some research suggests that DHEA might assist with the normal sexual functioning of postmenopausal women.[130] DHEA does not however appear to enhance the sexual responsiveness of younger, premenopausal women.[129] Because of the lack of research in this area, it's difficult to say how DHEA might impact sex drive in either men or women.

Is DHEA the Fountain of Youth?

One of the biggest urban legends about DHEA that refuses to go away is its mislabeled reputation as the "fountain of youth". This notion can probably be traced back to the often-quoted fact that DHEA levels are high in youth and decline as we get older. This is completely true. What is seldom mentioned though, is the fact that DHEA levels drop to almost undetectable levels shortly after birth, only to rise sharply at puberty.[127] Therefore, it is possible to be very young and have low levels of DHEA. This fact shoots a really big hole in the notion that "only young people" make lots of DHEA. Is it possible that there is a very good reason that DHEA levels decrease as we get older? Maybe. Regardless as to why we make less DHEA as we age, it seems unlikely that replacing it via supplements improves strength—a big factor in graceful aging. One study of seniors, 60-80 years of age, failed to show any improvement in strength following DHEA use for an entire year.[125]

While more research is needed, an aspect of aging where DHEA may possibly prove useful is our skin. Skin tends to become thinner as we grow older and research notes that DHEA may indeed increase skin thickness in older individuals.[132] Claims that DHEA is the fountain of youth however are essentially baseless. In other words, nobody has ever grown "younger" from using DHEA supplements.

DHEA & Wild Yams

Some fitness enthusiasts may eat wild yams in the hopes of boosting DHEA levels. Laboratories can make DHEA from chemicals in wild yams but our bodies cannot do this. If you like to eat yams, great—more power to you—they are a good source of phytonutrients and vitamins. However, eating wild yams to boost DHEA levels doesn't work.[454]

Side Effects and Concerns

While short-term use is probably without issues, the long-term consequences of DHEA supplementation is not without side effects, which can include hair loss, acne, changes in menstrual pattern, liver problems and hypertension, to name a few.

There are a few reports of people becoming highly excited following DHEA use, a condition clinically called *mania*.[95,96] This has been reported in individuals with no history of mental illness and may not arise until after months of DHEA use has halted.[97] Since this does not happen to everyone, it could be that only some genetically predisposed people may be affected by this.

Those with heart disease should use DHEA with caution. Some evidence suggests that DHEA can reduce good cholesterol (HDL) levels and increase the risk of heart disease.[100]

DHEA should not be used by anyone with cancer—especially prostate cancer, breast cancer, ovarian cancer and uterine cancer, which may be influenced by hormone levels.[451] This is prudent advice given that some research finds that DHEA can cause cancer in laboratory animals.[452,453] DHEA may also interfere with some anti-cancer drugs.[450]

DHEA may interfere with the normal breakdown and metabolism of some prescription medications. This might result in the levels of these drugs increasing to more than is needed. Related to this, DHEA has also been shown to aggravate some liver disorders.[128]

Until more is known, those with diabetes should be cautious about DHEA as it might interfere with the hormone insulin.[99]

Possible Side Effects of DHEA	
• Hair loss	• Acne
• Decreased HDL	• Liver problems
• Altered menstrual patterns	• Mania
• Possible increased heart disease risk	• Possible increase in cancer
• Altered breakdown of some medications	• Altered blood sugar levels

My Thoughts

I have said it before and I'll say it again: I am not a fan of do-it-yourself-over-the-counter hormone therapy. Despite the hype that sometimes surrounds DHEA, we have only scratched the surface in our understanding of this hormone. Even though DHEA is one of the most abundant hormones in the body we are still not sure what it does. DHEA has not been shown to improve or prevent any disease—and it is definitely not the fountain of youth. If you're looking to naturally boost your DHEA levels, try eating more vegetables. Some research notes that vegetarians have naturally higher levels of DHEA than us meat-eaters.[102] Being a vegetarian or just adding more vegetables to your diet will also go a long way in helping shed excess pounds, reduce a lot of disease risk factors and probably add to the quality of life as well.

DMAE

DMAE, which stands for dimethylaminoethanol, is a compound found in foods such as sardines and anchovies and is made in small amounts in the brain. In the body, DMAE is a precursor to choline which in turn is a precursor to the brain chemical *acetylcholine*. DMAE is advocated for a number of conditions, the most popular of which include skin wrinkling, Alzheimer's disease, and attention deficit disorder. Another term which is sometimes used in place of DMAE is *deanol*.

DMAE and Wrinkles

DMAE is thought to be a precursor to the brain chemical *acetylcholine*. Aside from working inside the brain, acetylcholine is also involved with sending nerve impulses from the brain to the muscles. Because of this, some advocate DMAE for the treatment of wrinkles.[381] The theory is that using DMAE topically on the skin will increase muscle tone and smooth out fine lines and wrinkles. For this reason DMAE may also be found in some anti-aging cosmetics. Preliminary evidence does find that a 3% topical solution of DMAE may hold merit in making the skin more firm.[382] While interesting, further research should be performed before these claims can be fully accepted.

DMAE and Alzheimer's Disease

The claims that DMAE may help Alzheimer's disease are also related to the brain chemical acetylcholine. In Alzheimer's disease, brain cells that make acetylcholine are damaged.[383] So, the theory is that if you can replace acetylcholine, Alzheimer's will improve. This is actually the premise of some Alzheimer's drugs, so it is logical to speculate that something like DMAE, might be effective.

Unfortunately, the research that has been performed so far does not show that DMAE can help Alzheimer's sufferers.[384,385] In fact, about 20% of the people in one of the studies referenced above experienced heightened confusion levels and increased blood pressures while using DMAE.[384] Based on these results it is generally felt that DMAE supplements would not help Alzheimer's sufferers or people with other forms of dementia.

DMAE and ADHD

Before DMAE, there was the DMAE-like drug called *deanol* which was marketed by Riker Laboratories.[386] Deanol was designed to help children with learning difficulties—what today might be labeled attention deficit hyperactivity disorder (ADHD). Riker Labs subsequently ceased making deanol in 1983 because of lack of evidence that it worked and lack of safety information.[394] With respect to DMAE, some older studies from the 1970s seem to show that it might help children with learning difficulities.[387,388,389] Another more recent investigation found that a combination of DMAE along with a vitamin and mineral supplement improved mood and feelings of well-being in adults. While this is intriguing, more research is needed to better understand if/how DMAE affects ADHD or other learning difficulties.

Side Effects and Concerns

DMAE supplements should be used with caution by those with schizophrenia or depression. In some individuals, DMAE may worsen these conditions.[391,392] Likewise, DMAE supplements should be avoided by people who have epilepsy or any seizure disorder as it may affect these conditions.[137]

People with Parkinson's disease may also be inappropriate for DMAE use. Theoretically, DMAE may decrease the effectiveness of drugs used to treat Parkinson's.[387]

Because spikes in blood pressure have also been noted in some who use DMAE, those with hypertension should exercise caution when using this supplement until more is known.[384]

My Thoughts

I think the jury is still out on DMAE. Until recently, it was an almost forgotten supplement and is only now starting to garner attention again. While probably safe in healthy adults, in others, DMAE may have some potentially serious side effects.

As a side note, I've occasionally noticed that DMAE is sometimes listed as an ingredient in weight-loss supplements. This may be due to the observation of slight weight loss that was noted in one DMAE study.[393] Whatever the reason, because some people who desire weight loss may be suffering from depression or have other medical issues, I think the use of DMAE in weight loss supplements is not warranted.

Dong Quai

Dong Quai, an herb common to Chinese medicine, is mostly used in America to treat issues surrounding menopause and PMS. Its scientific name is *Angelica sinensis*. Another name for Dong Quai which is sometimes used is *female ginseng*, a name which also makes reference to its predominate use by women.

Dong Quai and Menopause

Symptoms of menopause such as hot flashes, cramping and premenstrual syndrome (PMS) are common reasons why some women are attracted to Dong Quai. So far though, most of the evidence in support of Dong Quai helping menstrual-related issues is derived from anecdotal reports, and studies performed on laboratory animals. Additionally, the human research conducted on Dong Quai thus far has not shown positive results.[395] Research with ineffective results has used up to 4.5 grams of the herb a day. [395] Because of the lack of human research, it is difficult for anyone to say one way or another whether Dong Quai has merit in alleviating menopause-related symptoms.

Side Effects and Concerns

In healthy adults Dong Quai is probably safe for short-term use. Dong Quai should be used with caution by individuals who are using blood thinner medications. Dong Quai may enhance the effect of blood thinner medications such as Coumadin.[396]

There is some animal and laboratory evidence that hints that components of Dong Quai may stimulate the development of cancers that are sensitive to the effects of estrogen.[397,398] Examples of cancers which might be activated include cancers of the breast, uterus and ovaries.

My Thoughts

It seems that for the moment, there is not enough good evidence to recommend that women use Dong Quai for menstrual-related symptoms. With respect to speculation of its possible activation of some forms of cancer, little direct human evidence exists for this. Thus, how significant this issue is for people is not yet known. Even so, because of the lack of evidence that it works, and possible drug interactions, I can't give this herb a green light until more research is done.

Echinacea

Echinacea, a member of the daisy family of plants, is the most popular name for an herb which is used for its apparent abilities to fend off colds and infections.[399] In reality, echinacea refers to three different forms of the herb: *Echinacea angustifolia, Echinacea pallida* and *Echinacea purpurea*. Thus far, most of the research showing favorable results on colds have used echinacea purpurea; although the other species—pallida and angustifolia—also have some evidence in support of their efficacy. Other names that refer to echinacea include *comb flower* and *black sampson*.

Echinacea and Immunity

A number of studies and reviews of the herb have found that echinacea may reduce the duration and severity of common cold symptoms by about 10-30% when taken immediately at the onset of symptoms.[400,401,402] Currently, it is not well understood how echinacea affects infections. One of the ways in which echinacea seems to work is by stimulating cells of the immune system which go after and "eat" infecting microorganisms.[407,408] Other immune system cells such as lymphocytes which make antibodies also appear to be called into action following echinacea use. It is interesting to note that not all studies of echinacea find positive results.[404,405,406] This discrepancy may be due in part to a number of factors including, but not limited to, the species of echinacea used, the parts of the plant the echinacea supplement was created from, the number of people used in the study and even the overall quality of the echinacea supplement used.

Because of these discrepancies, individual success with this herb will probably vary.

Some people may take echinacea daily in the hopes of warding off colds before they start; however, there is no evidence that echinacea can prevent colds.[401] This may be due to echinacea's apparent lack of ability to stimulate the immune systems of healthy people.[409]

Several different amounts of echinacea have been used and it is generally recommended that several smaller dosages are better than one large dose. Some experts recommend using three 300 mg doses of echinacea per day.[137] In spite of this, it should be noted that the optimal amount of echinacea needed to impact the immune systems of cold sufferers has yet to be determined.

Side Effects and Concerns

Echinacea is generally free of any serious side effects in most healthy adults. Because echinacea may stimulate the immune system, in theory, it should not be used by people who are taking drugs to suppress the immune system. For example, people who receive new organs, such as kidneys, hearts etc., must take drugs to prevent their immune systems from attacking the transplanted organ. Taking echinacea might "wake up" the immune system, which then might attack their new organ.

People who have autoimmune disorders should also steer clear of echinacea supplements until more is known. Autoimmune disorders occur when the immune system, which normally only attacks invading microorganisms, gets *stupid* and begins attacking an area of the body. There is some evidence that immune-stimulating supplements may exacerbate the symptoms of autoimmune disorders.[403]   People who have autoimmune disorders should consult their physician before using echinacea or any nutritional supplement touted to boost the immune system.

Individuals who are infected with the HIV virus should consult their physician before using echinacea or any supplement reputed to stimulate the immune system. There is some thought that echinacea may aggravate HIV symptoms.[10]

My Thoughts

Most of the studies done to date seem to show that echinacea may modestly help improve cold symptoms and the duration of colds. This is good news for people who are opposed to taking medications as well as those whose symptoms are caused by a virus—which antibiotics are ineffective against. However echinacea is not a miracle cure and its effects are likely to be modest at best. How echinacea works is not well understood and it's very likely that there are several components of echinacea that work in concert to bring about its immune-stimulating effects. Most of the positive evidence for echinacea is obtained from using the above-ground portions of *echinacea purpurea*, such as the leaves, stems and flowers. Because some have found that echinacea may be contaminated with lead, it is recommend that you only do business with established companies that you trust.[410]

EGCG

EGCG stands for *epigallocatechin gallate*. You're probably saying to yourself, *what the heck is EGCG?* The fact is, you've probably heard of EGCG but call it by its more common name—*green tea!* More specifically, EGCG is one of the many components that make up green tea. Green tea has been used in the orient for centuries for a number of health-related reasons. In America, some drink green tea to assist with weight loss. The reasoning for this is that green tea contains caffeine, which has a mild weight loss effect. Other research hints that EGCG itself may also have a weight loss effect. Additional names that refer to green tea include *Japanese tea*, *Camellia sinensis*, *Camellia theifera* and *Thea viridis.*.

EGCG and Weight Loss

Emerging evidence suggests that EGCG may have some benefits in the battle of the bulge.[306] Other research also suggests that caffeine may enhance this effect.[307] The effect of EGCG on weight loss appears to be small and may take months before a noticeable effect is observed. Currently, it is unknown if supplements that contain EGCG work any better than drinking green tea itself. Because of the limited research on EGCG, it's not possible to make recommendations on amounts to use or even to say that it would work for sure. Consumers can estimate the amount of EGCG in supplements by looking at the Supplement Facts label of the products they use. Those ingredients listed at the start of the list are present in the highest concentration.

EGCG as an Antioxidant

Green tea is rich in phytonutrients called *polyphenols*. One of those polyphenols is EGCG. As such, EGCG is one of the compounds thought to be responsible for green tea's health benefits, although other polyphenols also seem to be involved.[305] Polyphenols are antioxidants, which might help reduce the risk of and progression of various diseases. For now though, the thing to remember is that the research on EGCG is not as plentiful as the research that exists for drinking green tea itself.

EGCG and Parkinson's Disease

For those who are diagnosed with the neurological disorder, Parkinson's disease, drinking tea seems to slow the progression of this syndrome. This is controversial and research is still in its infancy. Some speculate that this may have more to do with the caffeine content of tea rather than EGCG given that Parkinson's progression also appears to be slowed in those who drink coffee and caffeinated sodas.[326]

EGCG and Heart Disease

There is some evidence that people who drink green tea experience less heart disease than non-tea drinkers.[318,319] The evidence for EGCG is less strong than for drinking tea itself. Before a final judgment can be made, large numbers of people will have to be followed for many years, with some of those people taking EGCG supplements and others who don't.

EGCG and Cancer

Several investigations have noted that people who drink green tea have lower risks of various types of cancer. The cancers that seem to be the most reduced include cancers of the pancreas, bladder, stomach, breast, esophagus, ovary and cervix.[308,309,310,311] The effects of green tea on prostate and colon cancer are less clear.[316,317] The reasons why green tea might help some cancers but not others is not well known. The cancer-protective-effect is strongest for drinking green tea and not for EGCG supplements.

Side Effects and Concerns

Generally, green tea is well tolerated in healthy people so it shouldn't cause any significant side effects. Because of its caffeine content, green tea is not something to use right before bedtime—lest of course you want to be up all night watching old TV show reruns.

For people who use blood thinner medications, green tea may have either an opposing, counteracting effect or an additive effect, both of which may be undesirable.[321,323] In theory, green tea might also interact with some antidepressant medications.[322] In addition, green tea might also impact blood sugar levels, but this may have more to do with its caffeine content. [324,325]

My Thoughts

No doubt, green tea is a healthy drink and most likely contains a number of compounds that help protect us from disease. As such it's something to consider using.

At issue is whether studies on green tea can be applied to supplements that contain isolated extracts like EGCG? How drinking green tea appears to battle disease is unknown and probably has to do with the variety of and interaction between the many phytonutrients it contains, as opposed to any single ingredient like EGCG. So, based on the evidence, I'd give green tea two thumbs up but I'd hold off on concentrated green tea extracts like EGCG for now.

160

Enzymes

Right now, as you read these words, billions of chemical reactions are going on inside of your body. Crucial to the successful completion of most of these reactions are microscopic *machines* called enzymes. Enzymes take part in everything from helping you exercise and grow hair to even helping heal your big toe if you happen to bump it accidentally. Enzymes work by allowing a chemical reaction to occur much faster than it normally would. For example, it would take many decades to digest your breakfast if it were not for enzymes in your digestive system! Enzymes can be easily recognized because their names usually end in the letters "ase". While normally made inside us, enzymes can also be purchased as supplements. People use enzyme supplements for a number of reasons, including but not limited to, helping digestion, preventing disease, weight loss and even warding off the aging process.

Examples of Enzymes and Their Functions	
Enzyme	Function
• Lactase	Breaks down lactose in dairy products
• Superoxide dismutase	Neutralizes free radicals
• Sucrase	Breaks down sucrose
• ATPase	Breaks down ATP to release energy
• Protease	Breaks down proteins

Notice all enzymes listed end in the letters "ase"

Enzymes and Digestion

One of the most common reasons people will use enzyme supplements is to help with digestion. Sometimes people may suffer from enzyme-deficiency syndromes. *Lactose intolerance*, which results in the inability to digest lactose (milk sugar), is probably the most recognized condition of this type, affecting between 30-50 million Americans. While lactose intolerance can be dealt with by the use of over-the-counter products, other enzyme deficiency syndromes may require prescription drugs.

In supplements, common enzymes used to help with digestion include *bromelain* (found in pineapples) and *papain* (found in papaya). While such digestive enzymes may indeed help some people, in those with well-functioning digestive systems, enzyme supplements are unlikely to provide any additional benefit.[412]

Enzymes and Wellness

Some alternative health experts advocate using enzyme supplements in the hopes that extra enzymes will take stress off the body and promote healing.[411] Currently though, there is little convincing proof that this occurs in humans. Healthy people do not exhaust their supply of enzymes. Enzymes are indeed one of God's miracles of creation because they are not used up in the chemical reactions they facilitate.[146] In other words, enzymes can be used over and over again.[146] When an enzyme finally does wear out, an identical copy is made to take its place.

One criticism of enzyme supplement theory is that enzymes themselves are usually made of or contain protein. When you eat a piece of chicken, the protein that it is made of is digested and broken down into the amino acids that make up the chicken. The same thing happens with enzymes. The enzyme supplement is broken down to the amino acids that make up the enzyme, and your body will use those amino acids to do whatever it wants to with them, whether it is to help make more enzymes, incorporate them into helping growing hair or to make a cell in your pinky finger. Thus, it is unlikely that significant amounts of intact enzymes could pass undigested into the body when taken orally. Even if enzymes could somehow pass into the body undigested, it has not been proven that they do anything in humans.[412]

Problems with Enzyme Supplement Theory	
• The protein in enzymes are destroyed by digestion.	• Healthy people do not run out of enzymes.
• Little evidence that intact enzymes can make it into body.	• It's not proven that enzymes help alleviate stress.
• The enzymes your body makes are reusable.	• Little evidence that enzyme supplements help healthy people.

Side Effects and Concerns

Enzymes are relatively non-toxic in healthy adults and unlikely to cause any serious side effects. Common side effects include nausea, diarrhea and cramping. While not proven, in theory, bromelain, popular among people with digestive problems, may interact with some blood thinner medications.[414] Other drug interactions may also be possible.

My Thoughts

Protein-digesting enzymes like bromelain may indeed be of help to some people with digestive issues. So for those with digestive problems, bromelain or other similar digestive enzymes may be something to consider. Other than this, there is little concrete evidence that enzyme supplements promote weight loss, fight the aging process, reduce stress or prevent or reduce the risk of any disease. Some research from decades ago suggested that orally-taken enzymes may reduce pain from sports injuries.[413] That nice, but there is much more evidence that a bag of ice placed on the injured area also helps—and ice is cheaper! I have little doubt that quality-made enzyme supplements are safe for most people but until I start seeing studies of these products conducted on humans showing that they live up to their hype, I am of the opinion that they are not needed for most people.

Ephedra

Ephedra sinica or *ephedra* for short, is a plant that has been used by practitioners of Chinese medicine for thousands of years. Sometimes you will also see the name *ephedrine* associated with ephedra. Ephedrine is the drug which is found within the herb ephedra. Chemically, ephedrine is classified as a sympatho-mimetic drug because it *mimics* the effect of sympathetic (nerve-stimulating) hormones like adrenaline in the body.[103] While ephedrine is used in some over-the-counter cold and flu remedies, most people used ephedra supplements for weight loss. Another popular name for ephedra is *ma huang*.

Ephedra and Weight Loss

Research generally finds that ephedra is effective at promoting at least modest, short-term weight loss. Because of the controversy, potential side effects and popularity of this herb, the FDA commissioned the RAND Corporation, a nonprofit organization, to perform a comprehensive review of ephedra, consisting of only those studies that were of the highest caliber.[131,133] This report concluded that ephedra is effective at promoting an average loss of about 2 extra pounds per month than when compared to using nothing at all. This weight loss might be expected to continue for the first four to six months of use. Studies generally use 30-60 mg of ephedra when investigating weight loss. Because of possible negative side effects, it is wise to start at the lower end of this range, if not less, to see how you respond to ephedra. Don't assume more is better. Remember, the greater the amount used, the greater the risk of side effects occurring.

Sometimes ephedra is combined with other stimulants like caffeine and guarana to boost its effect. Regardless, for those considering ephedra, its important to use it in conjunction with a healthy, albeit reduced-calorie eating plan, as this is sure to enhance its effect.

Ephedra and Exercise

The effect of ephedra on exercise performance is controversial with little research specifically investigating the herb's effects under real life exercise situations. Some research finds that when used alone, ephedra is ineffective but when combined with caffeine, the ephedra-caffeine combination may provide modest improvements in short term exercise performance.[134] Whether or not ephedra alone might help improve athletic performance is unknown and needs more study.

RAND Report Summary

• Ephedra may result in the loss of about two extra pounds per month on average	• It is unknown if long-term ephedra use continues to improve exercise performance
• The weight loss effects may persist for up to 4-6 months	• Ephedra use is associated with a 2-3 times greater risk of side effects
• Ephedra + caffeine may provide a modest increase in ephedra's weight loss effects	• The longest well done ephedra study lasted 6 months
• Ephedra + caffeine may provide modest short term improvements in exercise performance	• The long term effects of ephedra use are unknown

Side Effects and Concerns

Ephedra is usually found to possess some potentially serious side effects when compared to other herbal supplements, especially when used carelessly and in high doses. For example, in a report published in the *Annals of Internal Medicine,* it was noted that while ephedra supplements accounted for less than 1% of herbal sales in the US in 2001, they resulted in 64% of all adverse and harmful reactions reported to poison control centers.[136] Looking at it from another angle, ephedra was found to be 720 times more likely to result in a negative report filed to poison control centers than was ginkgo biloba.[136]

Ephedra is well known to elevate both blood pressure and heart rate.[144] Ephedra can constrict blood vessels, reducing the space that is available for blood to squeeze though. This puts people with heart disease at greater risk of side effects. Ephedra may also produce alterations in the way the heart normally functions. This has been seen even in healthy persons with no obvious signs of heart disease.[144]

Individuals with diabetes should avoid ephedra-containing supplements. Ephedra can raise blood sugar levels.[142]

Glaucoma refers to several related conditions of the optic nerve of the eye which result in blindness. Ephedra can open up the pupils of the eye, which can make some types of glaucoma worse.[142]

Ephedra may make it difficult to urinate. Men with benign prostatic hyperplasia (BPH) most likely already experience difficulty urinating. The use of ephedra could possibly exacerbate the symptoms of enlarged prostate glands and those with BPH.

While controversial, some speculate that ephedra may exacerbate a rare form of cancer called pheochromocytoma which results in tumors of the adrenal glands. One of the side effects of this type of cancer is an increase in the production of adrenalin, a hormone that raises blood pressure and heart rate. Because ephedra also increases blood pressure and heart rate, its use by persons with pheochromocytoma might result in even greater side effects.[14]

Because ephedra seems to stimulate production of thyroid hormone, it should be avoided by individuals with overactive thyroid glands.

People with anxiety disorders should avoid ephedra. The use of ephedra in large doses has been associated with increased anxiety, and a worsening of anxiety symptoms.[142] Related to this, persons using antidepressant medications such as MAO inhibitors should avoid ephedra because it might elevate blood pressure to dangerous levels.[145]

Psychosis—a serious mental illness, characterized by changes in behavior and rational thought—has been reported in some people following the use of ephedra-containing supplements.[141] Psychosis has been found to develop after using ephedra for a short period of time as well as many months after ephedra is no longer used.[141] Usually people return to normal after stopping ephedra but in some cases supervision by a medical professional may be necessary. This seems to be a relatively rare side effect but it is worth mentioning because of the seriousness of the disorder.

Those with kidney stones or a history of kidney stones should avoid ephedra in light of evidence that ephedra may increase the chances of their development. Ephedra has even been found inside kidney stones.[143]

Pregnant women should stay away from ephedra supplements. Ephedra has been shown to stimulate contractions of the uterus.[145] This might result in premature birth of the growing baby.

Possible Side Effects of Ephedra

• Dizziness	• Hyperthermia	• Dry mouth
• Anxiety	• Heart attach	• Vomiting
• Personality changes	• Stroke	• Flushing
• Insomnia	• Seizures	• Rapid heart beat
• Increased thirst	• Death	• Higher blood pressure
• Nausea	• Irritability	• Heart rhythm changes
• Heartburn	• Poor concentration	• Brain hemorrhage
• Difficulty urinating	• Headache	• Loss of consciousness

My Thoughts

There is a reason ephedra is so popular with people looking to lose weight—it works, albeit modestly. That being said, ephedra can be a double-edged sword, helpful to some in small amounts, while potentially harmful in higher dosages, especially in those with medical issues. Proponents of ephedra sometimes state that the herb is only dangerous when used above the product's recommended dosage. However, sometimes inconsistencies are noted between what the label indicates and what the product actually contains.[138,139] In other words, the labels may not always be correct. While I personally feel the risks outweigh the benefits, for those who want to try ephedra, it's important to make sure you get a clean bill of health from your doctor first. Many supplements that once contained ephedra now contain a compound called *bitter orange*. See the section on bitter orange for a review of this supplement.

Epimedium

Epimedium is an herb that is mostly used as an aphrodisiac and cure-all for various sexual issues ranging from premature ejaculation to impotency. This explains the plant's more familiar and titillating name, *horny goat weed*. Some also view epimedium as a natural alternative to Viagra and other similar medications. It is noteworthy that epimedium refers to a family of over 20 related species of plants. Other names which also refer to epimedium include *Epimedium grandiflora, Japanese Epimedium, Herba Epimedii, Barrenwort* and *Yin Yang Huo*.

Epimedium and Sexual Function

Erections occur in part because of a vasodilatation or expansion of blood vessels in the penis. So, in theory, anything that could expand blood vessels might improve erections. A little research suggests that epimedium may have such properties.[461] Most of the evidence in support of this though currently stems from research that's either on lab animals or in test tubes. Very little concrete human evidence exists showing that epimedium can enhance sexual function or prowess in humans. Those who want to experiment with epimedium should make sure that supplements are derived from the leaves of the plant. This is where the active ingredients are thought to reside. Supplements may be based on Epimedium grandiflorum but other species may also have an effect.

Side Effects and Concerns

Short-term use of epimedium is probably safe in healthy adults. Some report symptoms of dry mouth, vomiting, nosebleeds and dizziness following use.[462] Because it might expand blood vessels, those with high blood pressure or heart disease should exercise caution with epimedium.[461]

My Thoughts

Epimedium has been used for thousands of years and continues to be a part of traditional Chinese medicine in the treatment of a wide range of syndromes. Despite its licentious nickname—horny goat weed—I highly doubt it has the ability to transform anyone into *Conan the Barbarian* in the bedroom. Sexual function and dysfunction are complex processes. This fact along with the lack of knowledge of active ingredients, the great number of species of epimedium that are known to exist and a host of other factors, probably makes obtaining a quality supplement hard (no pun intended) to find.

Evening Primrose Oil

Contrary to some diet myths, our bodies need fat to function optimally. In fact, some types of fat are so crucial that they are called *essential fatty acids*. Many reading these words are probably familiar with fish oil which provide essential fatty acids called omega-3s. This chapter will deal with a type of fat called gamma linolenic acid (also called GLA for short). Gamma linolenic acid is an omega-6 fatty acid. Other fats included in this family include arachidonic acid, and linoleic acid. While little GLA is normally consumed in the diet, we are usually able to make all that we need from its *cousin*, linoleic acid, which is found in vegetable oils. Some speculate that under some circumstances our need for GLA may increase. In this case, supplements might be needed. Here is where evening primrose oil comes in because it is a source of GLA. Evening primrose oil is usually derived from the seeds of a plant called *Oenothera biennis*, a flower whose pedals open up during the evening (hence the word *evening* in evening primrose oil). People supplement with evening primrose oil for a variety of reasons ranging from helping arthritis-related pain to improving symptoms associated with menopause. Other names that also refer to evening primrose oil include *GLA*, *EPO*, and *fever plant*.

Evening Primrose Oil and Arthritis

As was mentioned above, EPO is a source of gamma linolenic acid (GLA). In the body, GLA is converted to hormone-like substances called *prostaglandins*. Specifically, GLA is converted to prostaglandin E1. In the body, prostaglandin E1 can have a wide range of effects including some which are anti-inflammatory. Because of these anti-inflammatory properties, people might use EPO to help rheumatoid arthritis. Research has been conducted on EPO and its effects on arthritis but the evidence is mixed on this issue with studies finding that EPO may help and others that find no effect.[472,473,474,475] One study showing reductions in rheumatoid arthritis pain used 2.6 grams of EPO for six months.[476] If it works, EPO may take several weeks before people start to feel its effects. The extent to which EPO might improve arthritis may also be dependent on the severity of arthritis pain and the length of time one is afflicted with arthritis. Thus, positive results may vary.

Evening Primrose Oil and Osteoporosis

Some reseach suggests that EPO, along with fish oil, given over 18 months may lead to slightly thicker bones in seniors who have osteoporosis.[463] However, other investigations find that the combination of EPO and fish oils does not help.[464] Thus, more research is needed before EPO joins the ranks major bone builders like calcium and vitamin D.

Evening Primrose Oil and Menopause

Some women may be attracted to EPO because of claims that it will help reduce the symptoms of menopause and premenstrual syndrome (PMS). Unfortunately, because of issues regarding how some of the studies were done, it is not known how much EPO might impact these conditions although studies with positive outcomes have used between 2-4 grams per day. Some studies on this issue have been criticized because they may not last very long or because they contained inadequate numbers of participants. Still other studies may not have contained a placebo group to compare how EPO stacks up against taking nothing at all.[465,466,468] One thing seems certain though; if EPO is going to help, it may take many months before an effect is noticed.

One related area where EPO may be effective is in reducing *mastalgia* or breast pain which accompanies a woman's monthly cycle.[469,470] Research noting positive outcomes have used approximately 3 grams per day for several weeks.

EPO and Impotence?

Evening primrose oil, as was mentioned previously, can increase prostaglandin E1 (PGE1) which has anti-inflammatory properties. Prostaglandins, it turns out, have a wide range of effects in the body and PGE1 is no different. Studies show that PGE1 also can expand blood vessels, which can have an impact on erections. Because of this, some may make the claim that evening primrose oil can help men suffering from erectile dysfunction and impotence. Truth be told, PGE1 can produce erections in humans. There is one *tiny* drawback however: PGE1 must be *injected* directly into the penis prior to sexual intercourse! Evening primrose oil supplements are unlikely to have the same effect.

Side Effects and Concerns

Evening primrose oil is normally not associated with any harmful effects in healthy adults. Some express concern that the supplement should be avoided by pregnant women because it may complicate pregnancy.[478]

There is some speculation that EPO may increase seizures in people with schizophrenia, epilepsy or other seizure disorders.[479,480]

Because of possible blood-thinning effects, evening primrose should be used with caution by those using blood thinner medications or who have bleeding disorders.

My Thoughts

A lot of claims circulate on the Internet about evening primrose oil. Most of these claims need further study before they are formally accepted. It is noteworthy that some speculate that the American diet already contains too many omega-6 fatty acids (like EPO) and not enough omega-3 fatty acids (like fish oil).[477] A diet high in omega-6 fatty acids may predispose some to cancer and heart disease. This is food for thought before loading up on evening primrose oil or other supplements which boost omega-6 levels in the body.

Feverfew

Feverfew is a member of the same family of plants as daisies and has been used medicinally for centuries to treat a number of conditions ranging from colds and flus to menstrual problems. The name feverfew is thought to stem from the belief that the herb was able to reduce fevers but little evidence suggests this is true. Other research on this herb has focused not on the mitigation of fevers but rather on its ability to possibly reduce migraine headaches.[399] Additional names that also refer to feverfew include *Tanacetum parthenium*, *Featherfew* and *Featherfoil*.

Feverfew and Migraine Headaches

Several clinical investigations support the use of feverfew for reducing migraine headaches.[787,788] Studies find that 50 to 100 mg of feverfew taken daily over the course of several weeks may be effective at reducing both the number of migraine attacks as well as their severity.

How feverfew works is not well understood. Animal studies suggest that feverfew can help stabilize blood vessels, reducing their constriction. This might partially explain feverfew's improvement of migraine symptoms but the herb may also help in other ways.

Dozens of different constituents have been identified as possible candidates for feverfew's effect on migraines but there is little agreement on which is the active ingredient or ingredients. What is generally agreed upon, is that the active ingredient or ingredients reside in the *leaves* of the plant. Thus, feverfew supplements derived from the leaves would probably be more potent than those derived from other parts of the plant.

Some supplements may be standardized according to the amount of a feverfew ingredient called *parthenolide.* Usually this ranges from 0.2% to 0.3%. More research is needed to determine if parthenolide acts alone or in synergy with other feverfew components.

Feverfew and Arthritis

Feverfew is sometimes used by people who have rheumatoid arthritis. This rationale might be based upon the finding that feverfew might inhibit the function of cyclooxygenase 2 (COX-2), an enzyme that is involved in the production of hormone-like substances called prostaglandins. Some prostaglandins are involved in inflammation and pain, like that which typically accompanies rheumatoid arthritis. Thus, the reasoning for its use in arthritis may be that feverfew acts in part like popular prescription medications called "COX-2 inhibitors" but without the side effects. As intriguing as this sounds, clinical trials thus far have found feverfew to be ineffective for the treatment of rheumatoid arthritis. One natural alternative to feverfew which has repeatedly been shown to be effective for reducing arthritis pain is exercise. In fact, the effects of a sensible exercise program on arthritis improvement are so well known that the American Arthritis Foundation even has a program called PACE (People with Arthritis Can Exercise) to help those who are afflicted with this condition.

Side Effects and Concerns

Side effects observed with feverfew are usually minor and include ulcerations of the mouth and tongue from chewing feverfew leaves. Swelling of the lips and dizziness have also been reported, but in general, feverfew is well tolerated in healthy adults.[788] Some older research recommends that when no longer needed, feverfew supplementation be halted gradually. A *post-feverfew syndrome* characterized by muscle stiffness and migraine symptoms has been described following the abrupt stopping of feverfew in those who have used it for long periods. Whether or not this condition actually exists is open to speculation. For those who have used feverfew for many months to years and decide to stop, cut back gradually to be on the safe side.

Before experimenting with feverfew, people should make sure their headaches are indeed caused by migraines. Migraine-like pain can be caused by other conditions.

Some clinical research suggests feverfew may have a slight tendency to reduce blood clotting and thus might interact with drugs and supplements that also have anti-clotting properties.

There is speculation that feverfew may interact with the way a number of medications are metabolized in the body. Drugs that might be affected include those used to treat depression, high blood pressure, asthma and heart disease. This is mostly conjecture at this point and clinical studies have not shown feverfew to be associated with any serious side effects or drug interactions.

My Thoughts

Feverfew may prove to be of use in reducing the intensity and frequency of migraine headaches in some individuals. While not all clinical studies find feverfew effective, enough research exists to warrant trying the herb for a month or two to see if it works. Like all supplements, deal only with reputable companies to ensure you are getting a quality product. While feverfew is unlikely to result in fewer fevers, for some, it may be a natural path to fewer migraines.

Fish Oil Supplements

Fish oil contains polyunsaturated omega-3 fatty acids, which studies have shown may reduce the risk of heart disease. Specifically, fish oil supplements are likely to list two key omega-3 fatty acids—EPA and DHA. EPA and DHA stand for *eicosapentaenoic acid* and *docosahexaenoic acid,* respectively. Thus, the terms DHA and EPA are sometimes used interchangeably with fish oils.

Fish Oil and Heart Disease

Fish oils first came to public attention following research on Eskimos, who, in spite of the high fat diet they consumed, developed less heart disease than other groups of people. It turned out that Eskimos consumed lots of fish which were high in—you guessed it—fish oils.[497]

Fish oils are believed to exert their protective effects on the heart in a number of ways. One way they seem to help is by altering the mixture or ratio of hormone-like chemicals called *prostaglandins* in the blood. Fish oils seem to decrease the prostaglandin that makes blood sticky and increase the prostaglandin that makes blood less sticky. Overall, this makes blood less likely to clot and contribute to plaque formation. Other ways include lowering cholesterol and triglyceride levels and raising HDL (good cholesterol).[499] Fish oils might also slow the rate of progression of heart disease after it has started.[507] Additionally, fish oils also seem to slow the heart rate, which in theory might better stabilize a weakened heart.[498]

One of the new theories of heart disease is that it is caused by a long-term, inflammation in the body.[510] This inflammation can be determined by measuring a chemical called *C-reactive protein* (CRP). CRP levels increase during stresses like infections or surgery. Studies also find high CRP levels in those who have heart disease.[510] It is possible to have normal cholesterol levels and high CRP levels. Some research suggests that one of the ways in which fish oils may reduce the risk of heart disease is by lowering CRP levels if they are high to begin with.[511] This is probably related to the anti-inflammatory properties of EPA and DHA.

Most studies looking at fish oils and heart disease have used between 1 to 4 grams per day. More aggressive dosages (3 to 6 grams a day) have been found to modestly reverse heart disease in some—but not all—diagnosed with this condition. Such high doses should be reserved only for the worst of the worst and then used only in association with guidance from a physician.

Size Matters

Many people think of LDL cholesterol as the "bad cholesterol". While too much LDL in the blood is certainly nothing to smile about, new research is finding that not all LDL cholesterol is created equal. For example, it is now thought that bigger, more buoyant LDL cholesterol molecules may be less likely to clog blood vessels than smaller LDL molecules.[512] Emerging research finds that the fish oil, DHA, may be able to increase the size of LDL cholesterol.[512] This may be yet another way that fish oil supplements lower the risk of heart disease.

Fish Oil and High Blood Pressure

Having a resting blood pressure of greater than 140/90 for long periods of time is referred to as high blood pressure or *hypertension*. High blood pressure is also a contributor to heart disease. Some studies provide evidence that fish oils can moderately lower blood pressure in people whose blood pressure is high.[505] This effect is less pronounced in those with normal blood pressure. Research suggests that it may take about 4 grams of fish oil per day to achieve this blood-pressure-lowering effect.[506] This is actually quite a high dose and may increase the chance of side effects occurring. Because everybody is different, it is probably wise to start lower and adjust the amount accordingly. Because mild to moderate levels of exercise have also been shown to reduce blood pressure in those with hypertension, combining this with fish oil might also work.

Fish Oil and Cancer

Overall, eating fish on a regular basis seems to reduce the risk of getting a number of cancers such as those of the breast, colon, ovary and esophagus.[500] Translating this in terms of supplements, it appears that about 1 gram of fish oil per week is all that is required to reap this benefit. This is a relatively low dose and one that is easily obtained by eating fish itself.

Some intriguing studies suggests that high doses of fish oils might modestly slow cancer-related weight loss and improve appetite in those suffering from pancreatic cancer.[501,502] In theory, this might also hold true for other cancers although, definitive proof is still needed. While more research is needed to better define optimal dosages, positive results have been observed with about 7 grams of fish oils a day. This is a high dose and because of side effects it's wise to start at a lower amount and increase accordingly over time.

Fish Oil and Weight Loss

Some weight loss supplements may contain fish oils. This may be based on studies that find when people with high blood pressure are placed on a reduced calorie diet that includes fish, that they tend to shed about 5 pounds more compared to those who do not eat fish.[508,509] While intriguing, it's important to remember that fish and fish oil supplements are not the same thing. Fish contains much more than EPA and DHA that might account for this observation.

Fish Oil and Arthritis

Several lines of research have noted that fish oils may reduce joint stiffness in those who suffer from rheumatoid arthritis.[503,504] This may be due to the ability of fish oil to reduce inflammation. Research suggests that approximately 2 grams of DHA and 4 grams of EPA may be needed to significantly impact arthritis-related joint stiffness. Smaller dosages may help those with less advanced forms of arthritis. Fish oils do not appear to slow the progression of rheumatoid arthritis. The impact of fish oils on the more common, osteoarthritis, has not been well studied.

How Fish Oils Might Help	
• Lower Cholesterol	• "Thin" the blood
• Lower triglycerides	• Raise LDL size
• Raise HDL	• Lower joint pain
• Lower blood pressure	• Lower cancer risk
• Lower CRP levels	• Lower body weight

Side Effects and Concerns

Fish oil supplements are usually free from serious side effects in healthy adults, with bad breath, softened stools and gas being some of the more commonly reported consequences. Nevertheless, there are some things to consider before using fish oil supplements, especially in high doses.

Those using blood thinner medications or other supplements which might also affect the blood's viscosity should remember that fish oil supplements may have an additive interaction which might *thin* the blood too much. Supplements like vitamin E, ginseng and ginkgo are such examples which might interact with fish oil.

People who have immune disorders should exercise caution when using fish oil supplements. Some speculate that high amounts may of fish oil impair immune function.[513]

Because fish oil supplements may lower blood pressure, in theory, they should be used with caution by those who are using medications to treat high blood pressure.[505]

In dosages of 3 grams or more per day, fish oil supplements may raise blood sugar levels. This may be problematic for diabetics.

Some worry that fish oil supplements might be contaminated with mercury or other toxic chemicals. These fears appear to be baseless. Recent tests of the quality of fish oil supplements have not revealed any significant mercury contamination.[514,515] This was found to hold true for even less expensive brands.

Omega 3 Content vs. Mercury Levels in Commonly Consumed Fish[516]

Fish (3 oz)	Omega 3 Level (g)	Mercury (ppm)
Canned tuna	0.26 - 0.73	0.12
Shrimp	0.27	0
Salmon	0.68 - 1.8	0.01
Flounder	0.43	0.05
Pollock	0.46	0.06

My Thoughts

The old adage that fish is "brain food" notwithstanding, an impressive amount of evidence exists in support of consuming fish or fish oil supplements on a regular basis. Many experts now feel that the American diet does not contain enough omega-3 fatty acids and too many omega- 6 fatty acids. Eating fish or using fish oil supplements might help make this balance better. While higher doses may be required by those with special conditions, this is best undertaken with the involvement of a physician. For those who are healthy now, a few cans of tuna and one or two fish oil supplements a week might go a long way to helping keep us healthy for the long haul.

Flaxseed

Flaxseed refers to the seeds of the flax plant which has a long history of use dating back thousands of years. Flax-derived products have been used for purposes ranging from baked goods, laxatives and even chemicals used in various industries. Many reading these words are probably familiar with the popular flooring called *linoleum*. Linoleum is made from flax. Flax has even been used to make clothing! While used for eons, the introduction of flax to America dates back to the early 1600s. Today, Canada is the world leader in flax production. From flaxseed, three distinct compounds are usually mentioned: *flax fiber*, which is mostly a soluble fiber; *lignans*, a type of plant estrogen (phytoestrogen); and a third compound called *alpha linolenic acid*. Other names that also refer to flaxseed include *Linum usitatissimum*, *linseed*, and *flax*.

What is Alpha Linolenic Acid?

At the heart of many of the health claims for flaxseed and flaxseed oil is a polyunsaturated fatty acid called *alpha linolenic acid*. Alpha linolenic acid (ALA) is a member of the omega-3 fatty acid family of nutrients. ALA is found naturally in foods like salmon, soybeans, red meats, walnuts and dairy products. The richest source of ALA, however is flaxseed. Two other popular omega-3 fatty acids are EPA and DHA which are found in fish and fish oil supplements. In fact, when people use ALA about 10% of it is converted to EPA and DHA.

Flaxseed and Heart Disease

A number of clinical studies suggest that flaxseed may be effective at lowering the risk of heart disease.[789] Specifically, flaxseed has been shown to modesty reduce cholesterol and LDL (bad cholesterol) levels by about 10% and 20% respectively. This cholesterol-lowering ability appears to be due mostly to the soluble fiber content of flaxseed, which, like other soluble fibers such as pectin, have also been shown to lower cholesterol. To achieve these heart protective benefits, studies generally use about 40 grams of flaxseed per day.[789] It is probably wise to introduce flaxseed gradually into the diet to reduce diarrhea, one of flax's most common side effects. In contrast, most studies do not show that flaxseed improves HDL (good cholesterol) levels. Likewise, flaxseed's impact on triglycerides (blood fats) also appears to be insignificant.

Another way in which flaxseed may defend against heart disease lies with its ALA content. As was mentioned above, alpha linolenic acid can be converted to some extent to the omega-3 fatty acids, EPA and DHA. These, in turn, are involved in the production of hormone-like substances called *prostaglandins*. Some prostaglandins help keep blood cells from getting too sticky.

Flaxseed and Menopause

Postmenopausal women looking for a natural alternative to hormone replacement therapy may turn to flaxseed to reduce hot flashes and other symptoms associated with menopause. The logic in this is most likely based upon flaxseed's lignans, which appear to exert estrogen-like activity. Indeed, the use of flaxseed for this purpose may be warranted. While more research is needed, some evidence suggests that 40 grams of flaxseed daily may be as effective as hormone replacement therapy at reducing the severity of menopausal symptoms.[791]

Flaxseed and Osteoporosis

Osteoporosis is a devastating disease in which bones become fragile and break easily. Bone loss is accelerated after menopause when estrogen levels drop significantly. Anything that could elevate estrogen levels might be effective at preserving bone mass. Since flaxseed contains lignans, which are estrogen-like, it makes sense in theory that flax might help combat osteoporosis. While interesting, studies, though limited in number, have not found flaxseed effective for osteoporosis. In addition to calcium and vitamin D that are well known bone-builders, two other alternatives to flaxseed that might also have merit include soy and red clover, which are each reviewed separately in this book.

Flaxseed and Cancer

Flaxseed is sometimes used by postmenopausal women to help reduce the risk of cancer. Like that of osteoporosis described above, the basis for this reasoning lies with the lignans of flaxseed which are phytoestrogens. In theory, the use of such products might block estrogen receptors and reduce the risk of breast cancer. While this theory sounds plausible, the effect of flaxseed on cancer requires more study. Research hints that flaxseed may indeed be of benefit to those at risk for breast cancer but definitive research still needs to be conducted.

With respect to men, some—but not all—clinical studies suggests that *flaxseed oil* may promote the growth of prostate cancer.[790] Ironically, this may be due to the ALA content of flaxseed, which is usually touted for health reasons. This is a controversial issue that requires more investigation and there is no evidence that flaxseed itself is associated with prostate cancer. Until more is known, men with prostate cancer or a family history of prostate cancer may want to consider other supplements such as soy or fish oil which might be more prostate-friendly.

Flaxseed Oil

Flaxseed oil is a good source of omega-3 fatty acids and is usually an attractive option for those who don't like the fishy smell that sometimes accompanies fish oil supplements. The main omega-3 fatty acid in flaxseed oil is ALA which is different than EPA and DHA—the omega-3's found in fish. As was mentioned previously, the body can convert some ALA into EPA and DHA but this conversion is generally thought to be small. Flaxseed oil is also sometimes used to treat rheumatoid arthritis despite the lack of evidence showing it is effective. One important distinction between flaxseed and Flaxseed oil is that the latter generally contains no phytoestrogens (lignans) unless a manufacturer specifically adds them in during processing.

Side Effects and Concerns

Flaxseed is generally found to be safe for the vast majority of adults, with diarrhea being one of the most commonly reported side effects. This is related to the high soluble fiber content of flaxseed which acts as a laxative. Based upon what is known, the following things should be considered when using flaxseed.

Theoretically, flaxseed might interact with blood thinner medications because of its ability to affect blood platelet stickiness.

Some research suggests flaxseed may be able to lower blood sugar levels. If this is so, it could be problematic for diabetics.

Until more is known, men with a family history of prostate cancer and those who have prostate cancer should steer clear of flaxseed oil.

Pregnant women should suspend the use of flaxseed oil during pregnancy. While not well-studied, there is speculation flaxseed oil might promote contractions of the uterus.[10]

My Thoughts

While evidence suggests that both flaxseed and flaxseed oil may benefit various conditions, I am not yet convinced that either is better than eating fruits and vegetables along with fish or fish oil supplements. Studies show that flaxseed contains soluble fiber which can lower cholesterol. Soluble fiber is also found in oatmeal as well as the skins of many fruits, which have also have been shown to lower cholesterol. Flaxseed contains ALA which is an omega-3 fatty acid. ALA appears to exert at least some of its effects via its conversion to EPA and DHA, which are already found in fish and fish oil supplements. The lignans of flaxseed may also exert health-promoting effects via their estrogenic characteristics but how much is needed and for whom they might most benefit, we don't yet know. Also unknown is how the lignans stack up against other similar compounds like those found in soy. Further complicating this issue is the question of what's better, flaxseed or flaxseed oil? If I had to choose, I'd pick flaxseed, because it has everything as nature intended. And flaxseeds taste good—an added bonus. If you love flaxseed and are seeing improvements in your health, that's fine, keep using it; it has a long history of use and safety when used moderately. To improve their shelf-life, flaxseed and flaxseed oil should be refrigerated because both sun and heat can cause them to spoil.

Folic Acid

Folic acid is one of the B complex family of vitamins. Usually the terms folic acid and *folate* are used interchangeably. The subtle difference between them is that folate is the natural form of the vitamin found mostly in foods. Folic acid is the synthetic version that is usually found in supplements. A difference between the two versions is that folic acid is more absorbable by the body, hence its incorporation in supplements and fortified foods. Like all vitamins, folic acid participates in many vital chemical reactions including the making of red blood cells and the proper growth of developing babies. Folic acid also helps with the production of SAM-e, a compound reviewed separately in this book, that some people may use for arthritis. The RDA for folic acid for adults is currently 400 micrograms (µg). Like most vitamins, we do not have the ability to make folic acid and must obtain it from either food or supplements. Good sources of folic acid include *dark green leafy* vegetables, citrus fruits, whole grains and breakfast cereals.[496] Other names for folic acid include *pteroylmonoglutamic acid, folacin,* and *folate.*

Folic Acid and Heart Disease

Homocysteine is an amino acid made in the body that makes blood *sticky.* This in turn may to contribute to plaque formation and heart disease.[483] Many studies have noticed that people who have high homocysteine levels suffer more heart attacks than those with lower levels.[484,485] This may even hold true for those with normal cholesterol levels.[483] Studies find that folic acid, either from food or supplements, can reduce homocysteine levels.[486] For these reasons, folic acid supplements are often used by people to reduce their risk of heart disease. In addition to folic acid, vitamins B_6 and B_{12} also seem to lower homocysteine.[486] Because of this, these vitamins may be found in supplements designed to support healthy heart function. While not often mentioned, the fact that folic acid can reduce homocysteine, does not automatically mean that it also reduce the risk of heart disease. In fact, some research finds that this strategy doesn't work. Until more is known, people looking to cover all their bases should opt for a quality multivitamin that contains the RDA for folic acid, B_6 and B_{12} and combine this with other heart-healthy choices like regular exercise and a diet rich in fruits, vegetables and whole grains.

Folic Acid and Pregnancy

Many women reading these words are familiar with the popularity of folic acid during pregnancy. Folic acid used during pregnancy reduces the rate of defects to the *neural tube*, which eventually develops into the baby's nervous system. In other words, folic acid reduces birth defects and is the reason it is found in prenatal vitamins. Some advocate that women begin using folic acid at least two months prior to becoming pregnant to best reduce birth defects.[495] There is even some evidence that pregnant women who have the highest levels of homocysteine give birth to babies who weigh less—yet another reason for pregnant women to use folic acid.[482]

Folic Acid and Cancer

Studies hint that folic acid may reduce the risk of cancers of the breast, colon and possibly pancreas.[487,488,489] Folic acid is required for the proper functioning of DNA, our personal *software* program. A lack of this vitamin might, in theory, lead to errors in the way DNA directs the complex orchestra of chemical reactions needed every second of our lives to keep us healthy. Whatever its role in the curtailing of cancer, eating foods high in folic acid appears to be a wise preventive step. For those reading these words who currently are receiving treatment for cancer, the decision to use folic acid supplements should be discussed with a physician. Folic acid supplements may reduce the effectiveness of some drugs used to treat cancer.[490]

Folic Acid and Restless Leg Syndrome

For years, I have always known when it was time to go to bed. Whenever I became really tired, my feet seemed to develop an annoying *need* to move uncontrollably. This is referred to as *restless leg syndrome* (RLS). Some research suggests that folic acid may reduce RLS symptoms.[481] Folic acid might also appear in supplements alongside the mineral magnesium because of evidence that it, too, may help with the abatement of RLS. How folic acid appears to help RLS, is unknown. Until more is known, those with RLS should make sure they are getting the RDA of folic acid (and magnesium). This is easily obtained via a quality multivitamin and a healthy diet.

Side Effects and Concerns

Folic acid is usually free from serious side effects in healthy adults especially when used at the RDA of 400 micrograms (abbreviated as µg or *mcg* on supplement labels) per day. In very high doses (over 10 mg) folic acid may lead to irritability, excitability and confusion.[491] It is unlikely, though, that these levels would be reached by people eating food or by even combining a folic-acid-rich diet with a high potency multivitamin.

Seniors may sometimes suffer from anemia because of a deficiency in vitamin B_{12}. Folic acid may disguise the symptoms of vitamin B_{12} deficiency.

People who are using cholesterol-lowering drugs may need folic acid supplements. Some cholesterol-lowering medications may reduce the absorption of folic acid.[493]

My Thoughts

Folic acid has been a rising star in the battle against heart disease for the last several years despite concrete proof that it works. Until all the answers are in, the best advice for those wishing to reduce their risk are to use a quality multivitamin that has the RDA for folic acid, vitamin B_6 and B_{12}. This, of course, should be combined with a healthy lifestyle that's rich in fruits vegetables and whole grains, and also incorporates regular exercise. A component that's often missing from this recipe is to deal as well as possible with the negative, long-term stresses that, overtime, can weigh us down and contribute to this number one killer of Americans. Folic acid may one day prove effective at reducing heart disease, but just in case it isn't, taking these other steps is a much better and time tested way of covering your bases.

Forskolin

Forskolin refers to a compound found in the roots of the plant, *coleus forskohlii*, which is a member of the mint family.[145] While used for centuries in Ayurvedic medicine for a number of conditions such as asthma and respiratory infections, these days, one of the main reasons people might supplement with this herb is weight loss. Other names that also refer to forskolin include *Plectranthus barbatus*, *borforsin*, *coleus barbatus*, *coleanol*, *HL 362* and *makandi*.

Forskolin and Weight Loss

The theory of how forskolin might foster weight loss is full of technical jargon which you may or may not have heard of before. Forskolin is able to stimulate an increase in the production of an enzyme called *adenylate cyclase*. This enzyme in turn promotes a rise in another molecule called *cyclic AMP* (or cAMP for short). In the body, cyclic AMP is very important because it helps cells *talk* to each other. The body is sensitive to both increases and decreases in the level of cyclic AMP. When an increase or decrease in the level of cAMP is detected, it acts as a signal for the body to do something. One of the things that cAMP can do is produce an increase in an enzyme called *hormone sensitive lipase*—which breaks down fat. cAMP also stimulates the release of thyroid hormone which also helps burn fat.[455] So, the theory goes like this: forskolin stimulates fat-burning enzymes and hormones which, in turn, causes weight loss. The theory sounds good but does it hold any water?

Studies performed on laboratory animals hint that forskolin may promote the release of fat from fat cells. However, concrete proof that forskolin can promote weight loss in humans is currently lacking. This doesn't necessarily mean that forskolin doesn't work. Rather, it might mean nobody has gotten around to taking a serious look at it yet. This is unfortunate because forskolin supplements are heavily promoted on the Internet.

Side Effects and Concerns

When injected, forskolin is a vasodilator which means that it expands blood vessels. Theoretically, forskolin supplements might also expand blood vessels which could be a problem for those using medications for high blood pressure and heart disease.

Forskolin appears to have a *blood thinning* effect.[456] Thus, it might interact with medications and supplements that also have this property. Supplements which might interact with forskolin include vitamin E, ginkgo and garlic.

My Thoughts

Considering how much forskolin is promoted to fitness-minded people and others looking to lose weight, it's too bad the hype surrounding this herb seems to have leaped ahead of the evidence. Just because forskolin stimulates a rise in fat-burning enzymes doesn't necessarily mean it will significantly impact weight loss in people, although in theory it might if combined with a healthy, lower calorie diet and sensible exercise. While the theory behind forskolin is intriguing, I would like to see some human weight loss studies published first before I give it two thumbs up. I would also like it to be proven safe for long- term use as well. Just because the plant from which forskolin is derived has been used safely for centuries, does not mean that highly concentrated extracts of forskolin are safe.

Gamma Oryzanol

Gamma oryzanol refers to a plant steroid that is derived from rice bran oil.[517] Small amounts are also found naturally in some fruits and vegetables. One of the main reasons people supplement with gamma oryzanol is in the hopes that it might increase muscle size and strength. Other names that also refer to gamma oryzanol include *ferulic acid* and *rice bran oil*.

Gamma Oryzanol and Exercise

People who lift weights are sometimes intrigued by gamma oryzanol because of claims that it might heighten levels of the male hormone, testosterone.[517] More testosterone, in theory, might mean bigger, stronger muscles. In spite of its popularity among fitness enthusiasts in the 1990s, the evidence that gamma oryzanol raises testosterone or improves any aspect of exercise performance is limited at best. In fact, it is generally believed that gamma oryzanol possesses no significant ergogenic properties.[517,518] One study found that 500 mg of gamma oryzanol per day for 9 weeks was ineffective at raising testosterone, growth hormone or altering cortisol levels—even when it was combined with a strength training program.[518] The ineffectiveness of gamma oryzanol may be related to its poor absorption where it is estimated that only about 5% of what is ingested actually makes it into the body.[517,520] Some speculate that gamma oryzanol may actually reduce testosterone levels.[519,520] Regardless of its impact on anabolic hormone levels, based on the evidence to date, gamma oryzanol is unlikely to improve any aspect of exercise performance.

Gamma Oryzanol and Cholesterol

Some clinical studies find that gamma oryzanol may be effective at reducing cholesterol levels.[521,522] Studies generally find that 300 mg of gamma oryzanol per day might help those with high cholesterol levels. In theory, this might lower heart disease risk; In reality though, long-term use of gamma oryzanol for this purpose has not been adequately studied.

Side Effects and Concerns

Studies have generally found gamma oryzanol to be safe with no significant side effects.

My Thoughts

The evidence just isn't there for gamma oryzanol improving strength, decreasing body fat or increasing testosterone or growth hormone levels. While for some, gamma oryzanol may help lower cholesterol levels, any effects it may have are likely amplified when it is used as part of a comprehensive lifestyle change that includes eating better and getting more physical activity. Food for thought: If I had to choose between gamma oryzanol and exercise to reduce my cholesterol and improve the quality of my life, I'd pick exercise in a heartbeat!

Garcinia Cambogia

Garcinia cambogia is a plant that grows in Asia and which contains a compound called *hydroxycitric acid* (abbreviated as HCA). Thus, hydroxycitric acid and Garcinia cambogia are often used interchangeably. The major claim of Garcinia cambogia is weight loss. Other names that also refer to Garcinia cambogia include *hydroxycitrate, malabar tamarind, Garcinia cambogi* and *gorikapuli.*

Garcinia Cambogia and Weight Loss

Some theorize that HCA might assist weight loss by interfering with the process of making fat.[327] Indeed, some animal research has shown that HCA may be effective for weight loss.[328,329,457] The impact of HCA on reducing the waistlines of humans however has generally not been positive.[327,331,332] One study, while finding no weight loss following the use of 900 mg of HCA per day for two weeks, did observe a 15-30% reduction in food intake.[332] While interesting, how this affects long-term eating patterns is unknown. In addition, whether amounts less than 900 mg might have the same effect requires more study. Human studies using between 1000 and 3000 mg of HCA a day have not generally observed reductions in bodyweight. Whether amounts greater than these promotes weight loss in humans requires more study.

Garcinia Cambogia and Exercise

Emerging research hints that HCA may be of benefit to some athletes. At rest and during exercise the body usually burns a mixture of fat and carbohydrates. Fat breakdown is intimately dependent on a steady supply of carbohydrates (called glycogen). When the body exhausts its glycogen reserves, our ability to exercise declines precipitously. Runners sometimes call this situation "hitting the wall". In theory, anything that could reduce the breakdown of glycogen during exercise might prolong exercise time and enhance exercise performance. Some research hints that HCA may have such properties. Specifically, under some circumstances, HCA may lead to greater fat utilization and reduced glycogen use during exercise.[458,459,460] In theory this may be of use to athletes such as runners, cyclists and triathletes. Studies finding positive outcomes have used 250 mg of HCA per day.[459] Research suggests that supplementing with HCA for several days before participating in exercise might produce optimal results.[459]

Side Effects and Concerns

HCA appears to be safe in healthy adults. Currently, HCA has no known drug interactions or side effects.

My Thoughts

While interesting, the effectiveness of HCA for weight loss in humans remains open to speculation with claims based mostly on laboratory animal research. The effect of HCA prolonging exercise is also interesting and may be something athletes might want to experiment with. Because not all studies are in agreement as to its effectiveness, individual results will probably vary from person to person.

Garlic

Like that of many herbs, the use of garlic for medicinal reasons dates back to before the time of the Bible. Garlic is reputed to influence a wide variety of conditions ranging from heart disease and cancer to even the common cold. Today, two of the most well known chemicals in garlic are *alliin*, which, when chewed or broken down, produces the chemical *allicin*. Allicin, in turn, breaks down further into other chemicals. It is allicin which is mostly responsible for garlic's distinctive odor. Other names that also refer to garlic include *Allium sativum ali, ajo*, and *stinking rose*.

Garlic and Heart Disease

While garlic may be the herb of choice in Transylvania for warding off vampires, here in America, one of the primary reasons people use garlic supplements is for the reduction of heart disease risk—and for good reason. Several lines of research find that garlic may have a positive impact on several heart disease risk factors. For example, garlic has been shown to reduce the development of atherosclerosis (hardening of the arteries), "thin" the blood modestly, lower cholesterol and bad cholesterol (LDL), as well as reduce blood pressure and triglyceride levels.[523,524,525] These effects are probably best observed in those who have problems in these areas to begin with. Successful results have been found with 200-400 mg of garlic used three times a day. Garlic does not appear to significantly raise good cholesterol (HDL) levels. Individual success with garlic may vary from person to person. This caveat is reinforced by the fact that not all research agrees that garlic works.[532,533]

Garlic and Blood Sugar

Some people may be attracted to garlic because of claims that it stabilizes or normalizes blood sugar levels, something very important to diabetics. The impact of garlic on blood sugar in humans is still open speculation.[534,535] Food for thought: A tremendous amount of evidence exists for the power of exercise to lower blood sugar levels.

Garlic and Cancer

When scientists look at large groups of people, they sometimes find that those who eat the most garlic (anywhere from 3 grams to 30 grams a week) tend to get less cancer. Cancers that seem to be reduced by garlic consumption include colon cancer, stomach cancer, and prostate cancer.[526,527] Some speculate that garlic may act as an antioxidant in the body.[528] Whether this is responsible for garlic's actions on cancer requires more study. It is important to emphasize here that only garlic eaten as food appears to have this effect. The research on garlic supplements and cancer is sketchy and open to interpretation. When garlic is digested, it forms hundreds of chemicals, any of which might be responsible for its apparent anti-cancer effects. Concentrating one or a few key ingredients in garlic supplements may or may not act the same as eating the whole herb.

Garlic and Infections

Some research finds that garlic may have antibacterial and antiviral properties. For these reasons some may supplement with garlic in the hopes that it might ward off colds. One study noted that during a three-month period, people who used garlic supplements suffered only half the colds as those who did not use garlic supplements.[530] Those using the garlic supplement also seemed to recover faster from colds as well. More research is needed to determine how garlic appears to battle colds and to figure out the right amount to use.

Side Effects and Concerns

In healthy adults, garlic is usually considered safe. Besides bad breath, some of the more common side effects include mouth irritation, vomiting, body odor and diarrhea. In spite of its relative safety, some groups of people should consider the following points before using garlic supplements.

Some research hints that garlic might reduce the effectiveness of some HIV medications.[531] As such, people taking drugs to treat HIV infection should talk to their doctor before using garlic supplements.

Those with new organs or who have rheumatoid arthritis may be familiar with a drug called *cyclosporine* that affects the immune system and prevents tissue rejection. Some research suggests that garlic may interfere with *cyclosporine.*[531]

There is some concern that garlic supplements may reduce the output of thyroid hormone.[10] This could be problematic for those with under-active thyroid glands (hypothyroidism).

Garlic appears to "thin" the blood. Because of this, care should be exercised when combining garlic supplements with blood thinner medications and other supplements which might also have blood thinning effects.

People using high blood pressure medications should remember that garlic supplements may also lower blood pressure. The combination of garlic and high blood pressure medications may lower blood pressure too much.

Garlic May Interact With	
• HIV medications	• High blood pressure medications
• Blood thinner medications	• Supplements that *thin* the blood
• Arthritis medications	• Anti-tissue rejection medications

My Thoughts

A lot of evidence supports the notion that garlic is not just for fending off Count Dracula. While eating garlic from food definitely seems to have health-promoting effects, it is still not fully accepted that garlic supplements do the same thing, although research is supporting their use under some circumstances—like possibly warding off colds. While both alliin and allicin receive a lot of attention, remember that they are just two of hundreds of chemicals in garlic. Excluding any of these other chemicals during manufacturing may void any potential benefit of garlic supplements. Those who are frustrated by all of this can avoid the hassle of trying to find a quality supplement by just eating garlic and letting nature take its course.

Gelatin

Gelatin is essentially collagen, a connective tissue that is found in bones, skin and tendons. In fact, gelatin is most likely obtained by boiling the bones of cows. Aside from being a main staple of many a lunches in elementary school (as Jell-O®), gelatin is sometimes used by people to strengthen muscles, reduce arthritis pain and diminish bodyweight. Other names which also refer to gelatin include *hydrolyzed collagen* and *collagen hydrolysate.*

Gelatin and Exercise

Some supplements marketed to strength trainers and fitness-minded people may use gelatin as their main protein ingredient. Gelatin, though, is of lesser quality than other popular proteins like whey or soy because it lacks some of the essential amino acids, which the body cannot make on its own. Thus, the argument can be made that gelatin may not be the best choice for the individual looking for optimal muscle growth. Conversely, the argument can also be made that the amino acids contained within gelatin complement other proteins that are consumed in the diet. Regardless as to which philosophy you subscribe to, while a little gelatin is unlikely to be a problem for strength trainers, it should not be the main source of protein in the diet.

Gelatin and Arthritis

Some clinical research suggests that gelatin may be an effective tool in reducing the pain of osteoarthritis.[542] Thus, gelatin may be found in products alongside other supplements like glucosamine that also have shown promise in this area. How gelatin appears to work, as well as the amount that is best to use, is unknown. Some speculate that gelatin may stimulate the formation of new cartilage or decrease the breakdown of existing cartilage. Ten grams of gelatin used over the course of several weeks has shown some efficacy in the treatment of osteoarthritis-related pain.[542] More research is needed to compare how gelatin stacks up against other popular supplements like glucosamine and chondroitin.

Gelatin and Osteoporosis

Like arthritis mentioned above, the research on gelatin supplementation helping those with osteoporosis is preliminary and open to speculation.[542] Because of the paucity of research in this area, those who want to experiment with gelatin should probably use the guideline for arthritis (10 grams a day) until more is known. One thing is certain; any effect gelatin may have on strengthening bones is surely to be enhanced by the use of calcium and regular participation in a comprehensive exercise program that includes strength training.

Gelatin and Weight Loss

Some weight loss supplements may contain gelatin as their main ingredient. In spite of this, there is no published peer-reviewed evidence proving that gelatin speeds weight loss. Because protein contains less energy per gram than fat, any reduction in weight that might be had by consuming such supplements may be the result of simply eating fewer calories. Those trying to lose weight should definitely consume a little more protein, but it's probably wiser that they eat chicken, tuna, whey or other superior proteins than a supplement with lower-quality protein like gelatin. Unless it's used alongside a reduced-calorie eating plan that includes regular exercise participation, gelatin alone is unlikely to provide any healthy weight loss.

Side Effects and Concerns

Gelatin is usually well tolerated in healthy adults and is unlikely to cause any significant side effects. Because gelatin is often derived from the connective tissues of cows, there has been some concern about the possibility of *mad cow disease*. To date, no documented cases of mad cow disease have occurred via the use of nutritional supplements in the US. To minimize the risk, consumers should investigate the makers of gelatin supplements and specifically ask for information regarding safeguards to prevent mad cow disease transmission.

My Thoughts

The evidence just isn't there to support the claim that gelatin-based supplements can improve muscle size or strength or foster healthy weight loss. Gelatin was a big part of the protein fad diets of the 1970s which—because of their poor quality—resulted in the deaths of many people. Despite the hype in some circles, the research on gelatin improving arthritis or osteoporosis is in its infancy and a lot of questions need to be answered. For example, would eating *Jell-O*—which is probably in your kitchen cabinet right now—have the same effect as gelatin supplements? Maybe? It certainly can't hurt; it definitely tastes great, and, as one of my favorite commercials used to say, *there's always room for Jell-O!*

Ghrelin Blockers

If you have not heard of ghrelin, don't feel bad because you are not alone. *Ghrelin* (pronounced *gr-rell-in*) is a stomach hormone discovered in the late 1990s. One of the big reasons scientists study ghrelin is because it appears to affect the amount of food we eat and as such may play a role in weight gain and obesity. Conversely, blocking the action of ghrelin might, in theory, encourage weight loss. This is the main promise behind supplements that claim to block or inhibit the action of ghrelin.

Ghrelin and Weight Loss

Several studies have found that the hormone ghrelin makes people hungry.[536,537] When we are fed to our heart's content, ghrelin levels decrease and when we are hungry, ghrelin levels increase, causing us to eat again.[538,539] Also, when ghrelin is injected into people, they tend to eat more. Sometimes gastric bypass surgery (*stomach stapling*) is performed on morbidly obese people. There is evidence suggesting that one of the reasons that this surgery works is because it lowers ghrelin levels in the body. Thus, based on this evidence ghrelin appears to be a player in weight gain and weight loss. So, if we could block the effects of ghrelin, would people lose weight? Maybe, but to date there is no good evidence that any nutritional supplement can block the action of ghrelin and promote weight loss.

Ghrelin and Growth Hormone

Another action of ghrelin is that it stimulates the release of growth hormone, a major player in muscle growth. For this reason, some bodybuilders and fitness enthusiasts may be attracted to ghrelin supplements in the hopes of stimulating more growth hormone, which in theory might lead to bigger, stronger muscles. So far, research finds that ghrelin does not elevate growth hormone levels even when combined with a strength training program.[541] Ghrelin is a protein and like all proteins would probably be digested shortly after taking it orally.

Side Effects and Concerns

Little is known about how ghrelin supplements interact with other supplements or medications. The most consistent side effect noted following ghrelin use is an increase in appetite.[538]

My Thoughts

Ghrelin is a hot topic in research and its discovery literally caused the re-writing of medical books around the world. Supplements purported to block ghrelin or to augment its effects should be backed up by clinical studies performed on humans and published in medical journals to give validity to their claims. Claims not accompanied by this proof should be viewed with skepticism.

Ginkgo

Ginkgo, or *ginkgo biloba* as it is also called, comes from the ginkgo tree, the last remaining member of a once large number of related trees that were said to have existed for over 200 million years.[399] While cultivated in China for thousands of years, ginkgo is a relative newcomer to America with the first tree being planted in 1784 in a garden, just outside of my hometown in Philadelphia.[570] While advertised for a number of conditions, most people today use ginkgo for improving memory and concentration. This use is reinforced by the fact that in Germany, ginkgo is one of the treatments of choice for those suffering from dementia. Other names for ginkgo include *ginkgo leaf extract, GBE, EGb, ginkgoaceae* and *Japanese silver apricot.*

Ginkgo and Memory

A number of clinical investigations, published in respected medical and scientific publications have found that ginkgo can moderately improve mental function in some older people who suffer from an age-related decline in memory.[554,555,556] The optimal dosage to achieve this effect is still being investigated; Some research has found positive results with between 120 and 240 mg of ginkgo leaf extract per day.[429] So far, ginkgo has not been shown to benefit seniors who do not have memory impairment.[557] Ironically, for reasons that are not well understood, some research also hints that ginkgo may improve the attention span of younger people.[555,558]

Multiple studies have also noted that ginkgo appears to assist in retarding some of the effects of

Alzheimer's disease and other forms of senile dementia.[562] Studies in this area generally use between 120 to 240 mg spread out over the course of the day in three or four equal doses. It should be stressed that the improvements from ginkgo appear to be mild at best and may not work for everyone. Also, it is important to keep in mind that not all studies find that ginkgo works.[563] Whether long term supplementation with ginkgo by healthy people is effective at warding off dementia down the road is still open to speculation.

Ginkgo and Sexual Function

Ginkgo may find its way into supplements tailored to improve sexual function and performance. The rationale for this could be based on research that ginkgo (120 mg per day in two equal doses) may help erectile dysfunction in men using antidepressant medications as well as studies finding that the herb may expand blood vessels in the penis.[561,565] For now, more research is needed before it can say for sure if ginkgo improves erections in men who are not on antidepressants.

How Does Ginkgo Work?

Ginkgo is composed of a number of phytochemicals which are thought to have a variety of effects. This makes figuring out how ginkgo works difficult because all of its different ingredients may work both in concert and independently of each other. Several investigations have noted that ginkgo can improve blood flow to the brain, protect brain cells from damage, reduce the stickiness of blood, and act as an antioxidant.[559,560] These, plus other effects, might explain how ginkgo works.

Side Effects and Concerns

Ginkgo is usually well tolerated in healthy adults with some of the most common side effects being occasional headache, dizziness, and mild stomach upset. Because ginkgo has a blood thinning effect, it might *over-thin* the blood if combined with both blood thinner medications and other supplements having similar effects.

Some studies hint that ginkgo, when taken in high doses, may increase the risk of seizures.[10,566] What constitutes a "high dose" is not well known.

Over the years, there have been anecdotal reports of ginkgo possibly causing brain bleeding or *hemorrhages*. One of these reports occurred in a 56-year-old male who developed a hemorrhage after using 40 mg of ginkgo three times a day for 18 months.[569] A review of his case indicated that the only supplement he was using was ginkgo. This does not prove that ginkgo causes hemorrhages and this outcome might simply have been due to this persons unique physiology. Nevertheless, this is something to consider before supplementing with this herb regularly.

Some reports suggest that ginkgo may be inappropriate for diabetics because it may raise blood sugar levels and speed the removal of both insulin and other diabetic medications from the body.[567,568]

My Thoughts

Ginkgo appears to have a wide range of effects, some of which may benefit memory in older persons who may be having difficulty remembering. The problem is that older individuals may also be taking medications or have other health conditions which could interact with ginkgo. While ginkgo is probably safe for many people, those with health concerns should see their doctor first. If you are going to experiment with ginkgo, understand that no studies show that it will transform a person from a dementia-induced vegetable into someone capable of refuting *Einstein's Theory of Relativity!* This fact is buttressed by the story of a friend who once was taking ginkgo to improve her memory—and actually forgot where she kept it in her house.

Ginseng

Ginseng is a slow-growing plant that takes at least 6 years before it is usually cultivated.[399] In fact, the older the ginseng is, the more it can cost with people paying many thousands of dollars for ginseng roots that are decades old! Ginseng can be a rather difficult herb to get a handle on for a number of reasons. First, it's touted to improve a variety of conditions. For example, people use ginseng to improve energy levels, enhance sexual performance, reduce stress and to ward off disease. Another reason which adds to the confusion surrounding this herb is that different types of ginseng are available to consumers and each type goes by different names. Thus, picking up a bottle of "ginseng" may not give you the product—or results—you're looking for.

Types of Ginseng

While there are many different species of ginseng, three types are most popular. They are *American ginseng, Asian ginseng* and *Siberian ginseng*. All three belong to the same family of plant (Araliaceae); however, Siberian ginseng is kind of a *kissing cousin* to the other two because it belongs to a different genus. Below is an overview of the three popular ginseng types and some of their alternative names.

Ginseng Type	Also Known As
American Ginseng	Panax quinquefolius, Canadian ginseng, occidental ginseng
Asian Ginseng	Panax ginseng, Korean ginseng, white ginseng
Siberian Ginseng	Eleutherococcus senticosus, eleuthero ginseng, ciwujia, eleuthero ginseng

Because different types of ginseng are available, let's review each individually to get a better handle on claims, usefulness etc.

American Ginseng

The scientific name for American ginseng is *Panax quinquefolius*, a plant that grows in both America and Canada. Traditionally, American ginseng is used for a number of reasons such as improving exercise ability, promoting general health, improving sex drive and reducing stress. While American ginseng contains many different ingredients, the active parts are thought to reside in the root of the plant and are a family of related compounds called *ginsenosides*.[571] Ginsenosides are part of a larger family of compounds called *saponins*. So, you may see the words ginsenosides and saponins used interchangeably when researching ginseng.

What Are Adaptogens?

You can't get far into researching ginseng before you run into the word *adaptogen,* so it's best if we define it here. An adaptogen is a generic term for something that helps people cope with (in other words, adapt to) a stress. The stress can be anything such as physical stress (like exercise), emotional stress, pollution, cold temperatures, etc. Essentially, adaptogens are said to change the way they work according to what your needs are. Some feel that ginseng works by acting like an adaptogen in the body. It is important to remember that the term adaptogen does not refer to any specific molecule but rather was created to help explain the different effects that have been observed by users of ginseng. In other words, just like Bigfoot, nobody is sure if adaptogens really exist.

American Ginseng and Exercise

Because exercise is a type of stress, some may use ginseng in the hopes that it will help improve their physical performance in the gym or on the playing field. While this might sound logical, the role of ginseng improving any aspect of exercise performance is controversial and open to speculation. Some clinical studies have found no exercise benefit following ginseng use.[577,578] Others have also criticized the overall quality of studies that find positive outcomes.[579] For example, evidence supporting the use of American ginseng may inadvertently be derived from studies of Asian ginseng. Both American and Asian ginseng may appear with the prefix *panax*. While both plants are related, it is possible that they differ not only in the total amount of ginsenosides present but also in levels of the different types of ginsenosides that are known to exist.

American Ginseng and Nitric Oxide

Nitric oxide (NO) is a gas produced in the body that expands blood vessels and can lower blood pressure. Preliminary research does suggest that American ginseng may augment nitric oxide production.[580] As such, American ginseng may play a role in blood pressure reduction and indeed some research exists in support of this.[627] For this reason, ginseng may be found in supplements designed to boost levels of nitric oxide. Such products can range from "healthy heart" type supplements to those marketed to men suffering from impotence. Nitric oxide-boosting supplements may also be popular among strength training enthusiasts who seek fuller, more *pumped*, muscles. In all of these cases, the majority of evidence in support of ginseng is not based on concrete evidence. The bottom line is that more research is needed before ginseng's role in nitric oxide production is firmly tied to the reduction or improvement of any condition.

Ginseng and Cancer Prevention

Some may use ginseng in the hopes that it might help reduce cancer risk. Indeed, some studies suggests that this practice may be warranted.[583,584] Most of the evidence to date on this topic is derived from asking large numbers of people questions about their lifestyle practices. Those consuming ginseng report less cancer. While encouraging, it could be that ginseng users might have other healthy habits (i.e. didn't smoke, ate more vegetables, etc.) that contributed to their reduction in cancer. It should also be remembered that this benefit appears strongest for Asian ginseng rather than the other types. The effect of ginseng in those who currently have cancer is unknown. Some speculate that ginseng might interact with some forms of cancer, so it might be wise to steer clear of this herb until more is known. The bottom line of all of this is that for the moment, ginseng and cancer prevention is an open question, but one that is surely worthy of more study.

American Ginseng and Diabetes

Several studies have observed that American ginseng may lower blood sugar levels in some individuals who have type II diabetes.[572,574,575] Other research suggests that American ginseng may also lower blood sugar levels in people without diabetes.[572,573,576] While more research is needed, dosages of between 1-3 grams have been used to achieve this effect.

Side Effects and Concerns

In healthy people, American ginseng is usually found to be safe.

One group who should steer clear of American ginseng is pregnant women, where animal research suggests it may be linked to birth defects.[581]

People using blood thinner medications should consult their physician before supplementing with American ginseng as the herb may decrease the effects of blood thinners.[582] Likewise, those with bleeding disorders should also exercise caution with ginseng.

In test tubes, American ginseng seems to promote the growth of cancers that are sensitive to the hormone estrogen.[397] This may be tied to ginseng's apparent estrogen-like effects and may be an issue for women with a history of breast, uterine or ovarian cancers.

American ginseng may lower blood sugar levels.[572] Because of this, people with diabetes should monitor their blood sugar regularly if they supplement with ginseng.

Asian Ginseng

Asian Ginseng and Exercise

The scientific name for Asian ginseng is Panax ginseng. Like all types of ginseng, Asian ginseng is sometimes advertised to improve physical endurance and strength during exercise. However, several studies have been unable to substantiate this claim.[578,593,594,595] Likewise, Asian ginseng does not seem to elevate testosterone or growth hormone levels even in young men who participate in strenuous strength training programs.[593] Asian ginseng also seems unable to prevent cortisol from rising after exercise.[593] Cortisol, a hormone which has many different effects in the body is vilified in some fitness circles because of thoughts that it limits muscle growth. Asian ginseng neither appears to hinder muscle growth or facilitate it based upon the limited research available.

Asian Ginseng and Energy Levels

It seems that these days people are on the go from the moment they wake up until the time their head hits the pillow. Thus, one of the most popular reasons people use Asian ginseng is to boost energy levels to help them get through their hectic days. Unfortunately, there isn't much evidence that Asian ginseng supplements enhance energy levels.[587,588] Sometimes ginseng is combined with caffeine or other ingredients. This may explain why some say they have more energy after using ginseng.

Asian Ginseng and Brain Function

Studies show that even a single dose of Asian ginseng can affect brainwave activity.[589] Other research finds that Asian ginseng may enhance creativity and the speed at which we do simple arithmetic tasks.[590] Thus far, ginseng has not yet been found effective at improving memory.[591]

Asian Ginseng and Sexual Performance

Asian ginseng may be listed as an ingredient in some supplements touted to improve male sexual ability. This may be based on research finding that 900 mg used three times a day might help enhance performance in men with erectile dysfunction.[592]

Whether ginseng also is effective in those without erectile problems is open to speculation.

What is Red and White Ginseng?

The terms *red* and *white* ginseng refer to how the ginseng was prepared. Ginseng root is naturally white in appearance. When the root is steamed, the color of the root turns red and it is called red ginseng. When the root is simply air-dried and doesn't receive any further processing, it retains its natural color it is called white ginseng. Both red and white ginseng contain different levels of ginsenosides—the compounds many think are some of the herb's active ingredients.

Asian Ginseng and Menopause

Some women may use Asian ginseng as a natural alternative to hormone replacement therapy because of speculation that it acts similarly to the hormone estrogen and as such might help them cope with hot flashes and other symptoms of menopause. Currently, the ginseng-estrogen connection is controversial. In other words, there is evidence that it has estrogen-like properties and evidence that it doesn't. Regardless of how it works, the research so far tends to show that while Asian ginseng may not reduce hot flashes, 6 grams of Asian red ginseng may help alleviate depression and fatigue levels which sometimes accompany menopause.[596,597]

Asian Ginseng and Cancer

In studies performed in test tubes, Asian ginseng is found to possess anti-cancer characteristics.[598,599] Specifically, Asian ginseng seems to prevent damage to genetic material, which might make us more susceptible to cancer.[598] Studies of large populations of people also hint that those who consume the most Asian ginseng tend to get fewer cancers of the liver, lung, stomach and ovary.[600,602] As a rule, people who use supplements tend to also have other healthy habits, like not smoking, getting more exercise, etc. Thus, one possible drawback to observing the habits of large groups of people is that the effect of ginseng may be caused by either ginseng itself or the combination of ginseng with other healthy habits. The bottom line is that more research is needed before anyone can say if Asian ginseng prevents cancer.

Asian Ginseng and Radiation Protection?

Some laboratory research suggests that Panax ginseng may offer some protection against the effects of radiation.[626] Thus, Panax ginseng may be incorporated into cosmetics to protect the skin from sun exposure as well as supplements marketed to people hoping to reduce radiation-injury following national emergencies. How ginseng appears to protect people from radiation has not been well studied. One caveat to this might be that ginseng supplements may be counterproductive in those who are receiving radiation treatment for cancer. In other words, might ginseng reduce the effectiveness of radiation therapy? Nobody knows. Those undergoing radiation treatments should consult their oncologist before using ginseng.

Side Effects and Concerns

Like ginseng in general, Asian ginseng is usually free of significant side effects in healthy people. A few points to consider when using Asian ginseng are as follows:

In theory, Asian ginseng may lower blood sugar levels. Diabetics should monitor blood sugar levels closely when using Asian ginseng.

Asian ginseng seems to lower blood pressure in laboratory animals.[603] Because of this, Asian ginseng might alter blood pressure in humans.

In theory, Asian ginseng might interact with blood thinner medications.[604] People with heart problems of any kind should talk to their physician before using ginseng.

The idea that ginseng acts like the hormone estrogen is a matter of debate with evidence on both sides of the argument. Some studies suggest that ginseng may latch onto the estrogen receptors on breast cancer cells. In theory, this might not be good for the person who has breast cancer.[605] To be on the safe side, those with personal or family histories of cancer should steer clear of ginseng until more is known.

Siberian Ginseng

Siberian ginseng, which grows in Russia, China, Korea and Japan is not always considered "true" ginseng because it belongs to a different genus of plants than its relatives—Asian and American ginseng. Siberian ginseng is easily distinguished from its cousins by its scientific name, *Eleutherococcus senticosus*, which, in turn, gives rise to other frequently used names such as *eleuthero ginseng* or simply *eleuthero* for short.

Another name for Siberian ginseng that is popular in some circles is *ciwujia* (pronounced su-wa-ja). Like that of Asian and American ginseng, the roots of Siberian ginseng appear to be the source of its active ingredients. The active ingredients of Siberian ginseng are thought to be a variety of compounds collectively called *eleutherosides*.[608] Different types of eleutherosides are believed to elicit different effects in the body. Siberian ginseng may also contain other compounds which may exert influence in the body as well. Much of the research on Siberian ginseng was done in the former Soviet Union where a cheaper, faster-growing, yet equally effective alternative to Panax ginseng was desired for Soviet athletes.[607] Because of this, one of the big reasons people use Siberian ginseng is to improve exercise performance. Other claims for Siberian ginseng range from improving overall energy levels, decreasing mental stress and stimulating the immune system. Like other ginseng types, Siberian ginseng is also thought to be an adaptogen, changing the way it works according to the type of stress one is under.

Siberian Ginseng and Exercise

Because of research, mostly conducted in the former Soviet Union, some may opt to supplement with Siberian ginseng to improve aerobic and muscle endurance during exercise. In fact, Siberian ginseng may be an ingredient of supplements marketed to runners, cyclists and other aerobic endurance athletes because of research finding that it may improve both strength and endurance in humans.[611] Recently, the quality of these early Siberian ginseng studies have come under fire by others.[579,612] Adding to the controversy are the conclusions of other studies which fail to show that Siberian ginseng improves exercise performance in humans.[609,610] Studies finding no improvement in exercise capacity have use 1000 mg to 1200 mg a day for several weeks. Whether or not greater amounts than this might improve exercise performance requires more study.

The Ginseng-Cortisol Connection?

Since ginseng is said to decrease stress, and because exercise is a type of stress, some athletes may include ginseng in their daily supplement regimen. Some evidence hints that Siberian ginseng, when given at a dosage of 4 grams per day might *increase* cortisol levels in aerobic-endurance athletes.[619] Cortisol is a stress-related hormone, which in small amounts is needed for the proper functioning of the body. In theory, high levels of cortisol might decrease exercise performance. Interestingly, Asian ginseng has not been observed to increase cortisol (or testosterone) when given to strength trainers in amounts of 20 grams a day.[593] Arguably, the ginseng-cortisol connection deserves further research before anyone can say one way or another what is going on. For the moment, if you are going to use Siberian ginseng, do so in moderation—especially if you're a highly-trained athlete.

Siberian Ginseng and Memory

There is some evidence that Siberian ginseng may improve short-term memory in healthy persons.[613,614] The amounts which might achieve this effect are not well studied. Whether or not this means college students using Siberian ginseng will perform better on exams is also unknown.

Siberian Ginseng and the Immune System

People who have colds and flus may use Siberian ginseng because of research suggesting that it might augment some aspects of the immune system. For example, research finds that Siberian ginseng may alter *mast cells* which play a role in allergies.[618] On the other hand, not all evidence is positive for Siberian ginseng with some research finding no effect on the immune system.[617] At this point there is no compelling evidence that Siberian ginseng can prevent colds or flus.

Siberian Ginseng and Heart Disease

Some people may use Siberian ginseng to reduce or prevent heart disease. One of the components in Siberian ginseng is *beta sitosterol*, a plant steroid which has been shown to lower cholesterol levels as well as LDL ("bad" cholesterol).[628] It remains to be seen whether the lowering of cholesterol also results in a reduction in heart disease (food for thought: the same can be said for some cholesterol-lowering medications as well). For those investigating beta sitosterol itself, research generally finds that about 800 mg a day used in conjunction with a healthy, low fat diet and exercise may be required to alter cholesterol levels.

What About Standardized Ginseng?

In an effort to offer consumers a greater level of certainty as to what they are purchasing, some ginseng products are *standardized*—in other words, guaranteed to contain a specific amount of a product's active ingredients. A few issues should be considered when choosing standardized products. One. Ginseng—like many herbal products—contains several different compounds. In many cases we simply do not know which is the active ingredient, or ingredients. Two. Concentrating one or a few ingredients may alter any positive effects the herb might have. Three. Unfortunately, random tests of supplements continue to find that the amount listed on the label may differ from what the product actually contains. In one study, the actual eleutheroside content of Siberian ginseng was found to vary by as much as 200 percent from that listed on the label.[620] Standardized or not. There is still no better option for the consumer than to deal only with reputable companies.

Side Effects and Concerns

Like all types of ginseng, short-term use of Siberian ginseng appears to be safe, with few side effects in healthy adults. It is worth mentioning that the *German E Commission*, which is somewhat analogous to the FDA in America and which performs tests on herbs, recommends that Siberian ginseng not be used for more than 3 months at a time to limit side effects.[27]

One commonly reported effect is sleepiness, which is why some use Siberian ginseng to help insomnia. Because of this, Siberian ginseng should not be combined with sedative medications.

Diabetics should monitor their blood sugar closely because of research that Siberian ginseng may lower blood sugar.[623]

People who use blood thinner medications should consult their physician before using Siberian ginseng because of some older evidence that the two may *over-thin* the blood.[625]

Some research suggests that Siberian ginseng may elevate levels of *digoxin*, a medication used by some who have heart disease.[624]

My Thoughts

Like the legends of ginseng itself where it is said to act in a variety of ways under different conditions, the investigations of this herb are also somewhat contradictory, with some studies showing it works and other studies finding that it doesn't. These discrepancies could be due to a number of factors. So, for the moment until more is known, ginseng remains a mystery. However, this does not mean all hope is lost. If you are a person looking for something that will help you cope with stress better, give you more energy, battle colds, help you sleep better, reduce your risk of diabetes, cancer and a host of other diseases as well as improve the overall quality of your life, I do have an answer for you. It's not ginseng. It's a little *supplement* I like to call exercise. I'm not kidding! Let's look at the claims for ginseng and stack them up against the benefits that occur when you take part in a regular exercise program.

Ginseng vs. Exercise: How They Compare		
Claim	Ginseng (all types)	Exercise
• Improves energy levels	no	yes
• Lowers blood sugar	maybe	yes
• Raises testosterone	no	yes
• Improves immune function	maybe	yes
• Prevents cancer	unknown	maybe
• Lowers blood pressure	maybe	yes
• Improves mood	maybe	maybe
• Improves strength	no	yes
• Improves exercise endurance	maybe	yes
• Improves sleep	maybe	yes
• Improves sexual performance	maybe	yes
• Improves quality of life	unknown	yes

And, as an added bonus, there are fewer side effects with exercise!

Can ginseng have positive effects in the body? Yes, I think it can, but I also think we need to do more research to better figure out what those effects are and the right types and amounts of ginseng to use. Until that day arrives, you have the opportunity right now to achieve most, if not all, of the alleged benefits of ginseng by simply going for a brisk walk 3 or 4 times a week. So, what are you waiting for...?

Glucomannan

Glucomannan almost sounds like some sugary superhero; however, it's actually a fiber derived from the root of the *Konjac* plant which grows in Asia. One of the main reasons people use glucomannan is weight loss; Other names that also refer to glucomannan include *Amorphophallus konjac, konjac mannan* and *konjac.*

Glucomannan and Weight Loss

Glucomannan is an insoluble fiber that is said to expand in size due to its ability to soak up water like a sponge. Thus, glucomannan is thought to promote weight loss by absorbing excess fluids and speeding their departure from the body. Because the fiber expands in the stomach, some speculate that glucomannan may also assist weight loss by making people feel full for a longer period of time. Several small studies, mostly conducted during the 1980s and 1990s have had encouraging results observing that glucomannan, when combined with eating fewer calories, may lead to modest weight loss in humans.[630,631,632,633] An amount used in some studies is 1 gram of glucomannan taken three times a day before meals.[633] It should be noted that not all research finds that glucomannan is effective for weight loss, so individual results will most likely vary and would probably be enhanced if combined with a sensible exercise program.[629]

Glucomannan and Cholesterol

Several studies suggest that glucomannan may be effective at reducing both cholesterol and LDL in people with type II diabetes.[635,636,637] Amounts used in research range from 3 to 10 grams a day.[635,636] Other studies also imply that the combination of glucomannan and chitosan (reviewed previously) may be more effective at reducing cholesterol than either alone.[634] In addition, some studies also report reductions in blood pressure following glucomannan use. This effect may be related to glucomannan's effect on weight loss. Weight loss might also positively impact cholesterol levels as well.

Side Effects and Concerns

Aside from flatulence, diarrhea and abdominal pain, the studies to date find glucomannan safe in healthy adults. Because of its ability to expand in size, glucomannan—as well as any other supplement with similar properties—runs the risk of blocking portions of the digestive system.[638] This can be particularly dangerous if glucomannan swells up in the throat. Supplements in capsule or tablet form should be used with caution.

Because of the possibility of lowering blood sugar, diabetics should monitor their blood sugar while on glucomannan. Some recommend that glucomannan be used at least two hours before or two hours after medications because it may alter the absorption of the drugs you are taking.[10]

232

My Thoughts

Many nutrition experts routinely recommend eating a higher fiber diet for those desiring weight loss. This is sage advice considering that most Americans do not get enough fiber in their diet. Glucomannan is indeed a fiber. While research does find that glucomannan shows promise for weight loss when used in addition to a reduced calorie eating plan and exercise, I would like to see more research conducted. Is there anything special about glucomannan? Maybe, but then again it's hard to say one way or another at this point. It would be interesting to put 100 or so people on glucomannan and the same number of people on another type of fiber, have them eat the same number of calories and see what happens after several months. For now, all that can be said is that glucomannan is intriguing for cholesterol reduction, but how much of a player it is in the grand scheme of weight loss is yet to be determined.

Glucosamine Sulfate

Glucosamine is a natural compound made in the body from the sugar glucose and the amino acid glutamine. It is also extracted from the exterior skeletons of sea-dwelling animals like lobsters, crabs and shrimp. The main reason people supplement with glucosamine is for the reduction of pain associated with arthritis. When people talk about glucosamine, they are usually referring to *glucosamine sulfate*. However, other related forms also exist. Two other popular types of glucosamine include *glucosamine hydrochloride* and *NAG*. Other lesser known names that also refer to glucosamine sulfate include its scientific name *2-amino-2-deoxyglucose sulfate* as well as *G6S* and *chitosamine*.

Glucosamine Sulfate and Arthritis

Many studies conducted since the 1970s have documented that glucosamine can help reduce the pain of osteoarthritis.[643,644,645] While early studies were criticized by researchers for a variety of reasons, taken as a whole, these, as well as more well-designed investigations generally find glucosamine effective in many individuals. When stacked up against medications, studies generally find that glucosamine acts as well as aspirin or ibuprofen, but takes longer to work.[651] More specifically, when compared to medications, glucosamine may take up to two months before its effects are noticed. On the plus side, studies suggest that glucosamine may be effective at slowing the progression of osteoarthritis.[640,646] This is an advantage that glucosamine may have over aspirin, ibuprofen and other pain-relieving medications. The typical dosage used in studies is 500 mg taken three times a day.

234

Glucosamine and Chondroitin: Better Together?

Supplements for osteoarthritis may use a combination of glucosamine and another compound, called *chondroitin sulfate*. Chondroitin sulfate, like glucosamine, also has some evidence supporting that it may help osteoarthritis-related pain.[659] The rationale of using both compounds together is that they might work better together than either would by themselves. While this seems logical, more research is needed to confirm this.

Most research shows glucosamine is effective for osteoarthritis of the knee. While it makes sense that glucosamine would also work for other joints afflicted with osteoarthritis, this can't be said with certainty. Other investigations hint that glucosamine may not be effective for those who have had osteoarthritis for many years.[647,648,652] In other words, both the severity of pain as well as the length of time you have had osteoarthritis may dictate how effective glucosamine is for you. Further complicating the issue is that not all studies find that glucosamine works.

Aside from oral supplements, glucosamine (and/or chondroitin) may be also used in ointments that are applied to the skin's surface to alleviate arthritis pain. Currently, there is little proof that glucosamine or chondroitin can be absorbed through the skin so they may not be much help under these circumstances. Such ointments might likely contain other ingredients like capsicum, camphor or menthol that provide temporary relief by masking pain with sensations of cold or heat.

Glucosamine Sulfate and Rheumatoid Arthritis

Rheumatoid arthritis is thought to occur when the immune system attacks the joints, causing inflammation and pain. Rheumatoid arthritis is a different condition than osteoarthritis. This is an important distinction to make because there is no good evidence that glucosamine helps or treats rheumatoid arthritis.[649] Alternatively, a supplement which might help rheumatoid arthritis pain is fish oil, which is reviewed separately in this book.

How Does Glucosamine Work?

How glucosamine works is still being studied. Glucosamine is one of the key elements in formation of *proteoglycans*, molecules that help with the formation cartilage. Some scientists feel that glucosamine works by not only decreasing pain levels but also by slowing the breakdown of cartilage.[640]

It is generally thought by laypersons that glucosamine can re-grow joint cartilage. These claims may be traced to the speculation of researchers who conducted a study the early 1980s.[642] This study, though, has been criticized by other researchers.[643] Currently there isn't much proof that glucosamine re-grows cartilage that has already been destroyed or severely damaged.[641]

What About The *Other* Glucosamines?

As was mentioned previously, glucosamine sulfate is one of three popular glucosamine types on the market. The other two are *glucosamine hydrochloride* and *N-acetyl glucosamine* or "NAG" for short. Both of these alternative compounds have some evidence in support of their use in treating/reducing osteoarthritis-related pain. People considering a glucosamine supplement and confused about which type to use should remember that there is more research on glucosamine sulfate than either of these other related compounds.

Side Effects and Concerns

Glucosamine is usually well tolerated in healthy adults. Side effects sometimes mentioned in research include occasional abdominal pain, nausea and headache.[639]

Some research suggests that glucosamine may aggravate asthma.[658] This could be problematic for asthmatics.

Consumers might want to check the labels of glucosamine supplements for the presence of the mineral manganese. Manganese is sometimes used in glucosamine (and chondroitin) supplements because it plays a role in bone formation. That being said, too much manganese over time may negatively affect brain function.[660] The average American gets between 1.5-2.5 mg of manganese a day through the diet. The upper limit past which the potential for side effects might occur is set at 11 mg a day.

Glucosamine sulfate (and chondroitin also) may have weakly acting blood-thinning properties that might—in theory—interact with medications that have similar effects.[657]

Glucosamine and Blood Sugar?

Because glucosamine contains the sugar glucose, some have raised concerns that this supplement may be inappropriate for diabetics. Animal research has hinted that injected glucosamine may interfere with insulin secretion.[653] However, other research in both diabetics and non-diabetic individuals has found that glucosamine does not alter blood sugar levels.[654,655] To be on the safe side, diabetics should consult their physician before using glucosamine and monitor blood sugar levels closely.

Like all supplements, consumers are advised to deal only with companies that they trust. This is also true in the case of glucosamine where studies occasionally find differences between what the label indicates and what the supplement actually contains.[2]

My Thoughts

There is a lot of evidence suggesting that for some, glucosamine sulfate may decrease the pain of osteoarthritis. Glucosamine is not a cure for osteoarthritis, but rather should be viewed as part of a comprehensive program to improve quality of life. Another crucial part of this comprehensive plan is participation in a balanced exercise program, which also has been shown to improve arthritis-related pain. Before you try glucosamine, I suggest you check with your doctor to make certain you have osteoarthritis—the type of arthritis that responds to this supplement. It has been my experience that many people do not know which type of arthritis they have and use glucosamine for the wrong reasons.

Glutamine

Glutamine is an amino acid—one of the building blocks that make up protein. In fact, glutamine has bragging rights in that it is the most plentiful amino acid in the entire human body.[661] Glutamine serves a variety of purposes, being used by the digestive and immune systems, muscles, kidneys and liver. Glutamine is usually labeled a *non-essential* amino acid, because we have the ability to make it as needed. That being said, it appears that our need for glutamine may increase during certain conditions. It is for this reason that glutamine is sometimes called a *conditionally* essential amino acid. In other words, under some conditions, our need for glutamine may increase. People use glutamine for a number of reasons, some of the most popular of which include decreasing muscle breakdown following exercise, improving the immune system and treatment for HIV infection. Glutamine is formed from leucine, isoleucine and valine—which collectively are called the *branch chain amino acids*. Other popular names that also refer to glutamine are *L-glutamine* and *GLN*.

Glutamine and Exercise

Clinical studies find that the body's need for glutamine increases under stressful conditions. However, what is created by the body may not always be enough to meet our needs.[663] Because exercise is a type of stress, glutamine supplements are popular among many bodybuilders and strength training enthusiasts. One of the main reasons exercisers use glutamine is to reduce or prevent the breakdown of muscle that may occur following intense exercise. Research finds that there may indeed be evidence in support of this reasoning. For example, in some people who are seriously ill, giving glutamine intravenously has been shown to improve body weight and muscle mass and reduce the time one spends in the hospital.[663,664,665] Might these interesting results also apply to weightlifters who take glutamine supplements? Maybe, but so far, studies have not found that glutamine supplements make people stronger or improve athletic performance.[667,668,669]

But, what about the more interesting notion of glutamine reducing muscle breakdown following strenuous exercise? For the moment, this appears open to speculation. Most of the evidence for this case is extrapolated from research of *injected* glutamine used on severely ill people or studies conducted on lab animals or in test tubes. Research has found that orally-taken glutamine, when combined with the amino acid arginine and HMB has shown promise in reducing muscle loss in those with cancer and HIV.[192,193,194] Glutamine, arginine, and HMB are combined in the patented product called *Juven®*, a product made by Metabolic Technologies.[194] Healthy people are different than those who are very sick so whether this combination would be of benefit to strength trainers needs more study.

Glutamine and the Immune System

It is well documented that strenuous exercise like running a marathon, appears to increase the risk of getting sick in the days following the event.[662] Some research suggests that glutamine may be effective at reducing infections after marathons.[670] Glutamine is a favorite *food* of many cells of the immune system so in theory, giving your immune system more glutamine might explain its immune boosting effects. Positive results have been noted with 5 grams of glutamine given prior to exercise. Keep in mind that this is a controversial issue and not all researchers agree that glutamine helps reduce infections in athletes.[673]

Glutamine and Overtraining Syndrome

Overtraining syndrome refers to a series of related issues that can be traced to overdoing exercise. Typically seen in athletes or those involved in long periods of high intensity exercise, symptoms may include increased resting heart rate, difficulty sleeping, personality changes and lack of progress when working out. Some research finds low glutamine levels in those who regularly participate in high intensity strength training.[671] Does this mean glutamine supplements might reduce the risk of overtraining syndrome? Maybe. While more research needs to be done, glutamine might help bolster the immune system and alleviate some overtraining symptoms. That being said, the best defense, overall, is to eat right and get adequate rest between exercise sessions so the body has time to recuperate. Glutamine may be one component of many that can help reduce overtraining syndrome but should never be used in place of listening to your body and taking appropriate action.

Side Effects and Concerns

In healthy adults, glutamine is usually well tolerated with few side effects.

Some have raised concern that glutamine supplements may be inappropriate for those with *bipolar disorder*, a syndrome in which people alternate between feelings of depression and euphoria. In these individuals, glutamine might cause mania or hyper-excitement.[672] Until more is known, those with bipolar disorder should avoid glutamine supplements. Related to this, in theory, glutamine supplements may increase the risk of seizures in those with epilepsy by interfering with epileptic medications.[674] Epileptics should consult their physician before using glutamine supplements for the most up-to- date information.

My Thoughts

The research seems clear that under some circumstances the body's need for glutamine increases. The research is less clear that glutamine lives up to the reputation it has gained among some athletes who exercise intensely on a regular basis. So are the bodybuilders wrong about glutamine? It's difficult to say. Most of the research is on very sick people, who usually don't eat well to begin with. This is very different from someone like a bodybuilder or cyclist who exercises regularly and eats a nutritionally sound diet. The best advice to give at the moment is to look at the intensity and frequency of the exercise program you are involved in and weigh that against both the cost of glutamine supplements and any benefits you might obtain. For the professional athlete, glutamine might be something to try. If, on the other hand, you typically get to the gym 3 times a week for an hour or so at a time, how glutamine might help you is open to speculation.

Grape Seed Extract

Grape seed extract is just what the name says—an extract from grapes, usually red grapes. Grape seed extract contains a large number of ingredients, some of the most popular of which include a large class of compounds called OPCs which stands for *oligomeric proanthocyanidins*. OPCs are also found in other foods as well such as fruits, vegetables and even the best food of all—chocolate. Some people reading these words may be familiar with another compound called *pycnogenol* . It, too, contains OPCs and is derived from a species of pine tree. While people may take grape seed extract for a number of reasons, the treatment of heart disease is one of the most common. Additional names that also refer to grape seed extract include *Vitis vinifera*, *GSE*, and *grape seed oil*.

Grape Seed Extract and Heart Disease

When scientists look at large groups of people, they find that those who consume a little red wine on a regular basis develop less heart disease. Probably the most famous case of this occurs in the French who generally get less heart disease in spite of their high saturated fat diets. Since wine is made from grapes, some feel the same effect would be obtained from using grape seed extracts. In support of this idea, research in both animals and studies conducted in test tubes does indeed suggest that grape seed extract may be heart-protective.[546,547] While it makes sense that human hearts might also benefit, questions such as what's the optimal amount to use and does it work for everyone, still need to be answered.

Some people may suffer from a syndrome known as *chronic venous insufficiency*, a condition where blood flow from the legs back to the heart is impaired. This can result in swelling of the legs, leg pain and possibly varicose veins. Some research suggests that grape seed extract, used at about 700 mg per day for several months may be effective for this condition.[543]

Grape Seed Extract and Cancer

Several studies find that grape seed extract has antioxidant properties.[544,545] Grape seed extract has also been shown to raise antioxidant levels in healthy people.[545] There is also some evidence that grape seed extract might work against some forms of cancer when used either alone or in combination with traditional cancer therapies.[548,549,550] Conclusive evidence, that grape seed extract reduces cancer risk in humans is thus far lacking. These studies would be difficult to do, employing the service of thousands of people and carried out over many years.

Side Effects and Concerns

Grape seed extract is usually well tolerated in healthy adults with no serious side effects reported.[27] In theory, grape seed extract may interact with blood thinner medications.[10] Grape seed extract may also have an additive effect when combined with other supplements that also have blood thinning properties.

What is Resveratrol?

Resveratrol is another chemical in red grapes. It is also found in red wine and some types of grape juice. Scientists first became interested in resveratrol in the early 1990s when it was found in red wine. This, some thought, might explain the "French Paradox" which makes reference to the reduction in heart disease observed in French wine drinkers. Evidence suggests that resveratrol is an antioxidant; it might also *thin* the blood, and slow the spread of some cancers.[552,553] Research also finds that resveratrol is a weak-acting estrogen.[551] While the research on resveratrol is intriguing, most of the evidence is derived from lab animals or studies in test tubes. Thus, its applicability to reducing disease in humans is unknown. One issue that should be considered when using resveratrol is its rapid breakdown and excretion from the body. Because of its estrogen-like properties, resveratrol may be inappropriate for women with cancers (like breast and ovary cancer) that are sensitive to hormone fluctuations.[551]

My Thoughts

While intriguing, I feel grape seed extract deserves further study before I give it two thumbs up for everybody. It should be remembered that grape seed extract is just one of many phytonutrients in grapes. The same thing goes for resveratrol. One of my personal mottos is, "If it has color, eat it." Grapes certainly do have color and are fun to eat—especially when they are frozen! For the moment, I would stick to eating grapes and other colorful foods as opposed to focusing on any single ingredient whose effectiveness in people has not yet been fully determined.

Guggul

Guggul (pronounced, *google*, like the popular internet search engine) refers to the tree sap resin that comes from the small mukul myrrh tree that grows in India. Myrrh has long been valued for of its usefulness in making incense and perfume and was also given as a present on special occasions. For example, those familiar with the book of Matthew in the Bible know that gold, frankincense and myrrh were the presents given to the baby Jesus by the three wise men. Guggul, which comes from the myrrh tree also has a long history of use where it has figured prominently in Ayurvedic practices to treat a number of conditions. These days, guggul's most notable claim is its apparent ability to lower cholesterol. Other names that may also refer to guggul include *Commiphora mukul*, *Guggulsterone* and *Guggulipid*.

Guggul and Cholesterol

The active ingredients in guggul (called *guggulsterones*) appear to inhibit the manufacture of cholesterol. Guggul may also reduce levels of C-reactive protein which appears to play a role in heart disease risk. Thus, the theory behind guggul improving cholesterol levels and reducing the risk of heart disease seems logical. In support of this, guggul has also been used for centuries in India to treat heart disease and several studies have noted that guggul appears effective for this reason. Some reports have noted that 100 mg guggulsterones used over the course of several weeks can lower cholesterol and triglycerides by as much as 20%. Interestingly, one study has found that guggul was not only ineffective at lowering cholesterol but ironically observed that it might slightly elevate LDL (bad cholesterol).[792] These conflicting results could be due to several issues such as differences in dietary intakes among test subjects and the overall design of the research.

As was mentioned previously, guggulsterones appear to be the active ingredients in guggul. Current evidence suggests that the cholesterol-lowering properties of guggul may be due to the actions of a couple of specific types of guggulsterones (referred to as E and Z). Thus, supplements may be standardized according to the concentration of E and Z guggulsterones they contain. Like all natural products, guggul is composed of many different elements and the E and Z guggulsterones may rely on these other elements to function properly. Supplements may also be standardized according to the percent of total guggulsterones they contain (without regard to E or Z forms). Those who wish to try guggul are encouraged to have their cholesterol levels checked before and after starting the supplement to see how guggul is working.

Guggul and Arthritis

As was mentioned above, there is some evidence that guggul may reduce levels of C-reactive protein. C-reactive protein is an indicator of inflammation in the body and as such, increases during some disease states including arthritis. Thus, by lowering C-reactive protein levels, guggul may exert anti-inflammatory effects and be of help to those suffering with arthritis. For this reason, arthritis supplements may include guggul among their ingredients. Some evidence does hint that 1500 mg of guggul taken over the course of the day for several weeks might help osteoarthritis, but the lack of human research on this topic makes drawing definite conclusions difficult. Guggul's effects on rheumatoid arthritis are less studied.

Guggul and Weight Loss?

A few studies suggest that guggul might stimulate an elevation of thyroid hormone, which helps regulate metabolism. Metabolism can be thought of as the speed that we burn calories. So the question is, could elevations in thyroid hormone brought about by guggul supplementation lead to weight loss? Maybe. It is an interesting theory, but one that for the moment has more questions than answers. For example, it is not known how guggul stacks up against diet and exercise to achieve weight loss. This, combined with the lack of good evidence in humans probably makes guggul a crap shoot for weight loss at this point. In other words, it might work or it might not. People considering guggul to improve their existing thyroid problems should check with their doctor first.

Guggul and Acne

Some studies find that guggul supplements may have merit in reducing acne flare-ups and may be as effective as antibiotics, especially in those who have oily faces.[793] Effective results have been observed with 50 mg a day.

Side Effects and Concerns

No serious side effects are usually reported to accompany guggul supplementation in apparently healthy adults, with mild stomach upset and rash sometimes reported.

There is speculation that guggul might interact with a variety of medications including some used to treat cancer and high blood pressure. In addition, guggul may interact with drugs used by those with under-active thyroids.

One report links the use of guggul (900 mg a day) to the development of *rhabdomyolysis*, a potentially serious condition where the muscles break down, releasing their contents into the blood where they can cause kidney damage.[794] Interestingly, rhabdomyolysis is also an occasional side effect of some cholesterol-lowering statin drugs, which may lend further support for guggul's ability to impact cholesterol.

My Thoughts

Guggul has been employed for thousands of years in India where its use in Ayurvedic medicine is well known. Thus far, most of the studies on guggul have been conducted in India and the majority of them find that it may be effective for lowering cholesterol. That's good news for people who want to try a natural alternative to cholesterol-lowering drugs. The evidence for guggul's impact on other conditions like weight loss is less accepted and requires more study.

HMB

The letters HMB stand for a compound called *beta-hydroxy-beta-methylbuterate*. Now you know why they call it *HMB* for short! Small amounts of HMB are created naturally when we metabolize the amino acid leucine. In other words, you are making HMB all the time, just not very much of it. Small amounts of HMB are also found in citrus fruits, alfalfa and catfish. HMB is usually popular with two groups of people: those who exercise and those with severe illness. Research exists in support of HMB in both of these groups so let's look at each area separately.

HMB and Exercise

When people exercise—especially strenuously—muscle tissue can break down. While this is a natural part of the process of growing stronger, anything that could speed the rebuilding of muscle or prevent significant muscle loss following repeated high intensity training sessions might, in theory, improve exercise performance and strength. Leucine, an amino acid found in high concentration in muscle, is metabolized to HMB. HMB, in turn, is thought to be a signal that tells the body to slow down muscle destruction. So the theory is that more HMB might promote better muscle recovery following exercise.

Over the past several years, HMB has been the focus of scrutiny to determine whether it can help build muscle or prevent the loss of muscle following weightlifting. Some research does indeed find that when combined with a weightlifting program, 3 grams of HMB a day may be effective at increasing strength and reducing muscle breakdown following high intensity exercise.[675,676,678,679] Other research notes that HMB may also be effective in older adults who strength train as well.[677] In spite of these encouraging findings, the effect of HMB on increasing strength is controversial in that not everyone agrees that it works.[680,681,682,683] One of the points of contention with HMB supplementation is that it seems to work best in those just starting an exercise program. Its effects in highly trained athletes appear to be less pronounced.[684]

HMB and Severe Illness

One of the most intriguing areas of HMB research involves its use in those with cancer and HIV. Ongoing research finds that the combination of 3g of HMB, along with 7g of both the amino acids glutamine and arginine may be effective at reducing weight loss in those with HIV infection and cancer.[192,193,194] Both glutamine and arginine, reviewed separately in this book, do have some research to suggest that they may benefit people with severe illness. So, in theory, the combination of these three supplements might act better than either would by themselves. Currently most of the research in this area has been conducted on a product called *Juven®* made by Metabolic Technologies.[194] More research is needed before HMB and the Juven cocktail supplement are fully accepted within the scientific community for the treatment of muscle wasting associated with cancer and HIV.

How HMB Works

Currently more research is needed to better determine how HMB works. HMB does not appear to raise anabolic hormones such as testosterone.[686] Some speculate that HMB inhibits the breakdown of muscle while others think that it increases synthesis of compounds that reinforce muscle cells.[677]

Side Effects and Concerns

HMB is generally found to be safe in healthy adults. There are no known drug interactions or significant side effects.

My Thoughts

HMB brings to the table several well-designed studies published in highly respected scientific journals attesting to its effects. While the early interest on this supplement focused mainly on its exercise effects, HMB's most interesting area of research is in those with cancer and other conditions where muscle weakness and loss is a concern.

HMB can be expensive. Because it is derived from the amino leucine, it's possible that somebody reading these words might get the idea to just take the leucine in the hopes that this might increase HMB levels. Unfortunately, there is little evidence that this would significantly raise HMB levels.[685] If you were considering this—nice try. You get an A for effort.

Hoodia

In the Kalahari desert of South Africa resides a cactus-like plan, about the size of a cucumber, called Hoodia Gordonii. Because nourishment is scarce, it is said that the hunter/gatherer residents of this region eat the roots of the hoodia plant in order to curb their appetites during their long treks across the desert in search of food. This curbing of appetite has piqued the interests of some supplement and pharmaceutical companies. The idea is that if hoodia curbs appetite, might it also help people lose weight. Hoodia supplements are usually just called *hoodia* or *hoodia gordonii*. An additional name that also makes reference to hoodia is *P57*

Hoodia and Weight Loss

Hoodia gordonii first garnered attention as a possible weight loss supplement after it was discovered that the inhabitants of the Kalahari desert often eat the plant to stave off hunger during long hunting trips. The thought was that if it curbed appetite it might help people lose weight. That being said, very little published clinical research exists on hoodia supplements and how they might impact weight loss. In one study that was not published, overweight men using hoodia did tend to eat less food and loose more weight than those using a placebo (which shouldn't have any effect). While this is intriguing, other studies should be performed and published to better understand what is happening.

The ingredient in hoodia thought to be responsible for its apparent suppression of appetite is a compound called P57AS3 (also known as "P57") which appears to reside within the roots and stems of the plant. As such, hoodia supplements may be standardized according to the amount of P57 they contain. Exactly how P57 affects appetite is not known but some research suggests that the compound can increase ATP levels within the hypothalamus, the brain's appetite control center. In support of this, some research finds that lab rats eat less food when P57 is injected directly into their brains. Whether this effect is also observed when P57 is ingested orally by humans needs more study.

Side Effects and Concerns

There are no known side effects or drug interactions stemming from hoodia or hoodia supplements. The alleged active ingredient in hoodia (P57) appears to have similar properties to compounds called cardiac glycosides, which can have an effect on the function of the heart. This has the potential to be very serious. Little evidence one way or another exists on how hoodia supplements effect heart function and until more is known, those with heart disease should consult their physician before supplementing with hoodia.

My Thoughts

There is no doubt that nature is full of miracles and hoodia may ultimately turn out to be on of them. Hoodia definitely is an interesting compound that appears to have some evidence in support of its ability to suppress appetite. While future research will surely broaden our understanding of hoodia, for now, there are more questions than answers. When reading about and interpreting the claims and effectiveness of hoodia and hoodia supplements, consumers should keep a few questions in mind:

1. Is there any published clinical proof that hoodia aids weight loss in humans?
2. Is there any published clinical proof that supplements containing P57 promote weight loss in humans?
3. If hoodia supplements curb appetite in humans, does this mean they promote weight loss? Remember, people eat for many reasons other than being hungry.
4. If hoodia (and/or P57) promote weight loss in humans, how much has been clinically proven to work?
5. What are the short term and long term side effects of hoodia supplements? Keep in mind that just because hoodia has been safely eaten for centuries does not automatically mean hoodia supplements (or concentrated P57 supplements) are also safe for everyone.

Another issue that needs to be considered is that it takes several years for hoodia to grow to maturity. So, even if hoodia extracts are indeed found to be effective at helping shed excess weight, harvesting the plant before it matures could, in theory, result in a less effective product. Also, several species of hoodia are known to exist. Other species include *hoodia* officinale, hoodia *parviflora* and *hoodia rosea*. The early evidence suggests that hoodia gordonii might curb appetite when the root of the plant is eaten. The appetite suppressant effects of other species of hoodia are not well studied.

Hyaluronic Acid

Hyaluronic acid is essentially a fancy sugar molecule made naturally in the body. Hyaluronic acid supplements are usually marketed to people with arthritis, although they may be used for other reasons as well. If you have never heard of hyaluronic acid, don't feel bad; it's not as well known as other arthritis supplements like, glucosamine. Glucosamine however, is a part of the hyaluronic acid molecule. Other names that also refer to hyaluronic acid include *Glycoaminoglycan*, *Hyaluran* and *Hyaluronate*.

Hyaluronic Acid and Arthritis

Hyaluronic acid is found in high concentration in the joints where, like oil in a car, it acts as a lubricant and reduces friction. It also appears to function like a shock absorber. In 1997, the US Food and Drug Administration approved hyaluronic acid *injections* to help reduce osteoarthritis pain.[688] This fact may have lead to the development of orally-taken hyaluronic supplements which are also touted to improve arthritis-related pain. Little published peer-reviewed evidence however supports the efficacy of oral hyaluronic acid supplements for the treatment of osteoarthritis. Thus, how much it might help is open to debate. Because of the lack of evidence, the FDA has even sent warning letters to some companies that make unsubstantiated claims on the virtues of hyaluronic supplements.[689]

The FYI on CMO

People investigating alternative treatments for arthritis may have heard of *cetyl myristoleate* (CMO), a type of fatty acid. Interest in CMO began after researchers at the National Institutes of Health discovered that a certain strain of mice didn't get arthritis—when they purposely tried to produce its development. Subsequent studies isolated a compound from the mice that appeared responsible for the protective effect—what we now call CMO. Since then, some— but not—all studies have found that CMO might help people better cope with osteoarthritis-related pain. This appears true whether taken orally or even if applied topically to the painful area. Lesser evidence exists for CMO's effectiveness for rheumatoid arthritis. How CMO works is still being debated but some think it might act as a joint lubricant. The CMO used in supplements today may be derived from cows, which also naturally produce it, or synthesized from palm kernel oil or nuts. Research has had some success with 350 mg a day, used for a month, but lesser amounts might also work. In spite of its being touted on some Internet sites as a "cure" for arthritis, the human research on CMO should be considered ongoing and contradictory. Nevertheless, CMO may be something worth looking at especially if you use it with an open mind and not expecting miracles.

Hyaluronic Acid and Wrinkles

In the skin, hyaluronic acid assists with giving the skin moisture and shape. As we age, hyaluronic acid decreases, which contributes to the formation of wrinkles. In 2003, the Food and Drug Administration approved the hyaluronic-acid-based drug, *Restylane*, to temporarily reduce the appearance of facial wrinkles.[687] This drug must be *injected* into wrinkles to work. Whether hyaluronic acid applied topically to the skin or taken orally improves wrinkles is unknown and open to speculation.

Side Effects and Concerns

Hyaluronic acid supplements appear safe in healthy people with no known side effects or drug interactions.

My Thoughts

While some evidence supports the use of hyaluronic acid *injections* for the treatment of arthritis of the knee and temporary diminishing of facial wrinkles, lesser evidence exists for hyaluronic supplements. Currently there is little proof that orally-taken hyaluronic acid improves arthritis or wrinkles. This doesn't necessarily mean the stuff won't work, but rather that it hasn't been well studied. There is some evidence that glucosamine supplements might naturally raise hyaluronic acid levels. This is because glucosamine is needed to make hyaluronic acid. For those who can't decide what to use for arthritis pain—glucosamine or hyaluronic acid—remember that glucosamine is much more accepted by experts and has a lot more evidence to support its use. On a final note, I sometimes see hyaluronic acid supplements touted as the "fountain of youth". Trust me, it's not.

Kava

For many people in industrialized nations today, a typical Saturday night might include going to a local tavern for an alcoholic drink or two with friends. If you were a native of the South Pacific islands, however, your Saturday night might include the imbibing of another beverage—kava. For hundreds, maybe even thousands of years, kava was to the South Pacific islanders what alcohol is to westerners. To those living in the South Pacific—like Hawaii and Fuji— kava, was the drink of choice at parties, weddings and other social occasions. The reason for this is simple: like alcohol, kava relaxes people, making them feel more at ease with their surroundings and reduces tension. Kava may also coax people to into temporarily losing their normal inhibitions. In short, kava helps people *let their hair down*.

Kava is a member of the pepper family of herbs.[690] The name *kava* is taken from the Hawaiian term for *bitter* or *sour*, a reference to its unpleasant taste. While people may use kava for a number of different conditions, two of the main reasons are to reduce anxiety and promote sleep. Other names that also refer to kava include *kava kava*, *Piper methysticum*, *Kava pepper*, *Kava root*, *Ava*, *Kawa Kawa*, and *Intoxicating pepper*.

Kava and Anxiety Reduction

Because it helps people relax, kava may be found in supplements marketed to people with insomnia and those looking for help in dealing with stress. Several studies do find that kava can help reduce feelings of anxiety.[701,702] The chemicals in kava thought to ease nervous tension are called *kavalactones* (also called *kavapyrones*). These chemicals are usually isolated from the roots and underground stems of the kava plant. Positive results on reducing anxiety have been found with supplements containing 70% kavalactones.[701,702] Lesser amounts might also have similar effects. It should be noted that there are several types of kavalactones, all of which may exert different effects. The long-term effects of kava supplements are not known. Some recommend that kava not be used more than 3 months at a time to minimize any side effects that might occur.[27]

Kava and Liver Damage?

In recent years, reports have come to light linking kava intake to liver failure.[691] Thus far, about 80 people have been treated for liver failure, with some requiring liver transplants. A few people have died following kava use. These serious issues prompted several countries including the United Kingdom, France, Australia and Canada to either restrict or ban the sale of kava until it can be proven safe. In America, kava can still be purchased as a dietary supplement, although the FDA has issued consumer advisories to warn people about possible liver damage following kava use.[692] The FDA and other agencies are actively investigating whether kava really does cause liver failure or whether impurities in kava supplements or interactions between kava and other dietary supplements are to blame. Because of the seriousness of these allegations, it may be advisable to steer clear of kava until more is known.

Side Effects and Concerns

While studies generally find it safe in healthy adults, kava is controversial and some authorities do not recommend that people use it until more is known about its possible effects on the liver. Liver dysfunction has been noted to occur following the use of normal amounts recommended on supplement labels and within 3 weeks of starting kava.[696] The reasons for liver problems following kava use are not known. Some speculate that those who don't metabolize kava very well may be more at risk.[696] Interestingly, other research of heavy kava use by Australian aborigines in the 1980s also noted liver enzyme abnormalities.[697] This hints that the kava-liver connection may not be caused by modern manufacturing processes, but rather be a side effect of kava itself. Kava should not be mixed with alcohol or any drug that affects the liver. Other more common side effects may include dizziness, sleepiness and possible impairment of judgment.

Studies in the 1980s first documented an odd occurrence in Australian aborigines who were heavy users of kava. Specifically, the skin of these people developed a scaly rash that was especially prominent on the hands, feet, forearms and back.[693] Fortunately, this seems to be a reversible phenomena with symptoms clearing up when kava use is halted.

Some people who use kava may experience uncontrollable movements. In theory, this hints that kava might worsen symptoms of Parkinson's disease.[698]

While not normally thought to significantly impair coordination, like alcohol, some evidence hints that kava may negatively impact attention span. As such, driving under the influence of kava is not recommended. Sporadic reports exist of police arresting erratic drivers who consumed large amounts of kava.[694,695] Breathalyzer tests indicated normal blood alcohol levels. Kava should not be combined with alcohol or any medication or supplement with sedative properties.

Some evidence suggests that kava interferes with enzymes that are needed to utilize a variety of prescription medications.[699,700]

Passion Flower

At first glance, one might think the moniker passion flower (*Passiflora incarnate*) was coined for sensual reasons; however, nothing can be further from the truth. So named by the Spanish in the 1500s because the plant was thought to be a botanical reenactment of the sufferings of Christ at his crucifixion, passion flower is today used by some to ease stress and promote sleep. Studies conducted on passion flower do suggest that it might help people with anxiety disorders but not all research is in agreement on this. How passion flower works is not well understood but some speculate that it acts similarly to prescription antidepressants known as MAO inhibitors. At present, the ingredients thought responsible for its effects are not well known but appear to reside in the above-ground portions of the plant—the flowery parts. Side effects, based mostly on case studies of lone individuals, hint that in some people, passion flower may speed up heart rate and affect the way the heart normally functions. Passion flower might also interact with blood thinner medications as well as some sedatives.

My Thoughts

Centuries of "field-testing" by South Pacific islanders and others, as well as modern research, generally find that kava temporarily reduces feelings of stress, nervousness and anxiety. However, what kava won't do is address the root cause of these emotions. Those experiencing overwhelming, crippling stress and anxiety do not need kava. They need to deal with what is causing the stress, either by confronting it directly or by seeking out a trained professional who can help them. Regardless of its effects on stress, because of the possibility of liver damage in some, I feel caution should be exercised at this time. True, it appears that only a minority seems to be affected by liver problems, but the implications of liver failure are too great to ignore. If you are dead-set on using kava, I suggest having your liver function tested regularly by your physician to be on the safe side.

Lutein

Lutein is one of over 600 known types of *carotenoids* (a type of phytonutrient) that occur naturally in fruits and vegetables.[708] Foods that contain lutein include kale, spinach, mangoes, broccoli, romaine lettuce, corn and egg yokes to name a few. Another type of carotenoid that is often mentioned in the same breath as lutein is *zeaxanthin*. Lutein is a very popular eye-supplement because of research finding that it may help preserve vision. Lutein is the most popular name for this nutrient, although it is also referred to as *Xanthophyll* in some circles.

Lutein and the Eye

Lutein (and zeaxanthin) are found in high concentrations in the eyes, specially in the lens and in a region of the retina called the macula. The macula portion of the eye is important because it allows us to see fine details and colors. Some research finds that those who consume foods containing lutein have a reduced risk of a condition called *age-related macular degeneration* (AMD).[704,705] AMD is an incurable syndrome that mostly affects older people and results in a gradual loss of vision. Other research also finds that foods high in lutein may moderately slow the progression of cataracts, a condition where the lens of the eye becomes *cloudy*, blurring vision. How lutein helps reduce AMD and cataract risk is not fully understood but may be related to lutein's antioxidant properties, which neutralize free radicals. Most of the research on lutein protecting the vision involves the consumption of foods that contain lutein. How lutein nutritional supplements impact AMD, cataracts and other conditions is not well studied and more research is needed. It's also important to note that not all research finds that lutein helps AMD or cataracts.[706] How much lutein is needed to help reduce AMD and cataracts is also unknown but according to some research, may be somewhere between 7 and 12 mg a day. This is roughly the amount consumed in food by people found to have reduced AMD and cataract risk.

Foods Containing Lutein	
Foods	Lutein
• Kale (1 cup, cooked)	12 milligrams
• Spinach (1 cup, cooked)	10 milligrams
• Green beans (1 cup, cooked)	1.8 milligrams
• Broccoli (1 cup, cooked)	1.6 milligrams

Side Effects and Concerns

Lutein has been around as long as there has been food to eat. When consumed in amounts found in food, lutein is unlikely to have any significant side effects in healthy people. Little research has been conducted on the side effects associated with long-term use of lutein supplements.

My Thoughts

When scientists look at large populations of people, they notice less AMD and cataracts in those who eat a diet rich in lutein. Other evidence also hints that lutein may reduce the risk of colon cancer.[707] This does not necessarily mean that lutein supplements would have the same beneficial effects. They might, but nobody is sure yet. Lutein is but one of the may hundreds of carotene nutrients found in food. It might be that the positive effects described above are due to lutein's unique interaction with all of the other carotene nutrients (as well as with other substances in food that have not yet been discovered). For the time being, I would use what the bulk of the research shows works—foods high in lutein—and leave the lutein supplements alone for now.

Lycopene

Like lutein discussed previously, lycopene is another member of the carotenoid family of phytonutrients. Lycopene is found in a wide variety of fruits and vegetables with tomatoes being probably the most famous of foods known to contain this nutrient. In fact, lycopene is the reason tomatoes are red! Other lycopene-containing foods include pink grapefruit, watermelon and apricots. While lycopene is likely to be used for a number of reasons, the most popular is cancer prevention.

Foods Containing Lycopene	
Food	Lycopene
• Tomato paste (1 cup)	75 milligrams
• Marinara sauce (1 cup)	40 milligrams
• Tomato soup (1 cup)	25 milligrams
• Vegetable juice cocktail (1 cup)	23 milligrams
• Tomato juice (1 cup)	21 milligrams
• Tomatoes (1 cup)	4 milligrams
• Ketchup (2 tablespoons)	5 milligrams
• Watermelon (1 wedge)	13 milligrams
• Grapefruit, pink or red (1/2 cup)	1.8 milligrams

Lycopene and Cancer Prevention

Research generally finds that people who eat foods rich in lycopene appear to have a reduced risk of prostate cancer, ovarian cancer and lung cancer.[709,710] Much of the excitement about lycopene surrounds its apparent effect on prostate cancer (the most common cancer in men), where some studies show that diets high in this nutrient may reduce prostate cancer growth by over 80%.[711] While optimal amounts of lycopene needed to reduce these cancers requires more study, a ballpark range of 6 mg to 30 mg a day might help.[709,710] Most of the research so far in support of lycopene stems from observing the eating patterns of people over time, with those who eat the most lycopene getting fewer cancers. Lesser research exists on lycopene itself. In other words, would we also see reductions in cancer if thousands of people were tracked for many years with some using lycopene supplements and others using nothing? That would be a truer test of lycopene's power over cancer.

Lycopene: Cooked or Raw?

Lycopene tends to be poorly absorbed in the body in its natural state. Some studies find that lycopene in cooked foods, like tomato sauce, has a greater absorption than lycopene in raw foods.[712]

Side Effects and Concerns

Lycopene, when consumed in amounts normally found in food, is not known to cause any serious side effects.

My Thoughts

Lycopene is another in the long list of phytonutrients thought to promote health and battle disease. How lycopene appears to work is a mystery at this time. As a rule, people are always on the lookout for simple answers to complex problems. Whether or not lycopene supplements are found to be one of those simple answers is not yet known. What is known, is that lycopene is likely to be most effective when other lifestyle changes are also made. This includes not smoking, eating properly, and exercising. Some speculate that lycopene supplements might help, but all of the answers are not in yet. My gut instinct is that lycopene does not work alone but rather is helped by other food nutrients. This is supported by some research finding that lycopene in food works better against prostate cancer than lycopene supplements.[714] If your multivitamin has some lycopene added to it, that's fine, but make sure that you supplement that vitamin with eating foods that contain lycopene to get the best results.

Magnesium

Magnesium is a mineral that plays key roles in hundreds of vital functions such as helping maintain the beating of your heart, energy production, bone formation and the making of proteins—to name just a few. The recommended dietary allowance for magnesium for adult men and women is 420 mg and 320 mg a day, respectively. Good food sources of magnesium include fruits, vegetables, nuts, and cereals. Magnesium supplements are used by consumers for a variety of issues ranging from improving exercise performance, treating migraine headaches and regulating blood sugar levels. The chemical abbreviation for magnesium is *Mg*.

Types of Magnesium

Magnesium may come in a number of different forms, with some of the most common types listed below.

Common Types of Magnesium	
• Magnesium oxide	• Magnesium hydroxide
• Magnesium citrate	• Magnesium chloride
• Magnesium gluconate	• Trimagnesium dicitrate

Magnesium hydroxide is a common ingredient in many laxatives such as *Milk of Magnesia,* while magnesium oxide is sometimes found in antacids. Most forms of magnesium have about the same absorbability in the body.

Magnesium and Exercise

Marathon runners, cyclists and others who participate in long-duration aerobic exercise may sometimes use magnesium to reduce cramping that might occur as magnesium is lost through perspiration. This practice, though, might only be minimally effective, given that only a little magnesium is lost via this route, and magnesium supplements have not yet been shown to improve aerobic exercise ability.

At the other end of the exercise spectrum are strength trainers who may use magnesium supplements because they are aware of the fact that magnesium helps with the production of muscle tissue. So, the thought here is that more magnesium will help optimize muscle growth during strength training. One older study of magnesium supplementation combined with a weightlifting program did find that magnesium might improve strength compared to those who did not use magnesium; however other research finds magnesium does not help.[752] An issue with some studies assessing the effectiveness of magnesium is the lack of figuring out if magnesium levels are low to begin with. Muscle weakness is a sign of magnesium deficiency. If magnesium levels are low to begin with, then magnesium supplements might help improve strength. But, so, too, would eating foods that contain magnesium. Strength trainers as a rule tend to eat pretty well, making it unlikely that they would be deficient in this mineral. So far, the evidence that magnesium will be of significant help to strength trainers is little at best.

Magnesium and Diabetes

It is well known that magnesium takes part in the metabolism of carbohydrates (sugars). Low levels of magnesium have also been observed in people who have diabetes. Other research suggests that magnesium intake may decrease a women's risk of developing type II diabetes.[753] This has lead some to speculate that magnesium supplements may be beneficial for those suffering from diabetes. Intriguing as this is, the idea of magnesium helping to regulate blood sugar is still controversial. Until more answers are known, magnesium supplements used to treat diabetes should not be undertaken without consulting a physician. Overdosing with magnesium is not without side effects.

Magnesium and Blood Pressure

There is evidence that magnesium may lower blood pressure in people who have hypertension. As such, a magnesium-deficient diet might, in theory, adversely affect blood pressure. The effect of magnesium on lowering blood pressure appears modest but could be significant for those whose blood pressure is already elevated. As such, those with hypertension might want to see how a magnesium-rich diet works for them. With respect to amounts which might help, research hints that 600-1000 mg a day may be effective at reducing blood pressure in those with hypertension.

**Magnesium & Calcium:
Are They Better Together?**

In addition to magnesium, low dietary levels of calcium might also impact blood pressure. Because of this, some may use calcium-magnesium supplements in the hopes that both minerals might stabilize blood pressure better than either could alone. In theory, this makes sense, although the link between these minerals and hypertension needs more research before their use is fully accepted. Until more is known, those with hypertension might want to consider increasing their calcium and magnesium intake from food sources first and see how this helps their blood pressure.

Magnesium and Osteoporosis

Some have suggested that magnesium might increase the absorption of calcium and hence, may be of benefit to people with osteoporosis.[847] In support of this, research does find that magnesium may lessen bone loss in women past the age of menopause.[754,847] Other research also hints that 600 mg of magnesium along with 500 mg of calcium may preserve bone mass in women better than estrogen by itself. Taken as a whole this evidence suggests that eating a magnesium-rich diet and/or use of supplements appear to be a player in preserving bone mass and reducing the risk of osteoporosis. Other equally important healthy bone-preserving practices include eating a calcium and vitamin D-rich diet and most importantly, performing regular strength training exercises—particularly those that involve the large muscles of the body like the legs, chest and back.

Magnesium and Migraine Headaches

Migraine headaches are a severe, often debilitating type of headache that affects tens of millions of Americans, most of which are women. Some research does find that magnesium may help reduce the frequency of migraines by a pathway that has yet to be fully understood. Complicating things, though, is the fact that not all studies find that magnesium helps. This hints that positive results with magnesium for this purpose may vary from person to person. Some success with migraines has been noted, with 600 mg of magnesium used three times a day. Magnesium does not appear to work overnight, with at least a month needed before any reduction in migraines is noticed.

Side Effects and Concerns

Magnesium is safe when consumed in amounts found in food. Common side effects from too much magnesium include nausea and diarrhea.

People with blood pressure problems or heart disease should only use magnesium supplements under the care of a physician. Large amounts of magnesium might interact with drugs such as calcium channel blockers used to treat heart disease and high blood pressure.

My Thoughts

Most of the therapeutic claims for magnesium are based on only a few studies or extrapolated from research in which magnesium was injected into the body. Deficiency in magnesium is rare in Americans and usually occurs because of an inability to absorb magnesium or by the use of medications which hinder absorption. Emerging evidence does suggest that magnesium may be effective for a number of conditions like diabetes, fibromyalgia and migraine headaches. The optimal dosage of magnesium to affect these or any disorders needs more study. Before using magnesium supplements it is suggested that you have your magnesium level checked. A simple test will tell you if you are deficient or not.

Medium Chain Triglycerides

The word *triglyceride* means fat. Triglycerides are the form in which fat is stored in the body. In the world of chemistry, fat essentially look like long chains of carbon atoms. Each carbon atom that makes up the *chain* is linked to the others, much like the chain you may wear around your neck. Normally, the length of the carbon chains that make up fats are pretty long. Other types of fat also exist which are not too long and not too short. These fats we call *medium chain* triglycerides or *MCTs* for short. MCTs are found in small amounts in some vegetable oils and have been used since the 1950s to help people with medical problems and those who cannot digest regular fats. Healthy people might also supplement MCTs because of thoughts that they might improve exercise performance and help shed excess pounds. Another name which also refers to medium chain triglycerides is *MCT oil*.

Medium Chain Triglycerides and Weight Loss

Several studies of both lab animals and humans have noted that supplementing with MCTs appears to enhance fat loss and modestly elevate metabolism.[715] This is because MCTs can pass directly into the body where they can be used for energy almost immediately. Ketones which might be formed by long term use of MCTs might also decrease appetite. In theory, this means MCTs might benefit those who are overweight. Whether MCTs are indeed an effective treatment for weight loss or obesity requires further study. At present, research is split with some studies finding MCTs might help and others finding they don't.[715]   For now, most of the evidence stems from the use of large amounts of MCTs for short periods of time. Ironically, MCTs have been used medically for years to help seriously ill people *gain* weight. This is because MCTs are a compact source of calories with one tablespoon containing over 100 calories.

Going Coco for Coconuts?

At some parts of the Internet, coconut oil is highly touted as a weight loss aid. The reason for this is that coconuts are rich in MCTs, making up about 50% of the fat of coconut oil. So, the thought is that using coconut oil will elevate metabolism and promote weight loss in a manner similar to using MCT supplements. Whether or not this is true is deserving of more study. Coconut oil is a saturated fat which could affect cholesterol levels and clog arteries. Coconut oil is also high in calories, which, if used in excess, might put a dent in weight loss efforts.

Medium Chain Triglycerides and Exercise

During aerobic exercise, such as running a marathon, the body uses a mixture of fats and carbohydrates to power the exercising muscles. It turns out that the human body only has enough carbohydrates to run about for 20 miles. When the carbohydrates are exhausted, exercise stops. Runners sometimes call this unfortunate situation *hitting the wall*. Anything that could slow the use of carbohydrates might, in theory, help athletes exercise longer. Because MCTs are absorbed directly into the body they might spare carbohydrate breakdown and thus improve exercise performance. This would definitely be of benefit to athletes like runners and triathletes. While more study is needed, research so far has not conclusively shown MCTs improve aerobic exercise performance.[717]

Side Effects and Concerns

MCTs are usually deemed safe for short-term use in healthy people. The most common side effects from MCT supplements include diarrhea, nausea and abdominal pain. Some speculate that these symptoms might occur after consuming only 30 grams (about once ounce) of MCTs.[716] Other research has used close to 90 grams of MCTs without ill effects.[716] Those who experiment with MCTs might want to opt for a low level first, see how they feel, and adjust the amount gradually over time as they see fit.

MCTs contain no essential fatty acids (unless companies add them to their products). So, people who use a high MCT diet might need additional supplements containing these fatty acids to replace what they are not getting.

Diabetics should steer clear of MCTs because of the possibility of *ketosis*, a potentially life threatening condition resulting from the buildup of acid-like compounds called *ketones*.

My Thoughts

There is little doubt that MCTs might be of benefit to some with debilitating diseases like cancer. In healthy persons, the issue is less clear. For weight loss, it appears that if MCTs are going to help, they will have to make up a relatively large proportion of the diet. Adding a tablespoon of MCTs to your diet is probably not going to result in any significant effects. An issue that still needs to be better studied is whether MCTs enhance fat loss long term when a *normal* diet is consumed under real life conditions. One of the downsides of using MCTs may be the taste which isn't very good.

Melatonin

Melatonin is a hormone that is manufactured from the amino acid tryptophan. Hormones are protein-based chemicals that the body uses to transmit information from one area to another. Melatonin is made in the brain, in an area called the *pineal gland*. While people may use melatonin for a number of conditions, its impact on sleep is probably the number one reason. Some may wonder why a hormone, like melatonin, can be sold in stores. The reason for this is because small amounts of melatonin are found naturally in fruits, vegetables and meats. Because of this, current laws permit melatonin to be sold as a supplement. Other names that also refer to melatonin include *N-acetyl-methoxytryptamine* and *pineal hormone*.

Melatonin and Sleep

Melatonin is thought to promote sleep by regulating *circadian rhythms*, the internal body *clock* that adjusts the rising and lowering of mental alertness that occurs normally during a 24 hour period. The amount of light we are exposed to affects the quantity of melatonin we make. During daytime hours, we make little melatonin. As the sun goes down and light levels decrease, we make more melatonin. The fact that we make more melatonin at night is one of the reasons we get tired at the end of the day. Some research finds that melatonin taken 30 minutes to a few hours before bedtime may not only help people get to sleep faster but also might improve the quality of sleep.[718] In other words, melatonin may actually help us wake up a little better because of the improved sleep quality.

Jet lag is a common side effect of traveling from one time zone to another. Symptoms can include lack of concentration, fatigue and trouble sleeping. Several studies find that melatonin may help those who experience jet lag.[720] Not all studies though find that melatonin works.[721] Those thinking about experimenting with melatonin should keep in mind that studies generally use dosages ranging from ½ to 5 mg.

Can Tyrosine Help?

In addition to melatonin, the amino acid tyrosine might also be of benefit to people, but for different reasons. While melatonin tends to put people to sleep, some research finds that tyrosine may improve alertness. Thus, tyrosine may be of help to airline pilots, military personnel, truck drivers and even college students cramming for finals. This effect of tyrosine might be related to its involvement in the production of thyroid hormone and adrenaline. Another way that tyrosine might help keep us awake is by limiting the brain's uptake of tryptophan. Tryptophan helps make serotonin, a brain chemical that makes us sleepy. The research on tyrosine and alertness conducted so far suggests that about 150 milligrams per kilogram of body weight might be needed to achieve this effect. For a 180-pound person, this equals about 12 grams. Lesser amounts might also work. Tyrosine is found naturally in foods such as meat, fish, dairy products and nuts.

Melatonin and Cancer Prevention?

Some research hints that melatonin deficiency may be a cause of some forms of cancer. In studies of laboratory animals, the removal of the pineal gland, where melatonin is made, appears to increase tumor growth.[719] Giving melatonin to the animals has been shown to decrease this growth. Does this mean that a lack of melatonin can cause cancer? It is interesting to speculate that decades of being exposed to light from lamps and other modern conveniences might cause cancer by decreasing melatonin levels, but at this point it's just that—speculation. There is no concrete proof that melatonin supplements prevent any type of cancer.

Smoking is a major cause of cancer throughout the world. Some research finds that melatonin may be of assistance to those trying to kick the habit by decreasing cravings and other withdrawal symptoms associated with abstaining from nicotine.[724] The optimal dosage which might help is not well known but 0.3 milligrams a day has been used with success in preliminary research.

Melatonin and The Aging Process

Some advocate melatonin supplements as a means to reverse the aging process. This may be based upon early research finding that older people appeared to make less melatonin than younger people. Other research though appears to show no difference in melatonin levels between healthy older and younger persons.[723] Some studies do find that melatonin may play a role in decreasing damage to the *mitochondria*, the site of fat breakdown and a major area of research among anti-aging investigators.[722] The ultimate significance of this is unknown at this time. One thing that is certain, though, is that melatonin is not the *fountain of youth*. All claims that melatonin reverses the aging process should be regarded with the greatest degree of skepticism.

Side Effects and Concerns

Melatonin is probably safe for short-term use in healthy adults. Commonly reported side effects include drowsiness (obviously), abdominal cramps and lowered body temperature. It is important to remember that while melatonin is a naturally occurring hormone, little information of long-term side effects are known.

People with asthma should avoid melatonin supplements. There is research suggesting that melatonin might contribute to inflammation of the airways.

Women who desire having children should be aware of speculation that melatonin may inhibit ovulation.[10] Also, pregnant women should see their doctor before using melatonin. We do not know how melatonin supplements affect developing babies in the womb.

In healthy men, some research hints that melatonin may increase estrogen levels as well as alter the shape, concentration and swimming ability of semen.[725] This might have an impact on a couple's ability to have children, but more research is needed to confirm this.

Children should avoid melatonin supplements unless prescribed by a physician. Some evidence suggests that this hormone may affect the development of the testes. While there is no concrete proof, potentially, long-term use of melatonin by children might delay the onset of puberty.

Preliminary evidence suggests that melatonin may affect insulin levels, the hormone that lowers blood sugar.[726] This could be problematic for diabetics.

My Thoughts

Research suggests that melatonin might be of help to those with insomnia and possibly jet lag. Because melatonin is a hormone, it most likely has a wide range of effects that we are only now beginning to understand. To minimize any side effects that might occur, melatonin should be used only occasionally. Insomnia may be caused by a number of things like stress, anxiety, waking up later than usual, lack of physical activity and some medications to name a few. Those suffering from long term insomnia are better served by determining the root cause of the problem rather than self-medicating with melatonin or any over-the-counter sleep aid.

MSM

Like many things with small names, the letters in that name usually refer to something more difficult to pronounce. MSM is no exception to this rule because the letters stand for *methyl sulfonyl methane*. MSM is a naturally produced sulfur-containing compound, found in small quantities in a number of foods such as milk, meats, some fruits and vegetables and even chocolate! While MSM may be used for many reasons ranging from sports injuries to even snoring, it is usually most popular among people suffering from arthritis. Other less popular names that may also refer to MSM include *DMSO2* and *Dimethyl Sulfone*.

MSM and Arthritis

MSM is sometimes found in supplements designed to improve osteoarthritis, that results when the cartilage between bones wears away. Some research hints that MSM might help osteoarthritis pain but, the evidence for it is less conclusive than that in support of glucosamine. One study noted that 1500 mg a day of MSM tended to reduce pain levels in people with osteoarthritis—and that its effects were more pronounced when MSM was used in combination with 1500 mg a day of glucosamine.[727] For this reason, some products may combine MSM and glucosamine together. MSM needs more research before the optimal amount which might work is fully agreed upon.

MSM contains the mineral sulfur, a key ingredient in making cartilage, so in theory there could be a reason that it might work. Sulfur is also plentiful in many commonly eaten foods like poultry, meat, fish, milk and beans. So, it is unlikely that people eating these foods would be deficient in this mineral.

Before MSM There Was DMSO

DMSO stands for dimethyl-sulfoxide, an industrial chemical and one-time popular alternative arthritis treatment. Small amounts of MSM are formed when DMSO breaks down. For arthritis, DMSO would be rubbed on the skin and according to anecdotal reports would provide temporary relieve from osteoarthritis and rheumatoid arthritis. This could be due in part to the ability of DMSO to penetrate the skin. Because of this property, DMSO might also carry into the body impurities such as bacteria and other toxins, which in theory might result in harmful side effects. DMSO is not a nutritional supplement and is not sold in stores. The use of DMSO for arthritis is still controversial and it is recommended that people consult their rheumatologist first before experimenting with this drug.

Side Effects and Concerns

MSM appears safe with no serious side effects noted. Because of the lack of rigorous scientific testing, little is known about how MSM interacts with prescription medications as well as with other supplements.

My Thoughts

Based on the research so far, there might be something to MSM, but for the moment the degree to which it contributes to the improvement of osteoarthritis pain needs more study. Keep in mind that most of the support for MSM is for osteoarthritis. MSM does not appear to benefit rheumatoid arthritis. For those who have osteoarthritis and are looking for a supplement that might help, remember that glucosamine sulfate has more evidence. Like many natural alternatives, MSM may require weeks of continued use before a noticeable effect is observed.

Myostatin Blockers

Unless you're a professional athlete or hardcore strength trainer, you may have never heard of myostatin blockers, but because there is some intriguing research in this field, this topic is worth mentioning. *Myostatin* is a protein that is inside all of us. The interesting thing about myostatin is that one of its duties is to prevent muscles from growing too big. Yes—you read that right—-myostatin, inhibits muscle growth! While this may be surprising to some, this is actually is a good thing. Think about it; who would want muscles that grew so big that you couldn't find any clothes to fit, or worse yet, muscles that grew so large that they compressed vital organs and caused them to fail? In spite of its positive role in health, some fascinating research has been conducted over the past several years to see what might happen if the action of myostatin were blocked or neutralized.

Myostatin and Muscle Growth

Myostatin was discovered in the late 1990s. Research conducted on laboratory animals has found that when the influence of myostatin is blocked, muscles grow bigger and even appear to get stronger *without* exercise.[728,729] To athletes like bodybuilders as well as millions of other people who spend long hours in the gym trying to change the way their body looks, anything that could help muscles to grow bigger and stronger without working out would be like finding the *Holy Grail* of exercise! Based on the animal research, supplements which reported to naturally block the action of myostatin soon started popping up in some health food stores and on the Internet. But, do they work? To answer this question, one first must look at the way the research was conducted. In these studies, myostatin was neutralized by injecting a special type of antibody. This is much different than a supplement that is swallowed, because of the likelihood that the supplement would be broken down by digestion before it entered the body. Some myostatin blocking supplements contain extracts from a seaweed called *Cystoseira canariensis.* Research finds that extracts from Cystoseira canariensis do appear to bind to myostatin in test tubes, making it, at least in theory, an attractive ingredient for myostatin blocker supplements.[731] However, at least one investigation has found that 3 months of Cystoseria supplementation used at a concentration of 1200 mg per day was ineffective at increasing muscle size or strength or reducing body fat, when it was given to people who also performed a strength training program.[732]

Medical Implications of Blocking Myostatin

Some research finds higher levels of myostatin (which means smaller, weaker muscles) in men infected with the HIV virus.[730] This hints that myostatin may play a role in the loss of muscle associated with disease. Inhibiting the action of myostatin through medical intervention may one day prove an effective treatment for a number of conditions ranging from muscular dystrophy to the age-related loss of muscle mass and strength known as sarcopenia. No research, though, finds that Cystoseira canariensis is effective for these conditions in humans.

Side Effects and Concerns

The long-term effects of blocking myostatin—through medical interventions or supplements—are unknown. Some evidence hints that *Cystoseira canariensis,* which is in some myostatin-blocking supplements, may be inappropriate for those who are using blood thinner medications.[731]

My Thoughts

Myostatin is actually one member of a larger family of specialized proteins that appear to play a role in muscle development. We are only beginning to scratch the surface on what myostatin and its related proteins do in the body. While one day the inhibiting of myostatin through medical interventions may prove beneficial, that day is not yet here. Until that day arrives, people really interested in this topic may want to keep working out because some research suggests that exercise might be able to naturally lower myostatin levels.[733]

Niacin

Niacin is a member of the water-soluble B complex family of vitamins. Understanding niacin can be a little tricky because it comes in two different forms: *nicotinamide* and *nicotinic acid*. Both are commonly called niacin but each is appropriate in different situations. Like other B vitamins, niacin helps us produce energy from the foods we eat. Natural sources of niacin include chicken, turkey, tuna, beans, salmon, peanuts and cereals. Additional names that also refer to niacin include *niacinamide* and *vitamin B₃*

Can B Vitamins Give You More Energy?

The B vitamins are sometimes touted to boost energy levels and give people more pep. The reason for this probably has to do with the fact that B vitamins help us produce energy from food. In this way they might help boost feelings of vigor in people who are not eating a nutritionally sound diet. For those who do eat healthy, B vitamins would probably be less effective.

Niacin and Cholesterol

The effect of niacin on cholesterol levels is well known. Clinical studies show that high doses of niacin, (the nicotinic acid form) can lower LDL (bad cholesterol), triglycerides (blood fats) and raise HDL (good cholesterol) in those who have high cholesterol levels.[736] In fact, niacin is sometimes prescribed by physicians for this reason. It is worth noting that very high dosages of niacin—1200-3000 mg per day—are usually needed to affect cholesterol levels. Because such high levels may have side effects, self medicating with niacin is not advised. Nicotinamide—the other form of niacin—does not appear to affect cholesterol levels.

Other Supplements That Might Lower Cholesterol	
• Fish Oil	• Policosanol
• Red Yeast Rice	• Garlic
• Guggul	• Soy

Does Niacin Have Other Uses?

Some studies suggest that nicotinamide may be able to reduce blood sugar levels in diabetics and may also improve the functioning of the *beta cells*—the cells that make insulin—in those recently diagnosed with diabetes.[734] Other emerging research finds that people who eat a diet rich in niacin appear to have reduced rates for Alzheimer's disease. Lastly, niacin may hold promise in improving osteoarthritis-related pain.[735] All of these other possible uses for niacin should be considered preliminary until more · studies are conducted.

Side Effects and Concerns

In small amounts, usually found in food, or at its RDA of 14 to 16 mg per day for women and men respectively, niacin is safe. One of the most common side effects of niacin is a flushing of the skin that occurs because of niacin's ability to expand blood vessels.

High doses of niacin can damage the liver. For this reason unsupervised use of high-dose niacin supplements are not recommended.

Some research finds that high dosages (1 to 3 grams a day) of niacin may elevate homocysteine, a chemical that is linked to heart disease.[737] Until more is known, persons with heart disease should consult their physicians before using niacin supplements. Healthy persons using high-dose niacin might also want to get their homocysteine levels checked periodically.

Niacin might lower blood sugar levels. Diabetics using niacin should monitor their blood sugar closely when using this supplement.

My Thoughts

Much evidence supports the use of niacin (the nicotinic acid form) for the treatment of abnormal cholesterol levels. Niacin's effect appears less than that of prescription medications used for elevated cholesterol. The effects of nicotinamide are less well-known but published research does suggest that it also may have beneficial effects that are still being investigated. Niacin is found in a variety of foods and can be made in the body from the amino acid tryptophan. Because niacin is easily obtained from food, its unlikely that people living in industrialized nations are deficient in this vitamin.

Noni Juice

Noni is a small tree that is common to areas such as Polynesia, Hawaii and Australia. Interestingly, it was the leaves of the plant that were originally used topically to treat burns and other wounds. Noni fruit was seldom consumed because of its bitter, unpleasant taste. Noni contains a range of vitamins, minerals, carbohydrates and other plant chemicals that for the most part are only recently starting to be investigated. Other names that also refer to noni include *Morinda citrifolia, Indian mulberry, nhau,* and *hog apple.*

Noni and Cancer

Some scientific support exists that noni may have anti-cancer properties. For example, noni has been shown to possibly inhibit blood vessel formation around tumor cells.[739] This might mean that noni may be effective at cutting off the oxygen supply to cancer cells, which in effect would be like suffocating them. Some other research also suggests that extracts of noni may stop cancer from spreading. Noni contains a chemical called "noni-ppt" which has been studied in test tubs and lab animals for its anti-cancer effects.

As intriguing as all of the above possibilities are, it must be noted that little evidence to date has been conducted on humans. There is a big difference between how something works in a test tube and how it acts in human beings. The studies mentioned here are preliminary and a lot of questions need to be answered before noni is formally accepted as a viable anti-cancer therapy. For example, how much noni is needed to affect cancer? Many different types of cancer exist. Which types of cancer might noni be effective against? Does noni interact with prescription drugs? Does noni extend the lives of cancer patients who use it? At this point nobody knows the answers to these questions.

What We Don't Know About Noni and Cancer

• Is noni effective against cancer in people?

• How much noni is needed to affect cancer in people?

• What types of cancer might noni improve?

• Does noni interact with medications?

• Can noni extend the lives of cancer patients?

Can Noni Help Other Disorders?

Noni is touted to improve a wide spectrum of diverse afflictions. The evidence that noni is effective for any disorder is not strongly supported by peer-reviewed evidence.

Side Effects and Concerns

In amounts found in food, noni is probably safe. Noni is relatively high in the mineral potassium, which is an important player in a wide range of functions including muscle and heart contraction and the transmission of nerve signals. High levels of potassium, though, can be dangerous, producing a condition called *hyperkalemia*. The kidneys normally excrete excess potassium, but in the case of kidney damage, potassium levels might rise too much. Noni also contains carbohydrates which can add calories to the diet and may in theory cause weight gain if used in excess.

My thoughts

The early research is finding that components of noni may have beneficial effects; however a lot of questions remain to be answered. For healthy people who want to try noni, a few weeks of use is probably sufficient to see if it is helping or not. Noni is often said to help a wide range of disorders but most of these claims are based on testimonials of lone individuals. In other words, there may be something to it but for the moment there just isn't much good clinical evidence yet. Testimonials can be the jumping off point to further investigations but should never take the place of well-designed clinical research.

Pyruvate

Pyruvate is a molecule formed when sugar is used to make energy and is found naturally in small amounts in fruits and vegetables. Pyruvate is recommended usually to help reduce weight and improve exercise ability. Other names that also refer to pyruvate include *pyruvic acid, sodium pyruvate, potassium pyruvate* and *calcium pyruvate.*

Pyruvate and Weight Loss

Pyruvate was first employed as a means to prevent fat build-up in the livers of laboratory rats.[741] From this, it was speculated that pyruvate might also prevent weight gain and assist with weight loss. Several studies have been conducted on pyruvate and most all of them so far have found that it appears to work.[742,743] These results lead to a lot of hype surrounding pyruvate with some advertisements claiming that it could lead to large percentages of weight and fat loss. A closer look at the research behind these claims reveals that while yes, almost 50% greater fat loss may occur with pyruvate use, this 50% only amounted to between 1 to 3 pounds. Another issue relates to the subjects in the pyruvate studies. The people who took part in the research were usually overweight women (over 200 lbs) and they consumed a very low calorie diet. This makes one wonder how effective pyruvate would be for people eating a more normal amount of calories. In addition, a lot of pyruvate (almost 50 grams a day) was consumed in research, much more than the 6 to 8 grams usually found in supplements. Some research finds that smaller dosages of pyruvate (3-5 grams a day) may also promote weight loss; but, the effect appears less than when larger amounts are used.

Pyruvate and Exercise

Athletes such as marathon runners, cyclists and triathletes are sometimes interested in pyruvate because of research hinting that it might improve the endurance capacity of muscle.[744] The research to date on this issue is limited. Pyruvate supplementation has not been adequately tested under real life exercise situations like running a marathon. So, whether pyruvate is of significant help to exercisers is open to speculation.

Side Effects and Concerns

When used orally, pyruvate is not known to cause any serious side effects. Likewise, there are no known drug interactions accompanying oral pyruvate supplementation. The most common reported effects include occasional diarrhea and gas.

My Thoughts

Unlike the vast majority of weight loss supplements on the market, pyruvate has actual, peer-reviewed scientific studies, published in respected academic journals to back up many of its claims. In my opinion, this fact alone puts pyruvate ahead of 99% of all the other weight loss products out there. These very studies, though, show that pyruvate is far from the magic weight loss bullet that it is sometimes portrayed to be. To date, most of the claims are based on only a few studies that involved small numbers of overweight women who used large amounts of pyruvate. That being said, pyruvate might be something to take a look at especially if you are an overweight woman. Remember that whatever success might be found with pyruvate is likely to be maximized when it is coupled with eating fewer calories and exercising regularly.

Red Clover

Red clover is a plant that grows throughout Europe and has been used for centuries not only for its medicinal properties but also as food for grazing cattle. Its name is derived from the red color that adorns the flowering heads of the plant. Contemporary interest in this herb centers mostly around its use by women to treat hot flashes and other symptoms associated with menopause. Other names that also refer to red clover include *Trifolium pretense, wild clover, meadow clover and purple clover.*

Red Clover and Menopause

Like soy, which will be discussed later, red clover also contains the estrogen-like isoflavones, *genistein* and *daidzein.* It is these chemicals that make red clover attractive to women suffering from hot flashes and other symptoms of menopause and premenstrual syndrome. Women who use red clover for this purpose should know that the evidence for this herb helping reduce symptoms of menopause and PMS is mixed with some studies finding it may work and others finding it doesn't.[748] While there are no guarantees, some research has been successful, with 40-160 mg of red clover isoflavones taken daily for several weeks.

Red Clover and Osteoporosis

Bone loss, leading to osteoporosis is a major concern for women after menopause. Because red clover contains plant-derived estrogen compounds (isoflavones), some speculate that this herb may be of help to women suffering from osteoporosis. Indeed, some evidence does find that components in red clover may inhibit the cells which *eat* bone. Anything that might inhibit these cells (called, osteoclasts) as well as other degenerative processes affecting bone as we get older, might reduce osteoporosis. As intriguing as this is, red clover is still controversial for this purpose. Some research finds that red clover might help and other research hints that it doesn't.[747] Red clover should not be used as a substitute for a healthy lifestyle (that includes bone-strengthening exercise) and eating well. While the optimal amounts of red clover isoflavones to use is not well known, some success has been found with 40 mg of red clover isoflavones taken over the course of several months.[747]

Red Clover and the Prostate

Red clover is typically of interest to women although there may also be cause for some men to also take notice of this herb as well. While controversial, research stemming mostly from laboratory animals finds that red clover may be of help to men who suffer from prostate cancer and those with an enlarged prostate gland—common problems among men as they age.[745,746] For this reason, red clover may be an ingredient in supplements designed for prostate health. More research is needed to determine if red clover is indeed effective in humans for these conditions. For men considering red clover for prostate problems, keep in mind that much more favorable research exists for *saw palmetto*, an herb which is reviewed separately in this book.

Side Effects and Concerns

Red clover is typically seen as a safe herb. Like all natural products, some side effects are theoretically possible. For example, Red clover appears to have a blood thinning effect and as such should not be combined with blood thinner medications or supplements with blood thinning properties.[10] Red clover might also interfere with the normal breakdown of prescription medications. Red clover should probably not be combined with hormone replacement therapy because of the unknowns associated with how they interact with each other. Related to this, it might not be wise for women who have cancer of the uterus, breast, or ovaries to use red clover. Because of its possible estrogen-like activity, red clover might, in theory, aggravate these conditions.

My Thoughts

Some support exists that red clover may be of benefit to women seeking relief from menopause symptoms; but, not all research is in agreement on this. For healthy women, red clover is probably safe. Unfortunately, investigations of the quality of red clover supplements have sometimes found that they may not always contain the amounts of the reported active ingredients (isoflavones) that their labels indicate. This is all the more reason to investigate who you do business with. It's important to also remember that red clover, like all natural products, contains hundreds of diverse molecules that may work together. The isoflavones of red clover do receive a lot of attention but in my opinion, focusing only on these compounds amounts to missing the forest for the trees.

Red Yeast Rice

In China, red yeast rice has been used medicinally to treat a number of conditions for over a thousand years.[749] More recently, red yeast rice is usually used by people to help lower cholesterol levels. Additional names that also refer to this supplement include *Monascus purpureus, red yeast, monacolin K.* and *Cholestin.*

Red Yeast Rice and Cholesterol

Clinical studies have documented that taking red yeast rice orally over the course of several weeks can lower cholesterol levels significantly. Some research finds that red yeast rice might be able to reduce total cholesterol, triglycerides (blood fats) and bad cholesterol (LDL cholesterol) by as much as 20-30% after several weeks of use.[749] Red yeast rice accomplishes this by interfering with the body's production of cholesterol. At the heart of red yeast rice's power over cholesterol appears to be one of its naturally occurring ingredients, a compound called *monacolin K,* which also goes by the name *lovastatin.* Lovastatin is also a prescription statin drug that is used medicinally to lower cholesterol. So, red yeast rice acts almost like a natural statin drug. Most research finding favorable results with red yeast rice supplements have used amounts ranging from 1 gram a day to about 2.4 grams a day.[749] It is important to note that red yeast rice contains many other compounds which also appear to impact cholesterol levels. For example, some supplements may mention a related red yeast rice-derived compound called *xuezhikang,* which also appears effective at helping reduce cholesterol.[848]

Side Effects and Concerns

Red yeast rice supplements are probably safe in healthy people. Red yeast rice has been used for centuries and research on these supplements has so far has not noted many negative side effects when used in the doses noted above. Many of the proposed side effects of red yeast rice supplements are derived from what we know about the side effects of lovastatin and similar cholesterol-lowering drugs. The following is a list of potential issues or worst-case scenarios that might arise when using red yeast rice supplements.

Red yeast rice, in theory, may interact with a number of prescription medications.

Drugs containing lovastatin may cause muscle weakness and pain due to depletion of coenzyme Q_{10} levels. This is very serious. Individuals who use red yeast rice and experience these symptoms should see their physician immediately and discontinue using the supplement.

In theory, grapefruit or grapefruit juice may augment the effects of red yeast rice (and the risk of negative side effects). This is due to the *grapefruit effect* which was discussed at the beginning of this book. To be on the safe side, avoid grapefruit and grapefruit juice while using red yeast rice products.

What About Policosanol?

Policosanol, a compound made from sugarcane, is also found in some supplements advertised to lower cholesterol. Research notes that 5-20 mg of policosanol a day may be effective at lowering cholesterol, triglycerides and bad cholesterol (LDL), as well increase good cholesterol (HDL)—something red yeast rice doesn't seem to do.[751]

My Thoughts

The research pretty well affirms that a quality red yeast rice supplement may help lower cholesterol levels in some individuals. As such, this supplement might be an attractive option for those opposed to medications. Because of differences in the concentration of lovastatin, xuezhikang and other ingredients, all brands of red yeast rice may not work the same and some experimenting may be needed before you find a product that works for you. In addition, it is important to remember that heart disease is a complex process and cholesterol is but one piece in the puzzle. You might be surprised to learn that many people have heart attacks in spite of having "normal" cholesterol levels. This speaks volumes for the need to attack heart disease from a holistic approach. Red yeast rice can be a part of that approach but keep in mind that the word *holistic* does not mean just popping a pill. Holistic is bigger than that and involves other healthy practices like coping better with stress (a major problem that does not get the attention it deserves), not smoking, eating well and yes, exercising on a regular basis. Reducing cholesterol by way of a red yeast rice supplement is definitely a step in the right direction but regardless of how your cholesterol changes, your health and quality of life are sure to improve if you focus on the *whole you* rather than just one piece of the big picture.

Ribose

Ribose is a type of sugar that is found in all cells of the body and plays key roles in several important chemical reactions. Two areas that ribose is involved in is the manufacture of ATP, our prime energy molecule and DNA, our genetic *software* program, if you will. Ribose supplements are usually popular among athletes who desire quicker recovery following exercise. This nutrient is found naturally in ripened fruits and vegetables, but in insignificant amounts. Thus eating these foods is unlikely to significantly raise ribose levels. Ribose is also normally made in the body from the sugar glucose. Other names that refer to ribose include *D-ribose* and *Beta-D-ribose*.

Ribose and Exercise

Ribose is one of the building blocks of ATP, the energy-rich molecule that is ultimately responsible for supplying our muscles with the energy needed to exercise. In theory, by providing the building blocks for ATP, one might be able to replenish energy levels faster during exercise and speed recovery time, thus allowing for enhanced exercise performance. This ability might be of most benefit to athletes who push their bodies to the limit day after day like those who participate in the *Tour de France* or weightlifters who train in the gym several days a week with heavy loads and little rest.

The research on ribose to date hints that there may indeed be something to it. During high intensity exercise, ATP levels inside muscles decrease. Furthermore, it may take several days before muscle cell ATP levels return to normal. This might limit exercise performance. Taking ribose also appears to raise muscle ATP levels.[780] Anecdotal evidence from people who have used ribose supplements, as well as some preliminary studies suggests that ribose may help improve strength. However, other studies do not find that ribose helps.[778,779] Because of this controversy, it is difficult to say one way or another whether ribose is effective for everybody or not. Questions such as what's the best time to take ribose, how much to use and is it better to take ribose once or several times a day, still need to be investigated.

Ribose and Heart Disease

Athletes probably first became interested in ribose as a performance booster because of research performed on people with heart disease. In these individuals, some studies show that ribose can improve heart function and extend the time people can walk on a treadmill before angina sets in.[781] Two issues here is that the effect has not been widely studied and according to one study, a lot of ribose was needed (up to 60 g taken over the course of the day).[781] Lesser amounts might also work and reduce any possible side effects. Because people with heart disease are likely to be taking medications to treat this and other conditions, it is highly recommended that a physician be consulted before experimenting with ribose.

Ribose and Fibromyalgia

There is some cause to speculate that ribose may help fibromyalgia, a type of arthritis of unknown origin that is characterized by muscle tenderness, fatigue and insomnia.[777] In a case study reported in the journal, *Pharmacotherapy*, a patient with fibromyalgia began using a ribose supplement in addition to normal therapies and noticed diminished symptoms after a few weeks. To test if ribose was indeed helping, the supplement was purposely stopped. After a short time, fibromyalgia symptoms worsened. After ribose use resumed, the symptoms decreased. As a double check, ribose was purposely halted once again. This was subsequently accompanied by the return of fibromyalgia symptoms. Upon resuming ribose, the symptoms again subsided after a few weeks. This is very interesting and more research is needed to better understand what is happening. For those with fibromyalgia who want to try this approach, note that favorable results in this case study were observed when 5 grams of ribose were used twice a day.[777]

Side Effects and Concerns

Ribose is generally safe with few adverse effects reported. General side effects sometimes reported include nausea and diarrhea. Because ribose is a sugar, there is some speculation that it may be inappropriate for diabetics.

Avoid "L-ribose". This type of ribose does not appear to have the same positive effects as D-ribose.

My Thoughts

For the moment, ribose goes in the *iffy* category with respect to exercise because there is disagreement as to whether it works or not. If it helps, ribose might be of most benefit to healthy athletes who are engaged in repeated sessions of high intensity physical activity day after day or during bouts of strenuous activity with little rest. Athletes reading these words should experiment with ribose before their official competition, to gauge how their bodies react to it. This is sage advice for all supplements as well.

St. John's Wort

St. John's wort is an herb which has been used for centuries to treat a number of conditions ranging from bug bites and burns to even helping people fall asleep. Over the last several decades, however, St. John's wort has been mostly used as a natural treatment for depression. Some may wonder where this herb obtained its curious name. Well, the term *wort* is old English for plant. The other part of the name—*St. John's*—is a reference to St. John *the Baptist,* of Bible fame. This is because the plant is most plentiful around June 24th, which is typically thought to be the birthday of John the Baptist.[399] Other names that also refer to St. John's wort include *Hypericum perforatum* and *Tipton Weed.*

St. John's Wort and Depression

Numerous studies carried out over the last several years have noted St. john's wort may improve mood and reduce feelings of anxiety associated with mild to moderate levels of depression.[755] Some studies find St. John's wort to be more effective than using nothing (a placebo) and others show it to be as effective as some antidepressant medications.[755] Research finds that St. John's wort is most effective in those who suffer from mild to moderate levels of depression. St. John's does not appear to help those afflicted with severe or debilitating depression. Some people tend to get depressed in the winter months. This condition is called *seasonal affective disorder* (SAD for short). Some research also finds that St. John's wort may be effective at easing depression symptoms associated with SAD. Like many herbal remedies, the effects of St. John's wort do not occur over night but usually require at least four weeks before any improvement in depression symptoms is noticed.

How Does St. John's Wort Work?

How St. John's wort works is not completely understood. Early research speculated that St. John's wort acts like some antidepressant medications by blocking a brain chemical called *monoamine oxidase*. This enzyme in turn increases levels of a brain chemical called *serotonin*. While St. John's wort has been shown to raise serotonin levels in test tube studies, not all research finds that it does this in the human body. It is possible that St. John's wort works by not only elevating serotonin levels but also by altering other aspects of brain chemistry as well. Regardless of how it works, the active ingredients of St. John's wort appear to reside in the flowering parts of the plant. Thus, supplements derived from this area of the herb would probably work the best.

Some St. John's wort supplements may list the amount of *hypericin* they contain. Hypericin is one of the chemicals in St. John's wort and has been found to inhibit the brain enzyme *monoamine oxidase* in a similar fashion to some antidepressant medications such as MAO inhibitors. Thus, hypericin was thought for a time to be the key active ingredient responsible for the herb's antidepressant effects. However, hypericin doesn't always seem to work in the body the way it does in the laboratory, leading some to speculate that other chemicals may be involved. We now know that hypericin is one of many different compounds that make up St. John's wort. Another chemical in the herb that receives a lot of attention is *hyperforin*. Hyperforin also appears to exert antidepressant effects that are separate from the actions of hypericin. Regardless as to whether hypericin or hyperforin are the actual active ingredients in the herb, they appear to be good indicators of a supplement's potency and effectiveness. Favorable results in research have been found with using three 300 mg doses of St. John's wort spread out over the course of the day.[755] Some research suggests that each dose should contain about 0.3% hypericin or hyperforin. Also, keep in mind that not all studies find that the herb is effective for depression. Thus individual success with St. John's wort will likely vary from person to person.

Side Effects and Concerns

St. John's wort has been used for centuries and when done so in small amounts for short periods of time is usually found to be safe in adults. Common side effects are usually minor and may include insomnia, headache and vivid dreaming.

St. John's wort may interact with a number of prescription medications ranging from drugs used to treat heart disease, cancer, epilepsy and AIDS. St. John's wort may reduce the effectiveness of drugs to treat these conditions.[755] In addition, the herb may also interfere with drugs used to treat ulcers, cholesterol and blood pressure.

One case study suggests that St. John's wort may worsen symptoms in people who have Alzheimer's disease.[833]

St. John's wort should not be combined with prescription antidepressant medications. In theory, this combination may cause serotonin levels in the brain to rise too much, resulting in a condition called *serotonin syndrome*, a potentially life-threatening condition.

Those who use certain antidepressants called MAO inhibitors have dietary restrictions to prevent elevations in blood pressure. This usually involves the avoidance of foods that contain the amino acid, tyramine. While unlikely to occur, those using St. Johns wort should use similar restrictions to minimize this effect.

People who have received new organs may suffer from depression and look to St. John's wort to help. There is some concern that St. John's wort may interfere with the effectiveness of anti-rejection drugs.[834]

Depression comes in many forms. Some may suffer from a condition where their mood alternates between the extremes of deep depression and high excitement. This situation is called a *manic depressive disorder or bipolar disorder.* Some studies note that St. John's wort may increase overly-excited feelings in those with bipolar disorders.[757] This is also a possible side effect in those who suffer from depression (without mania) as well.

Studies show that being exposed to bright lights may help depression. As such, it's possible that those suffering from depression may look to in-door tanning salons to help. Studies show that some people using St. John's wort may experience skin rashs or increased burning or blistering of the skin upon exposure to sunlight. This may be more pronounced in fair-skinned people. To reduce this effect, minimize direct exposure to sunlight and refrain from tanning while using this herb.

Emerging research hints that St. John's wort may interfere with some birth control pills.[835] This may result in an unwanted pregnancy.

New mothers should know that St. John's wort has been found in breast milk.[835] How this might affect the nursing baby is not known.

Not all St. John's wort products may be created equal. As was mentioned before, the active ingredients of St. John's wort seem to reside in the flowers and leaves of the plant. Consumers should contact the makers of the product they are considering if this information is not disclosed.

My Thoughts

It can't be stressed enough that the evidence strongly indicates that St. John's wort appears to work best in those who have mild to moderate levels of depression. In other words, if you're feeling a little blue or if things just seem out of kilter, then St. John's wort might help. If, on the other hand, you're reading these words while standing on the ledge of a building, getting ready to jump, then St. Johns wort is not for you! All kidding aside, all of us—myself included—get depressed from time to time. I've seen my share of difficult times as I'm sure you have as well. While it's tempting to self-medicate with substances like alcohol, drugs or even a supplement like St. John's wort to make the stresses of our life disappear, it goes without saying (but I'll say it anyway) that this effect is only temporary. People struggling with real life problems are best served talking to a friend or qualified professional to support them and help guide them through life's difficult moments. Yes, St. John's wort might help but it is no substitute for good advice, words of encouragement and the shoulder of a good friend to lean on.

SAM-e

SAM-e (pronounced "sammy") is short for *S-Adenosyl-methionine*, a sulfur-containing compound that is found in all cells of the body and which takes part in over a hundred biological reactions. SAM-e is created by combining the amino acid *methionine* with the energy-rich compound, *ATP*. SAM-e may be used to treat a number of different conditions but it is usually purchased to help two distinctly separate conditions: depression and arthritis. Both have multiple studies supporting SAM-e's role in these syndromes and in fact, in some countries SAM-e is actually available as a prescription drug to treat both depression and arthritis. Other names which also refer to SAM-e include *Ademetionine*, *SAMe* and *Sammy*.

SAM-e and Depression

Several studies find that SAM-e may be effective for improving mood in those who suffer from depression.[758] Many early studies were small, employing few people and have been criticized by other researchers, but most generally find SAM-e to be modesty effective for depression.[758] Some research has noted that SAM-e appears to work as well as a class of antidepressant medications called *tricyclics* and other studies show that it seems to work faster than St. John's wort. Unlike St. John's wort which has much research supporting its role for mild to moderate levels of depression, SAM-e has shown promise for *major depression*, which refers to severe, debilitating episodes of sadness and hopelessness that may follow traumatic life episodes like the loss of a spouse or loved one, for example.[837] While many studies have been conducted where SAM-e was *injected* into the body, taking SAM-e orally also seems to help depression.[837] How SAM-e improves depression is unknown. SAM-e does appear to increase levels of brain chemicals like *serotonin* and *dopamine* which are probably involved with its antidepressant effects, but whether it also helps in other ways needs more study. Research showing positive effects for depression have used between 400-1600 mg per day.[837]

SAM-e and Arthritis

SAM-e was first speculated to help arthritis after people who had been using it for depression began reporting improvements in joint pain associated with osteoarthritis. Since that time, multiple studies have been published on SAM-e showing that when taken orally, it appears to be more effective than using a placebo (which should have no effect) and just as effective as anti-inflammatory medications like as aspirin or ibuprofen. Some research finds that SAM-e may also work as well as some prescription anti-inflammatory drugs.[761]

One drawback to using SAM-e for arthritis is that it may take about a month before it is fully effective. This is longer than over-the-counter medications like aspirin. SAM-e is also more expensive than over-the-counter pain medications, a factor to consider for those on a budget.

How SAM-e helps osteoarthritis is not well understood. SAM-e appears to have anti-inflammatory properties which may partially explain its effects on osteoarthritis. Some speculate that SAM-e may be important for the production of proteins that help repair and re-grow joint cartilage, although more research is needed to verify this.[849] While the optimal effective dose of SAM-e has not been determined, studies finding positive effects for arthritis have used between 600-1200 mg per day.[838]

SAM-e and Fibromyalgia

Fibromyalgia is a form of arthritis in which people experience muscle tenderness and pain at specific parts of the body most, if not all, of the time. Because of its ties to arthritis and the success of SAM-e in helping osteoarthritis, some fibromyalgia sufferers may also look to SAM-e for help. Since the 1980s, a few studies have found that SAM-e may be effective at reducing some of the symptoms of fibromyalgia, while others show no effect.[759,760] Some of this research actually involved injecting SAM-e into the body.[760] Overall, it's open to speculation whether SAM-e helps this condition or not. Research finding that oral SAM-e has helped fibromyalgia has used between 600-800 mg per day.[759]

Side Effects and Concerns

SAM-e is generally considered safe with minor stomach upset usually reported. Most studies do not report any serious side effects. The following is a list of things to keep in mind when using SAM-e supplements.

Unless specifically prescribed by a physician, SAM-e should not be combined with prescription medications used to treat depression. SAM-e appears to elevate the brain's concentration of a chemical called serotonin. Because some antidepressant medications also raise serotonin levels, in theory, the combination of both may result in *serotonin syndrome*, a potentially life-threatening condition. This is a controversial topic and more research is needed to understand how SAM-e interacts with antidepressant medications.

Individuals who suffer from manic-depressive disorders should avoid SAM-e. In theory, SAM-e might cause mania in these individuals.

SAM-e shouldn't be combined with other supplements such as St. John's wort, touted to have antidepressant effects. It is not known how SAM-e interacts with other supplements also regarded as natural antidepressants.

People who have heart disease should have their homocysteine levels checked regularly when using SAM-e. In theory, SAM-e might raise homocysteine although research has not shown that this occurs. Ironically, some research finds higher rates of heart disease in people with low SAM-e levels.

There is some concern that SAM-e might decrease the effectiveness of the medication L-dopa, used to treat Parkinson's symptoms.

The Stability of SAM-e Supplements

SAM-e can be quite unstable and tends to break down easily especially when exposed to moisture or heat. Thus, SAM-e supplements must be created under strict conditions. In addition, supplements are often combined with other products that help stabilize and lengthen the time in which SAM-e is most potent. These stabilizing agents are either found listed on the label in parenthesis right next to SAM-e or on the supplement's ingredients list. Two common stabilizing compounds are *tosylate*, and *butanedisulfonate*. While needed to ensure quality, these stabilizing compounds can make it difficult to interpret how much SAM-e the supplement actually contains. For example, a 200 mg supplement may not contain 200 mg of SAM-e but rather some combination of SAM-e and the stabilizing agent. Unless it is made clear on the label, consumers should contact the maker of the supplement to find out how much SAM-e their product contains.

My Thoughts

SAM-e was discovered in Italy in the early 1950s and has been available in other countries as a prescription drug for decades. In the US, SAM-e has only been available as a supplement since the 1990s. A lot of research finds SAM-e effective for depression and osteoarthritis-related pain in some people. SAM-e does not however appear to benefit healthy people. Levels of SAM-e tend to decrease as we get older so it may be found in some "anti-aging" supplements; In spite of this, there is no good proof SAM-e slows or reverses aging in humans. SAM-e may also be combined with other products like glucosamine to treat osteoarthritis but the usefulness of SAM-e in combination with other supplements has not been well studied. Using a SAM-e supplement that is enteric coated might be best because it should enable SAM-e to pass from the stomach to the intestine unscathed, where it can be more easily absorbed.

Saw Palmetto

Saw palmetto is a small palm tree that that grows in California, South Carolina and Florida. Traditionally used for a number of reasons relating to bladder infections, it is sometimes also employed to treat other conditions such as sexual dysfunction and even baldness. The most popular use of saw palmetto, however, is its effect in men who have prostate problems. The most common name that usually shows up on supplement bottles is *saw palmetto*. Other terms that also refer to this herb include *Serenoa repens*, *LSESR*, *Sabal* and *Dwarf Palm Tree*.

Saw Palmetto and the Prostate Gland

The prostate is a small gland, about the size of a walnut that forms a portion of a man's reproductive system. As men grow older, one of the changes that may occur is an enlargement of this gland, what is referred to as *benign prostatic hyperplasia* or BPH for short. Because the prostate gland encircles the urethra, the tube through which urine flows from the body, an enlargement of the prostate can result in a stoppage of the urine stream. This can result in difficulty empting the bladder and frequent urination. Other common symptoms of BPH can include an urgent need to urinate (which usually disrupts sleep) and painful urination.

Over a dozen studies exist finding that saw palmetto is effective for alleviating symptoms such as painful and frequent urination that are frequently associated with BPH.[763,764] Other investigations also show that saw palmetto may be effective at slowing the growth of the prostate but it does not appear to shrink prostate size.[10] Taken as a whole, this means that saw palmetto appears to be an effective natural treatment for some men with BPH. Specifically, the research shows that saw palmetto is most effective for men who suffer from mild BPH symptoms.[764]

The cause of BPH is not fully understood. One of the most widely held theories advocates BPH may be due in part to a hormone called *dihydrotestosterone* (DHT). DHT is actually a form of the anabolic hormone, testosterone. In fact, in the prostate, an enzyme transforms testosterone into DHT. Some evidence suggests that saw palmetto works by inhibiting this enzyme (it's called *5 alpha-reductase*). Thus, by limiting the buildup of DHT, saw palmetto might reduce prostate problems. Others speculate that saw palmetto works through additional pathways. For example, saw palmetto appears to have anti-inflammatory properties, which might also explain its effects. When investigating saw palmetto, remember that not all research finds it effective for enlarged prostates. Thus, individual success with this herb may vary from person to person.

While the ingredients responsible for saw palmetto's effects are not well understood, it is generally thought they reside in the ripened fruit of the plant.[764] This means that saw palmetto supplements should be derived from the plant's berries or extracts of the berries.

Studies noting positive effects for BPH symptoms have generally used 1-2 grams of saw palmetto berries a day or 320 mg of saw palmetto extract per day.[27] Improvements in prostate function do not occur overnight and may take up to eight weeks of continued use with further improvements possibly occurring many months thereafter.

Saw Palmetto and Prostate Cancer

Prostate cancer is the second leading cause of death in American men, resulting in over 30,000 deaths each year. Men, armed with this information, sometimes opt to use supplements like saw palmetto to help reduce the risk of getting prostate cancer. However, there is little proof that saw palmetto is effective for this reason. A better option in this case might be the mineral *selenium,* where low dietary intakes have been linked to increased rates of prostate cancer.[766] On the plus side, saw palmetto does not appear to alter *prostate specific antigen* (PSA) results, a commonly used test for prostate cancer. For men at risk of prostate cancer, saw palmetto can't hurt and might help especially when combined with other important lifestyle changes such as eating less saturated fat and exercising more. This is sage advice, given that small changes like eating better and getting more active also tend to make big impacts on reducing other diseases as well.

Does Saw Palmetto Reduce Muscle Growth?

Testosterone, as many know, is the hormone mainly responsible for helping muscles get bigger and stronger. Since saw palmetto reduces a form of testosterone (DHT), athletes—in particular weightlifters—occasionally wonder if the herb also lowers testosterone levels which in turn might limit optimal muscle growth. Fortunately, the answer to this question appears to be no. While research on strength trainers needs more study, saw palmetto does not seem to affect testosterone levels and is thus probably ok for strength trainers to use.[765]

Saw Palmetto and Hair Loss

It appears that some hair follicles are sensitive to DHT, the same chemical implicated in benign prostatic hyperplasia. Thus, high levels of DHT might also promote hair loss as well. So a logical conclusion would be that if you could block the enzyme that makes DHT, hair would grow back – not a bad side effect if you were taking saw palmetto for prostate problems! In theory, there might be something to this, especially when at least one drug designed to treat prostate problems is also approved to help men with thinning hair. It's important to bear in mind that hair loss is actually a very complex issue (that's why nobody has cured it yet) and DHT is only one player in the game. No studies have proven that saw palmetto re-grows hair. For men who want to try it, saw palmetto might at most be mildly effective at slowing hair loss but its ability to re-grow hair that is already gone is probably wishful thinking at best.

Side Effects and Concerns

Saw palmetto is generally considered safe with side effects rarely found. Side effects that are sometimes mentioned are generally mild and include stomach upset, nausea and headache. The effects following long-term use (many years) of saw palmetto have not been well documented. The following are some things to keep in mind when using saw palmetto:

Men who experience symptoms that they think are due to benign prostatic hyperplasia should see their physician before self medicating with saw palmetto. Symptoms resembling BPH may also be caused by other things such as prostate cancer.

There is some speculation that saw palmetto may lengthen bleeding time. Thus, saw palmetto (like all supplements) should be discontinued prior to surgery. In theory, saw palmetto might also interact with blood thinner medications.

My Thoughts

In general, saw palmetto brings to the table a lot of evidence backing up its usefulness for helping benign prostatic hyperplasia. Whether or not saw palmetto can prevent BPH from occurring in the first place is unknown. Some supplements may combine saw palmetto with other herbs, vitamins or ingredients to boost its effects on the prostate. Little research exists as to whether this is a better approach than using saw palmetto alone.

Shark Cartilage

Shark cartilage is just that—cartilage derived from sharks. Supplements of shark cartilage are usually marketed to people who have cancer and those who wish to reduce cancer risk.

Shark Cartilage and Cancer

Cancer—like all living things on earth—needs oxygen, to survive. If we could somehow cut off its oxygen supply, cancer cells would suffocate and die. In a nutshell, this is the premise behind the use of shark cartilage for the treatment of cancer. Blood vessels are needed to transport oxygen and other nutrients to cells so that they can live. For years, doctors have noticed that cancer is less likely to occur in areas of the body that contained *cartilage.* Because of this apparent link between cartilage and less cancer, some people started to wonder if cartilage might contain a substance that inhibited the formation of blood vessels. If this substance existed and could be isolated, it might make a big impact on our ability to ward off cancer.

Researchers have indeed identified some substances in shark cartilage that may be effective at retarding the growth of blood vessels. Another compound isolated from shark cartilage appears to interfere with chemicals made by tumors that might facilitate the spread of cancer. Most of this evidence in support of shark cartilage, however, is derived from test tube studies or those conducted on laboratory animals. Tests of shark cartilage in people who have cancer have not been promising. For example, some research finds that shark cartilage supplements do not appear effective at lengthening or improving the quality of life of cancer patients.[767] When given to mice that had cancer, shark cartilage did slow the speed that cancer spread but did not cure it.[768] At this time, there is no evidence that taking shark cartilage supplements prevents cancer from forming in the first place. Most cancer experts regard shark cartilage as having more testimonials than hard facts to back up its claims.

Shark cartilage is basically protein and the compounds that make up shark cartilage also tend to be at least partially composed of protein. Critics of these supplements contend that the protein portion of the shark cartilage extracts would be destroyed by the stomach during digestion, rendering them ineffective.

Shark Cartilage and Arthritis

Osteoarthritis results when the cartilage cushioning between bones wears away over time. Some have speculated that shark cartilage may help replenish this cushioning or at least help decrease osteoarthritis-related pain. As of yet, there is very little research on how shark cartilage impacts arthritis and even less is known about how it interacts with other arthritis-related supplements like glucosamine.

Side Effects and Concerns

Cartilage is in all of us and if you have ever eaten *gristle*, you have eaten cartilage. Thus, shark cartilage is safe to use for most people. No significant drug interactions or side effects have been observed from using shark cartilage.

My Thoughts

The odds are that some people reading these words have unfortunately had their lives touched in some way by the ravages of cancer. I understand your plight because I, too, have experienced those feelings of utter impotence as you watch a loved one slowly fade away from this horrible disease. Placed in this situation, it is perfectly natural to wonder if there might be something out there, besides surgery, chemo or radiation that might also help. While shark cartilage supplements are unlikely to hurt anyone, they are equally unlikely to significantly impact cancer survival. Most of the evidence for shark cartilage stems from studies in test tubes and laboratory animals. Nobody has ever documented someone who was cured of cancer by using shark cartilage supplements. In theory, isolated extracts derived from shark cartilage may one day prove useful in the battle against cancer but unfortunately, that day is not today.

Shark cartilage first came to widespread public attention in the early 1990s following the publication of a book which claimed that sharks didn't get cancer. It turns out that sharks do indeed get cancer and they even get cancer of the cartilage.

Soy

Soy is derived from soybeans, which were first cultivated in China over 5000 years ago. While used for centuries in the East, soybeans didn't make it to America until the early 1800s where they languished in obscurity until almost the 20th century. Over time, soy's popularity in America slowly grew due in large part to the efforts of the famed chemist George Washington Carver, who developed hundreds of uses for the laudable legume. Henry Ford, who revolutionized American life by mass producing the automobile even had a suit made out of soybeans! Today America is the number one producer of soybeans in the world.

While popular for years among vegetarians, because it's a good source of protein, soy has gained widespread appeal because of research finding that it appears effective at staving off a number of diseases and conditions. Other terms that also refer to soy include *glycine max, tofu, tempeh, soybeans, genistein* and *daidzein*.

Soy and Heart Disease

Of all the claims for soy, its impact on the reduction of heart disease risk factors is most studied. Multiple investigations find that the addition of soy to the diet for only a few months can significantly reduce total cholesterol, bad cholesterol (LDL) and triglycerides.[769] On average, soy tends to lower total cholesterol by about 13% and LDL and triglyceride levels by about 10%. In addition, soy appears to make blood vessels more flexible which can also help reduce the risk of a heart attack. Soy's effects on HDL or good cholesterol are mixed with studies finding it either helps boost HDL or has no effect.[769] Its effects on HDL notwithstanding, the consumption of soy-containing foods on the reduction heart disease risk factors is impressive. Because of the evidence, in the US, foods high in soy are permitted to display the following message. *Diets low in saturated fat and cholesterol that include 25 grams of soy protein a day may reduce the risk of heart disease.* Most studies find that soy helps reduce cholesterol, LDL and triglycerides when an average of 25-50 grams per day is consumed. This is the reason 25 grams is used on the health claim found on soy-containing foods. In other words, it gives people a starting number to shoot for.

Soy and Menopause

Soy contains isoflavones, compounds that are similar to estrogen and appear to act like weak estrogens in the body. Because of this, women who are going through menopause are sometimes attracted to soy as a natural alternative to hormone replacement therapy (HRT), which research has linked to cancer in susceptible women as well as an increased risk of heart attacks and strokes. When scientists look at Asian countries where soy is a main staple of the diet, less hot flashes and other symptoms associated with menopause are observed. This has led investigators to study soy to see if it might help menopause. So far, research on soy alleviating menopause symptoms is mixed with some research being favorable and other research finding no effect.[772] While the isoflavone genistein, when used at about 50 mg per day does appear to reduce hot flashes, the research on this issue is strongest for a soy-rich diet as opposed to soy supplements. If soy supplements help, the optimal amount to use remains elusive. Those studies finding that soy can reduce hot flashes have used anywhere from 20 to 60 grams of soy protein per day or between 30 and 70 mg of soy isoflavones per day. Soy probably won't work overnight, with evidence that a few months may be needed before a noticeable effect is observed.

What Are Soy Isoflavones?

At the heart of many of soy's claims are elements called *isoflavones.* Isoflavones are not hormones but are weakly acting estrogen-like compounds. In other words, soy isoflavones have estrogen-like ability but their effects are weaker than that of the hormone estrogen. Isoflavones belong to a larger class of compounds called *phytoestrogens.* The popular soy constituents, *genistein* and *daidzein* are examples of soy isoflavones and receive much attention in the media. Research shows, for example, that genistein appears to help prevent the corrosion (oxidation) of bad cholesterol and may even help protect blood vessels from damage—both of which are important for reducing the risk of heart disease. While genistein and daidzein seem to exert positive influences, it should be remembered that soy contains a number of additional compounds that also may help explain its therapeutic effects. In other words, consuming just genistein or daidzein may not have the same effect as consuming soy itself. There is support for this with some research finding that concentrating soy isoflavones in supplement form may not give the same results as eating soy itself.[770,771] This is actually in line with the majority of evidence for soy. That is, soy's healthy reputation is largely based on what we observe happens when people eat soy as opposed to taking soy supplements.

Soy and Osteoporosis

Osteoporosis affects more than 25 million Americans with the majority of sufferers being older women. Estrogen has a protective effect on bones by reducing bone loss. When estrogen levels drop after menopause, the loss of bone is accelerated, speeding the onset of osteoporosis. Some estimate that this drop in estrogen can result in the loss of 10 to 20 percent of total bone mass within the first five years following menopause. Multiple studies of how cells respond in test tubes, animal studies, human studies as well as those which look at the diets of large numbers of people, generally find that soy either slows bone loss or may even help build bone. In Asian countries where soy is consumed, women tend to experience less hip fractures. Studies also find that both genistein and daidzein suppress the action of bone-eating cells called *osteoclasts*.[773] Because of these facts, soy has become quite popular among postmenopausal women. Its popularity not withstanding, the issue of how soy helps bone is still unknown. Some speculate that soy's protective effects are derived from its isoflavone content (genistein and daidzein) while other research hints that soy protein itself may have some bone protecting effects that act independently of isoflavonoids. Soy also contains a good amount of calcium which probably also helps bones.

One thing that seems certain is that if soy is going to be of help in battling osteoporosis, then it must be used in quantities larger than that which is typically consumed by most Americans. Studies generally use at least 40 grams of soy protein per day or about 80 milligrams of soy isoflavones per day to reduce bone loss.[839]

Does Soy Affect Muscle Growth?

Some athletes—especially those who lift weights—sometimes avoid soy protein because of a belief that soy's plant estrogens (isoflavones) might reduce muscle growth. For the moment there isn't much research on this topic. Some, but not all evidence does hint that soy may lower testosterone levels in animals.[776] Other research, though, finds that soy protein is of equal value to whey protein at building muscle during a strength training program.[814] In fact, because of its antioxidant properties, soy may even be a little better than whey![814] For the moment there is no compelling evidence that soy protein is detrimental to muscle growth. While more research is needed to resolve this controversy, those who exercise and enjoy soy protein but who are concerned about it affecting their muscle mass, may want to have their anabolic hormone levels checked periodically, if for nothing else, than to help them sleep better at night.

Soy and Cancer

In women, estrogen can be a double-edged sword. On one hand it is indispensable to women; For example, estrogen helps build bone and prevent its loss. Estrogen also helps the growth and development of breast tissue and is a key player in a woman's menstrual cycle. Estrogen also helps keep cholesterol levels in check, reducing the risk of heart disease. On the other hand, through its role in promoting cell growth, it is thought that estrogen can also be harmful by promoting the formation of some types of cancer. It is important to note that estrogen itself does not cause cancer. Rather cancer is thought to occur as a result of genetic changes (mutations) that occur in cells that grow rapidly in response to the actions of estrogen.

In order for estrogen to do anything, it must first attach itself to *estrogen receptors*. This is where soy comes in. Soy isoflavones are also able to bind to estrogen receptors. When the estrogen receptors are all filled up with isoflavones, there is little place for estrogen to latch on to, which in theory, means reduced cancer risk. This is how we think soy might help prevent cancer.

Soy is thought to reduce the formation of three types of cancer: breast cancer, endometrial cancer and maybe prostate cancer.[772] Currently, most of the evidence in support of soy's role in cancer reduction stems from looking at what happens when large number of people use soy. For example, soy is thought to reduce breast cancer because in countries where a lot of soy is consumed, less cases of breast cancer are reported. This may or may not be definitive proof of soy's power over cancer and currently this aspect of soy's effects is controversial.[772] Clinical studies are underway to better figure all this out but until more is known, consumers should opt for eating soy itself rather than soy supplements, which may contain only one or a few of soy's many ingredients. It's very likely that soy contains substances besides the popular genistein and daidzein that account for its effects.

Quick Reference: How Much Soy Might Help?	
Condition	Amount
• For cholesterol reduction	25-50 grams of soy protein per day
• For menopause symptoms	20-60 grams of soy protein or 30-70 soy isoflavones per day
• For osteoporosis	40 grams of soy protein or 50-60 milligrams soy isoflavones per day
• For cancer reduction	unknown

Side Effects and Concerns

Soy is considered very safe when used as a food and has few reported side effects. Soy supplements are probably also safe but do not have the long term track record that soybeans have because they have not been around as long. Those with special issues should adhere to the following points when considering the use of soy and soy supplements.

Some concern has been raised that soy may alter the clotting capacity of blood. In theory, this might be problematic for people using blood thinner medications.[774]

Some research suggests that soy isoflavone supplements, when used for several years, might slightly raise the risk for a condition called *endometrial hyperplasia,* which is a non-cancerous condition resulting from the growth of the endometrium. More research is needed to understand the implications of this observation. While research continues, diets rich in soy do not appear to cause this condition.[772]

Soy supplements—but not foods made from soy—should be halted during pregnancy. While open to speculation, the long-term effects of high levels of isoflavones on developing babies is not known and probably won't be for many years.

The impact of high levels of soy isoflavones on male fertility needs more study. Men who have fertility issues or erectile dysfunction should refrain from soy supplements until more is known.[776]

One of the most controversial areas of soy research revolves around speculation that under some circumstances soy might promote cancer.[775] Because some cancers—like that of the breast and endometrium—are sensitive to estrogen levels, soy's isoflavones might, in theory, activate the cellular processes of unrestrictive growth that characterizes cancer. The thing to keep in mind with this issue is that no one is in a position one way or another to state categorically that soy supplements can cause cancer in susceptible women or not. Women who are using soy for other reasons such as lowering cholesterol, and are having good results with it, are encouraged to continue using soy. While the risk is probably small, until more is known, women with a history of breast cancer or cancer of the endometrium should consult their physician before using soy-based supplements that contain concentrated isoflavones.

My Thoughts

Soy has been used by millions of people over many thousands of years and is generally considered a very safe and nutritious food. Because of research on its possible therapeutic effects, soy has skyrocketed in popularity such that a variety of soy-based foods and supplements are now available in supermarkets and health food stores around the world. While this is a book about nutritional supplements and not food, with the case for soy, the two are sometimes intertwined. Soy is a good food to use for a number of reasons and has a 5000-year track record of safety. My concern is what happens when components of soy, which are normally present in low levels in nature, start being concentrated to higher levels in supplements. In my opinion, soy is a better option than soy supplements because it contains the entire spectrum of soy's ingredients, just as nature intended. Those wanting to use soy isoflavone supplements are encouraged to keep the isoflavones to no more than 60 milligrams per day, which according to research should be more than sufficient to impact most conditions.

Tribulus

Tribulus is a plant that is found throughout the world, especially in warmer climate regions. While used in the past for a number of reasons, in America, tribulus is often marketed to two groups of people—those who want bigger muscles and those looking to increase their libido. Other names that also refer to tribulus include *Tribulus Terrestris* and *puncture vine*. The term puncture vine is derived from rumors that the plant's thorns are able to puncture bicycle tires. Tribulus, likewise, is Latin for "to tear", another reference to the plant's ability to do damage. In fact, the term tribulus also refers to a medieval weapon called a *caltrop* that was thrown on the grown during warfare to stop enemy horses from advancing. The caltrop was the forerunner of what we today know as tire spikes, used by law enforcement agencies around the world to stop motor vehicles.

Tribulus and Exercise

Tribulus is another member in the long list of supplements marketed to bodybuilders and others who desire bigger, stronger muscles. The general theory behind tribulus is that it is supposed to elevate luteinizing hormone which, in turn, sends instructions to the testes causing them to make testosterone. More testosterone might mean more muscle growth if combined with exercise. In theory, it all sounds plausible; the problem is that most experts don't think it works. While the amount of good studies that have been conducted on tribulus are few in number, they tend to show that it doesn't increase strength, decrease body fat or improve sports performance—even when it is combined with a strength training program.[782] In other words, even if tribulus could significantly elevate testosterone levels—which is debatable—it's irrelevant because that doesn't seem to translate into the real reason people use it—to make them stronger. Studies have used between 110 to 250 mg of tribulus per day without any significant exercise-related effects noticed.[782] If tribulus does indeed help muscles grow, then more research is needed to determine optimal amounts to use.

Tribulus and Sex

Because of its alleged effects on testosterone, tribulus is sometimes found in supplements purporting to improve issues of impotence, sexual performance and libido. Preliminary research in rodents does hint that tribulus may have some role in sexual arousal.[783] Other research hints that components of tribulus might expand blood vessels, which in part, is responsible for erections. Currently, though, how tribulus affects sexual desire or performance in people has not been adequately studied.

Side Effects and Concerns

Tribulus appears to be safe in healthy adults. Because of the lack of quality research on tribulus supplements, its interactions with medications and other supplements have not been adequately studied.

<u>My Thoughts</u>

Tribulus is a popular ingredient in some bodybuilding supplements, despite the lack of good research that it makes people stronger. The effects of tribulus on sexual performance, likewise, deserve more investigation. Research on rodents, while interesting, does not guarantee that it works in people. For those wanting to try tribulus or a supplement that contains it, remember that while it's probably safe, its ability to turn you into the *incredible hulk* in the gym—or the bedroom—is debatable.

Tryptophan & 5-HTP

This chapter is really about 5-hydroxytryptophan (5-HTP); however, it is not possible to delve into 5-HTP without also mentioning its forefather, tryptophan.

Both tryptophan and 5-HTP are related compounds. Tryptophan was a one-time popular sleep aid because it is converted to the brain chemical serotonin which has calming, tranquilizing effects in the body. Before tryptophan can be made into serotonin, it must first become 5-HTP. In other words, when we eat foods, like turkey, that contain tryptophan, 5-HTP is formed, which in turn makes serotonin. Tryptophan is not currently available as a supplement in the US due to evidence of its involvement in a rare blood disorder called *eosinophilia myalgia syndrome*, which resulted in the deaths of 37 people in the late 1980s.[586] Even though they are related, tryptophan and 5-HTP are not the same thing and the ban on tryptophan does not impact the sale of 5-HTP supplements. Unlike tryptophan, which was mostly used as a natural sleep inducer, 5-HTP has been investigated for the treatment of issues such as weight loss, depression and fibromyalgia. Supplements of 5-HTP are usually extracted from the seeds of *Griffonia simplicifolia,* a plant that grows in Africa. Another name that also refers to 5-HTP is *oxitriptan*.

5-HTP and Depression

Research links some depression to low levels of the various neurotransmitters that brain cells use to communicate and relay instructions with. Serotonin is one such example where low levels are linked to depression. In fact, many antidepressant medications work by reducing the rate that serotonin is broken down, an effect which essentially keeps the concentration of serotonin higher in the brain for longer periods of time. Since 5-HTP is converted to serotonin, in theory, using this supplement might also be effective for depression. While research on 5-HTP has hinted that it may indeed be effective for depression, studies in general tend to be hampered by problems that limit their acceptance by some in the scientific community. Issues such as not containing an adequate number of test subjects and not comparing 5-HTP's effects to that of a placebo (which should have no effect) are examples of problems with some 5-HTP studies. One analysis of 108 studies of the effectiveness of both tryptophan and 5-HTP for depression, revealed that only two studies were of sufficient quality to lend credence that they might indeed help.[784] Thus, evidence does suggest that 5-HTP may be effective for at least mild levels of depression in some people. The issues that deserve more attention are how effective is it and for which types of depression might it work the best. While more research is needed, studies that have obtained favorable results on depression have used 150 mg of 5-HTP. Lesser amounts may also work and might also reduce possible side effects.

5-HTP and Weight Loss

Understanding the reasons people might use 5-HTP for weight loss brings us again to the neurotransmitter, serotonin. Some research finds that low levels of serotonin might stimulate appetite. Thus, if serotonin levels could be kept high in the brain, appetite might decrease. This is actually the reasoning behind some prescription drugs to treat weight loss. Studies show that 5-HTP is effective at elevating serotonin levels when taken orally. Research also hints that giving 5-HTP supplements to overweight people may indeed help control appetite and promote modest weight loss.[785,786] While more research is needed to better pin down optimal dosages, studies on this issue have used 900 mg a day with favorable results.[786] Research also hints that this amount might also increase negative side effects.[786] To decrease the risk of side effects, starting with a lesser amount, and progressing upward slowly is probably a wiser choice than starting with a much larger amount.

5-HTP and Fibromyalgia

Some research suggests that there may be a link between low levels of serotonin and symptoms associated with fibromyalgia.[786] Indeed, previous research has noted low levels of serotonin in fibromyalgia sufferers.[786] Some research suggests that 5-HTP (100 mg three times a day) may help improve symptoms such as pain, morning stiffness, sleep quality and fatigue in those with fibromyalgia.[786] Overall, the amount of research investigating the efficacy of 5-HTP for fibromyalgia is not much. This makes it difficult to draw conclusions on how effective it might be. Also, several of the studies on this matter are older, dating back to the 1980s and early 90s. While significant negative side effects were not noted in clinical trials, studies tend to last only one to three months. Thus, the long-term side effects of 5-HTP for those with fibromyalgia is unknown.

Side Effects and Concerns

5-HTP is generally well tolerated in clinical studies, with nausea and stomach pain commonly reported. Most investigations of 5-HTP do not last longer than a few months, so questions regarding side effects following long-term use remain unanswered.

Much of the controversy surrounding 5-HTP revolves around its similarity to tryptophan which was implicated in the outbreak of eosinophilia-myalgia syndrome (EMS) in the late 1980s. To date, 5-HTP has not been found to cause EMS and unlike tryptophan, can be sold over-the- counter as a supplement. The debate continues though, because until the late 1980s tryptophan was not known to cause EMS either.

Another point of concern about 5-HTP involves its ability to elevate serotonin. *Serotonin syndrome* is a condition that occurs when serotonin levels rise too much. In theory, this can be lethal. 5-HTP does elevate serotonin levels. When used in combination with drugs or supplements that also raise serotonin, the risk of serotonin syndrome may be increased. Until more is known about its drug interactions, 5-HTP should not be used in conjunction with antidepressants such as MAO inhibitors, SSRIs or other medications that affect serotonin concentrations.[786] Supplements such as St. John's wort, SAM-e and possibly tyrosine might also be inappropriate to use with 5-HTP.[786]

Serotonin Syndrome Symptoms	
• Confusion	• Rapid heart beat
• Agitation	• Muscle twitches
• Restlessness	• Elevated blood pressure
• Sweating	• Elevated body temperature

My Thoughts

The connection between 5-HTP supplements and the development of EMS is almost as controversial as alleged sighting of UFOs and Bigfoot. This is not to diminish the possibility that EMS could result from using 5-HTP supplements but rather that it requires further investigation. The real issue with 5-HTP, I believe, lies in its capacity to raise serotonin levels. This ability, I feel, makes 5-HTP a double edged sword, possessing qualities that may be both therapeutic and potentially unsafe. For this reason, 5-HTP supplements can't be recommended unless under medical supervision.

Though often mentioned, and potentially very serious, the link between the amino acid tryptophan and EMS is still unresolved. For example, after the original EMS outbreak in the late 1980s, most cases could be traced back to a contaminated batch of tryptophan. However, not everyone who consumed tryptophan from the tainted batch developed EMS. Also, EMS had been reported in persons who consumed tryptophan that didn't appear to be contaminated.[586] This hints that only susceptible individuals may be at risk for tryptophan-induced EMS. Regardless, because of the potential seriousness of EMS, the US ban on tryptophan supplements is still in effect.

Valerian

Valerian, which is native to Asia, Europe and America grows between one and five feet in height and bears white to pinkish flowers. The herb has been used for over a thousand years mostly to treat issues of anxiety and sleeplessness. In Great Brittan, during World War II, it is rumored that valerian was given to people to combat stress resulting from their frequent air raids. In its natural state, valerian is a rather smelly plant, an odor that is said to be attractive to rats; in fact, according to legend, the *Pied Piper* used valerian to lure rodents out of the town of Hameln.[399] Other names that also refer to valerian include *Valeriana officinalis*, *setwall*, and *garden heliotrope*.

Valerian and Insomnia

Several clinical studies on valerian carried out over the last several decades find that 400-800 mg taken about an hour before bedtime, is effective at helping people fall asleep.[795] Because of this, valerian is likely to be found in supplements advertised as natural tranquilizers. Unlike some tranquilizer medications, valerian doesn't appear to reduce alertness or make people feel groggy the next day. On the downside, valerian usually takes about a month before any improvement in sleep is noticed. Valerian appears to be most effective for those with mild to moderate levels of insomnia.

It is important to note that there are over 250 species of valerian. The species that has been most studied is *valeriana officinalis*. Valerian supplements should list *valeriana officinalis* on their label so consumers know which species the supplement comes from.

The question as to how valerian works is still under investigation. One theory, which is often mentioned, states that valerian increases levels of a brain chemical called GABA, which has calming and sedative properties. Thus by increasing GABA, valerian might promote sleep.

Also unknown are valerian's active ingredients. Valerian supplements may be standardized according to the amount of *valerenic acid* they contain. Some research finds that valerenic acid can have a soothing effect on the body (by affecting GABA in the brain) but this does not necessarily prove that it is the key active ingredient. It's possible that there may be many parts of valerian that are responsible for its sleep-promoting effects. What is generally agreed upon, though, is that the active ingredients reside in the roots of the plant.[399] Thus valerian supplements should be derived from the roots.

Side Effects and Concerns

Valerian is usually thought of as a rather harmless herb with no serious side effects reported in studies. Vivid dreams, dry mouth, headache and ironically, insomnia have sometimes been reported following valerian use.

Because of its sedative properties, valerian should not be combined with tranquilizers, like valium or alcohol. Likewise, while it has not been shown to impair reaction time or alertness, driving is not recommended when using valerian.

Some studies hint that valerian may interact with a number of medications such as those used to treat high cholesterol and cancer. This interaction might result in medications being expelled faster from the body or by reducing their excretion, both of which might impact the effectiveness of the medication.

Still unknown is how valerian interacts with other supplements like melatonin, 5-HTP, kava and similar products that are also used to calm the body and improve sleep quality.

Rumors of valerian causing liver damage when used long-term continue to be debated.[399] No study to date has clearly shown that valerian negatively alters liver function. Even so, those with liver problems may wish to refrain from valerian until more is known. Getting periodic checks of liver function is probably also wise as well.

My Thoughts

Several studies, as well as centuries of use, provide evidence that valerian appears to have merit as a mild-acting natural sleep aid. While used since the time of Hippocrates, we still don't know how valerian works, how effective it might be for everyone or what its active ingredients are. It's important to remember that valerian appears to work best when used over several weeks. Thus, the herb might prove most valuable to the chronic insomniac as opposed to those who only occasionally spend the night channel surfing in front of the TV.

Vanadyl Sulfate

Vanadium is a silvery-grayish metal that is used industrially to improve the strength and corrosion resistance of steel. While presumably needed in small amounts by humans, in high doses vanadium is toxic. Vanadyl sulfate is one of the most popular forms of vanadium found in supplements and is often of interest to people who desire to get stronger and reduce weight. More recently, vanadyl sulfate may also be on the radar screens of diabetics, who are looking to help stabilize blood sugar. The name vanadium is derived from Vanadis, the Scandinavian goddess of beauty. Good natural sources of vanadium include breakfast cereals, mushrooms, shellfish and soy.

Vanadyl Sulfate and Exercise

Strength trainers sometimes may use vanadyl sulfate because it appears to function like insulin. The hormone insulin, while mostly recognized for its effects on lowering blood sugar, also has a slight anabolic effect by helping with the uptake of amino acids. So, by using vanadyl sulfate, strength trainers hope that it will enhance muscle protein formation which, in turn, might increase muscle mass and strength. Despite its popularity in some circles, there is no good evidence that vanadyl sulfate improves muscle strength, size or enhances exercise performance.[796]

Vanadyl Sulfate and Weight Loss?

Because vanadium appears to work like insulin, and insulin is involved in how we process carbohydrates (sugar), vanadium may be found in some weight loss supplements. The theory is that if our desire to eat carbohydrates were curbed, then our blood sugar levels would be better balanced and we might eat less and lose weight. This sounds plausible but as of yet, there is no good evidence for it. In addition, there is no credible proof that the amount of vanadium in weight loss supplements curbs appetite in humans.

Vanadyl Sulfate and Diabetes

Diabetics either don't make insulin or can't make use of the insulin they produce. These are usually called type I and type II diabetes, respectively. Some evidence suggests that vanadyl sulfate may help improve the body's sensitively to insulin and thus may be effective for some type II diabetics.[840] Studies have used 100 mg a day with success. This is a rather high amount of vanadyl and might increase the risk of negative side effects. Vanadyl sulfate is not often recommended for type II diabetics unless monitored closely by a physician. Vanadyl sulfate's impact on type I diabetes is less clear, with some evidence that it may not help.[840]

It's possible to be overweight and have trouble keeping your blood sugar in check—yet not be classified as "diabetic". This group of people may also be attracted to this supplement. The research however, hints that vanadyl sulfate may not work for overweight, non-diabetic individuals.[840]

Side Effects and Concerns

Most of what we know about vanadium's side effects stems from animal research and studies conducted in test tubes. Based on this, the amount at which the potential for toxicity might occur is 1.8 mg per day. Most people consume much less than this in the diet.

Just as hemoglobin makes our blood red, vanadium makes the blood of some sea-dwelling animals green. In fact, one of the classic signs of overdosing on vanadium is a green color on the tongue. Other signs of vanadium overload include fatigue, abdominal cramps and altered kidney function.

My Thoughts

When animals are fed a vanadium-deficient diet, their offspring are born with weaker bones and tend to die off sooner. Thus, in small amounts, vanadium is almost assuredly an essential nutrient.

Many people who are interested in vanadyl sulfate are attracted by the lure of a natural way to stabilize blood sugar. While research finds that vanadyl sulfate may help in this respect, the amounts needed to achieve this effect may overlap with the amounts that might be harmful. Because of this, and because it doesn't seem to work for everybody, high doses of vanadyl sulfate cannot be recommended.

Vitamin B-12

Like all vitamins, vitamin B-12 is involved in a multitude of chemical reactions needed for optimal health. For example, it is required for the manufacture of red blood cells which carry oxygen in the body. Vitamin B-12 also plays critical roles in the functioning of the nervous system. This vitamin is even needed for the manufacture of SAM-e, a molecule, discussed previously, which some may use to treat depression and arthritis. Vitamin B-12 is found naturally in foods that come from animals like chicken, steak, milk, eggs and turkey. Foods like breakfast cereals may also be fortified with vitamin B-12. The recommended dietary allowance (RDA) for vitamin B-12 is 2.4 micrograms per day. Additional names that also refer to vitamin B-12 include *cyanocobalamin, B_{12}* and *methylcobalamin.*

How *Vitamin* Got its Name

The history of vitamins is replete with men and women whose early investigations into the science of nutrition laid the foundations for practically everything we know today. One such person was the Polish biochemist, Casmir Funk, who, around 1912 discovered a nitrogen-containing compound that halted the progression of a disease he was studying called polyneuritis. Funk called this new compound "vitamine" because it was *vital* to life and because the word *amine* is the scientific term for something that contains the element nitrogen.[799] Funk originally thought all vitamins contained nitrogen; today we know this is not so. Therefore, the letter "e" was dropped from the end of vitamine, yielding the more familiar word *vitamin!* And now you know the rest of the story...

Who Needs Vitamin B-12 The Most?

Vitamin B-12 is one of the many nutrients needed to make red blood cells which carry oxygen throughout the body. If we are deficient in B-12, we make fewer and less effective red blood cells, creating a condition called anemia. *Pernicious anemia* is the name given to the type of anemia that results from an inability to absorb vitamin B-12. *Pernicious* means deadly and makes reference to the fact that this condition used to be fatal, until we learned that vitamin B-12 could cure it.

Strict vegetarians who do not eat any meat or other foods that contain vitamin B-12 are at risk of deficiency. While it may take many years to occur, in time, their vitamin B-12 reserves can eventually become depleted. Thus, vegetarians should at least use a multivitamin that contains the RDA for vitamin B-12. Vegetarians who consume milk and eggs may not require extra B-12 because they are getting it in the foods they eat.

Senior citizens are another group who may be in need of supplemental B-12. Occasionally seniors may even go to their doctor and get an injection of this vitamin. The reason for this is because as we age, we may not eat as much vitamin B-12-containing foods. Some may also find it harder to digest food properly which makes absorbing vitamin B-12 difficult.[797] Still others may also have an inability to absorb this vitamin. Getting an injection of B-12 bypasses the stomach and sends the vitamin directly into the body where it can be used.

Vitamin B-12 and Heart Disease

Clinical studies show that the addition of as little as 0.5 mg of vitamin B-12 can help lower homocysteine levels which are thought to play a role in the development of heart disease.[797] This effect of vitamin B-12 can be even more pronounced when combined with folic acid and vitamin B-6, which also lower homocysteine. Thus, vitamin B-12, along with folic acid and vitamin B-6 may appear together in supplements marketed to people interested in heart health.

It's important to remember that while vitamins B-12, B-6 and folic acid will all lower homocysteine, it is folic acid that usually receives most of the attention. The reason for this is that vitamin B-12, unlike most B vitamins, is usually stockpiled in the body for many years before it runs out.[797] Thus, healthy people who consume meat, poultry, dairy and B-12-fortified foods may not be deficient in this vitamin. Vitamin B-12's ability to lower homocysteine is most effective in those who are not getting enough of this nutrient in their diet.

Vitamin B-6 is usually not recommended as the first line treatment for high homocysteine because high doses are associated with altered liver function and nerve damage that is reversible upon halting the use of the vitamin.

Readers should remember that heart disease is a complex process and simply lowering homocysteine by the use of vitamin B-12 (or folic acid or B-6 for that matter) may not necessarily also reduce the risk or progression of this condition. Like most medical issues outlined in this book, the best defense against heart disease is prevention.

Vitamin B-12 and Depression

Some reports estimate that a significant number of depressed people may also be suffering from a vitamin B-12 deficiency.[797] As was mentioned earlier, vitamin B-12 is required to make SAM-e, which is used by some people for the self-treatment of depression. So, the question then becomes, is it possible that low levels of B-12 leads to decreased SAM-e which, in turn, fosters depression? It's possible but for the moment nobody knows for certain. Could it be that deficiencies in B-12 and depression are totally unrelated? This also is possible. Can it be that medications used by depressed people deplete B-12 from the body? Maybe. For those suffering from depression and looking for answers, the best advice for now is to make sure you are getting adequate vitamin B-12 from food and/or supplements. Other useful strategies in addition to this include addressing the root cause (if you know it) of your depression, maintaining contact with friends, seeking counseling, getting outdoors and yes, getting some exercise. Depression is complex and can have many causes. Attacking it from a multi-pronged holistic approach is probably more effective than any single avenue alone.

More Vitamin Trivia

Believe it or not, vitamins were first discovered in milk—although back then, nobody called them vitamins. Instead, they were known as *accessory growth factors*.[799] When they were first discovered, all that was known about these growth factors was that there seemed to be two of them. One growth factor, found in the creamy portion of milk, was named "A" (this later turned out to be vitamin A). The other growth factor was called "B". Later it was discovered that the B growth factor really was made up of an entire family of distinct compounds. As more were discovered, they were named in order B-1, B-2, B-3, etc...—what we today know as the *B-Complex* family of vitamins.

Side Effects and Concerns

Vitamin B-12 is usually regarded as a safe supplement with little side effects in healthy adults. Because no supplement is perfect for all people under all circumstances, the following are issues to consider when using this nutrient.

People afflicted with type II diabetes and who are using medications to treat their condition, might benefit from vitamin B-12 or a multivitamin that contains it. Some orally taken medications, like *glucophage* might diminish vitamin B-12 levels.[798]

Because ulcer medications may reduce stomach acid secretions which are needed to help absorb vitamin B-12, in theory, long-term use of drugs prescribed for the treatment of ulcers may lead to a deficiency in this nutrient.

Some people may suffer from a rare genetic eye disorder called *Leber's disease* that causes blindness. In these individuals, vitamin B-12 can make this condition worse.

Symptoms of a vitamin B-12 deficiency might be eclipsed by folic acid. For example, strict vegetarians who eat plenty of foods high in folic acid, yet consume no B-12- containing foods or supplements may eventually develop a B-12 deficiency and not know it.

My Thoughts

Because they are so well studied, vitamins in general are the only supplements where we have good information on their long-term side effects. Some of the strongest evidence for B-12 besides its well documented effects on helping anemia, is for lowering homocysteine, which appears to play a role in heart disease. Whether or not reducing homocysteine also reduces heart attacks and strokes needs more study. As an extra measure of protection, use homocysteine lowering supplements in conjunction with a healthy diet and lifestyle for optimum results.

Vitamin C

Vitamin C, along with all of the B vitamins, makes up what are collectively known as the *water-soluble* vitamins. Soluble means dissolvable. Water soluble vitamins are called water soluble because they dissolve well in water (as opposed to fat soluble vitamins that require a fatty environment to dissolve properly). A nutrient is usually labeled a vitamin when it satisfies one of two conditions; either we do not make the nutrient naturally in the body or when a lack of the nutrient is associated with a disease. The classic disease associated with a lack of vitamin C is scurvy, which plagued sailors a few hundred years ago. Scurvy was a big problem among all sailors until the British discovered that scurvy could be cured if they consumed limes and other vitamin-C-rich citrus fruits during their sea voyages. It's of historical value to note that it was because of their consumption of limes that British sailors came to be nick-named *Limies*. Besides citrus fruits, other good food sources of vitamin C include potatoes, broccoli and strawberries. The RDA for vitamin C is currently set at 90 mg for men and 75 mg for women. Many of the virtues of vitamin C were popularized by the late Dr. Linus Pauling, who advocated large doses of this nutrient to treat and reduce the risk of a number of conditions ranging from the common cold to cancer. Among his many achievements, Dr. Pauling had the distinct honor of being the only person ever awarded two unshared Nobel prizes; one for chemistry in 1954 and the Nobel Peace Prize in 1962. Other names that also refer to vitamin C include *ascorbic acid and ascorbate.*

Vitamin C and the Common Cold

One of the most popular reasons people use vitamin C is to help prevent colds and flus. This is actually an issue that has been well researched but unfortunately, still hotly debated. Many, but not all, studies find that the consumption of larger than normal doses of vitamin C (about 2 grams a day) is associated with a modest decrease in the duration and severity of colds.[800] On average the duration of colds tends to be reduced by about 2-3 days. The reasons for this effect are not well understood. In large doses, vitamin C appears to function like a natural antihistamine and seems also to stimulate some of the cells of the immune system.[800] Vitamin C is also a well-known antioxidant, which might further help explain its effects.

Related to this, there is evidence that vitamin C may benefit some athletes. It is well known that those who participate in marathons, triathlons, military basic training, and other similar, exhaustive exercise regimens tend to suffer more infections in the days following the event than those who take part in less-grueling physical activity. Specifically, studies find that 500-1000 mg of vitamin C taken several days prior to exhaustive physical activity might reduce infections by as much as 80%.[801]

Vitamin C and Cancer

How cancer starts is still a mystery. One of theories behind its development maintains that it is the result of cellular attack by free radicals. Free radicals are unstable atoms and molecules that disrupt normal cell operations. Vitamin C is a well known antioxidant. Antioxidants are compounds that neutralize free radicals, preventing them from doing us harm. So, vitamin C as a preventative step to reduce cancer, makes sense in theory. Most of the evidence in support of using vitamin C for battling cancer stems from studies that observe the eating habits of large groups of people over long periods of time. In these observational studies, it is found that people who eat fruits and vegetables tend to get less cancers.[800] This is not necessarily evidence in support of vitamin C supplements though because fruits and vegetables contain many other nutrients besides vitamin C which might explain their protective effect. People who eat healthy also tend to exercise and not smoke, which also probably helps with reducing cancer risk.

While separate issues, a possible flaw in the reasoning of those who single out vitamin C as cancer-protective could be likened to the case for beta carotene. Beta carotene (another antioxidant) was once thought to be one of the key common dominator nutrients responsible for the healthy effects of fruits and vegetables. That issue was laid to rest when it was discovered that beta carotene supplements (but not beta carotene in food), tended to increase lung cancer in smokers.[297] Again, these are two totally different topics but it reminds us all of an important point often not talked about; namely that individual nutrients, isolated from their natural environments (i.e. food) and concentrated to higher levels than that found in nature, do not always act the same way as when they are in their natural surroundings.

So what's the verdict on vitamin C and cancer? Well, the issue continues to be controversial. Factors such as to how much vitamin C might help, the stage of cancer that it might be most effective, the type of cancer studied and other lifestyle habits all cloud the issue. Until more is known, questions such as whether vitamin C supplements prevent cancer in healthy people or whether vitamin C supplements can prolong the lives of those with cancer are still open to debate.[801]

Vitamin C and Heart Disease

The information regarding vitamin C improving heart disease or reducing its occurrence is intriguing but far from complete. For example, at 500 mg dosages, vitamin C appears to dilate (open up) blood vessels, which might help blood move through the body more freely.[800] This may in part be related to the nutrient's ability to improve levels of nitric oxide, a known blood vessel dilator. Vitamin C is also an antioxidant and as such can protect cells from attack by free radicals, which might contribute to heart disease. Vitamin C also appears to help reenergize and reform vitamin E, another well known antioxidant. This vitamin may also help by reinforcing weakened blood vessels via its key role in the production of collagen, a major part of blood vessel architecture.

Growing evidence suggests that heart disease may be due in part to a low-grade widespread inflammation of the blood vessels. Because of this, doctors may choose to test for the presence of a compound called *C-reactive protein* (CRP), a marker of inflammation. While not conclusive, some studies find low levels of vitamin C are correlated with higher CRP levels.[803]

Most of the evidence so far on the issue of vitamin C and heart disease stems from looking at the eating habits of people. Examining what people eat is far different than, for example, giving vitamin C to ten thousand people and watching what happens for the next 5 years. Vitamin C probably does play some role in maintaining the integrity of the cardiovascular system. Whether or not vitamin C supplements are as effective as eating foods rich in vitamin C deserves more study.

Vitamin C and Bioflavonoids

Bioflavonoids, or simply flavonoids, as they are also called, are plant nutrients that some evidence suggests may exert health-promoting effects. As such, vitamin C supplements that contain citrus-derived bioflavonoids do exist. The reasoning behind this is that the vitamin-C-bioflavonoid combination would be superior to vitamin C alone. Emerging research on bioflavonoids does hint that they may impact health and may even do so independently of their interaction with vitamin C. For example, the bioflavonoid *quercetin*, found in grapes, appears to act as an antioxidant and may even help protect blood vessels from clogging. Most of the research on bioflavonoids is still pretty new and is ongoing. This makes it difficult at the moment to tell whether a vitamin C-bioflavonoid complex is superior to vitamin C alone.

Vitamin C and Muscle Soreness

When muscles are worked harder than normal or in a fashion that they are not used to, they tend get sore 24 to 72 hours later. This phenomenon is called *delayed onset muscle soreness* (DOMS for short). Because damage to the connective tissue surrounding muscles has been observed in those with DOMS and because vitamin C is needed to produce connective tissue, some might use this nutrient to decrease the occurrence of DOMS. The theory sounds plausible but because the evidence is mixed, more research is needed before anyone can say for certain if it helps or not.

What Are Rose Hips?

Rose hips are the tiny red colored fruits that form on rosebushes after the petals fall off. Because rose hips are a good source of vitamin C, they are popular among people who prefer natural over synthetic vitamins. Regardless of which you prefer, research generally shows that the human body cannot tell the difference between natural and synthetic vitamin C.[800]

Side Effects and Concerns

Vitamin C, like all vitamins, are safe for the vast majority of people especially when consumed in food as well as when used in amounts found in many supplements. As was mentioned previously, the RDA for vitamin C is 90 mg a day for men and 75 mg for women. Dosages greater than 2 grams of vitamin C a day have been associated with diarrhea and stomach problems, two of the most common complaints of over-doing this nutrient. Kidney stones have also been reported in people who consume large amounts of vitamin C.

Several medications may interact with vitamin C. For example, some oral contraceptives and aspirin have been shown to reduce vitamin C levels.

Large doses of vitamin C might alter the results of some laboratory tests. Individuals should disclose their use of vitamin C to their physician so this can be taken into consideration when interpreting laboratory test results.

It is well known that smoking reduces vitamin C levels.[800] This depletion may be due to vitamin C working overtime to neutralize the large amount of free radicals and other pollutants produced and inhaled by smoking. Because of this, some estimate that smokers may need up to 200 mg of vitamin C a day to maintain adequate levels of this nutrient.[841] This is, of course, no guarantee that vitamin C reduces cancer or other ill effects in smokers. There is still no substitute that's better than not smoking at all.

Vitamin C enhances the absorption of iron. Iron is an essential nutrient. In those who have the rare genetic condition called *iron overload disease,* vitamin C can make the condition worse.

The use of vitamin C by those with cancer is controversial. While not proven to occur in humans, the use of antioxidants in general by cancer patients, in theory, might reduce the effectiveness of some cancer therapies. Further blurring the issue is the observation that vitamin C levels are sometimes found to be higher inside cancer cells.[801] Does this mean that cancer cells may be using vitamin C? Or, is the higher uptake of vitamin C evidence that the nutrient is infiltrating cancer cells and helping to destroy them? Both of these questions needs more study. People with cancer should discuss the use of vitamin C (and all supplements) with their oncologist for the most up-to-date information.

My Thoughts

There is no doubt that vitamin C (like all vitamins) are needed to keep us healthy. The *sixty-four-thousand-dollar question* is whether more vitamin C above the

RDA is better. The studies conducted to date are definitely intriguing but not yet conclusive enough to recommended mega doses of vitamin C for everybody. The big issue to address is whether vitamin C itself is better than foods that contain vitamin C. While this nutrient appears to carry some possible therapeutic effects, for the moment I feel the evidence is stronger for eating more vitamin-C-rich foods. Those who don't feel they have the time (or desire) to eat more vitamin C-containing foods may want to consider juicing. Now, the juicing I'm talking about is a little different from what you may be used to. Many quality juicers are on the market but most of them tend to remove the fiber-rich pulp from the juice. To overcome this problem, I prefer to mix a variety of fruits and vegetables in a blender. One of my favorite recipes involves the following: red and white grapes, frozen strawberries, blueberries, raspberries, one orange (minus the peel), a cup of water and a handful of baby carrots. Drinking this concoction provides not only vitamin C but also a host of other nutrients (like bioflavonoids, discussed previously) and fiber. As an added bonus, it tastes great and fills you up so you are less likely to snack in-between meals. Give it a try and see what you think.

Vitamin D

Vitamin D, along with vitamins A, E and K, make up the fat-soluble family of vitamins. Vitamin D is unique because it is the only vitamin that can be made by the body. Specifically, we make vitamin D when we are exposed to sunlight. Hence, the other name for this nutrient is the *sun* vitamin. Ultraviolet radiation from the sun (UVB rays specifically) stimulate the skin to make vitamin D. While often thought of as a single vitamin, there are actually two separate but related versions of this nutrient. Vitamin D-2 (*ergocalciferol*) is sometimes found in vitamin supplements and is derived from plants. Vitamin D-3 (*cholecalciferol*) is the type that is made upon exposure to sunlight. Both types can be used by humans although cholecalciferol, made from sunlight, appears to be better at raising vitamin D levels.

While mostly known as the vitamin that helps keep bones strong by enhancing our absorption of calcium, vitamin D also appears to have other functions, many of which are only now starting to be understood. If you take a look at the foods in your kitchen right now you'll soon notice that vitamin D can be rather difficult to get into the diet unless it is purposely added to foods. For example, milk that has been fortified with vitamin D is one of the most common dietary sources of this nutrient. Vitamin D is also found naturally in fatty fish such as tuna, mackerel, sardines and catfish. Many multivitamins are usually also a good source of vitamin D. Other names that refer to this nutrient include *25-hydroxycholecalciferol* and *1,25-ihydroxycholecalciferol.*

Vitamin D and Bones

It is well known that a lack of vitamin D can lead to impaired calcium absorption. Two classic vitamin D deficiency syndromes are *rickets,* which normally occurs in children and *osteomalacia,* which is common in adults. Both conditions result in weakened bones that break easily. The reason why lack of vitamin D harms bones is made clear when it is realized that calcium is important to many biological functions besides helping keep bones strong. In the absence of adequate vitamin D, our absorption of calcium drops. In this situation, the body begins to pull calcium from the bones to help meet its other calcium needs. Over time, this continual draining of calcium weakens the bones and eventually can contribute to osteoporosis.

How Much Vitamin D is Needed?

Vitamin D intake is currently based on age with 200 IUs normally recommended for healthy persons up to the age of 50. This number increases to 400 IUs for those age 50 to 70. Lastly, for persons over 70 years of age, 600 IUs are generally recommended. Many general purpose multivitamins contain 400 IUs of vitamin D.

Vitamin D and Older Adults

As we get older, our skin becomes less efficient at producing vitamin D. This, coupled with the tendency by many to spend less time outdoors, might precipitate a deficiency in seniors. For these reasons, vitamin D is sometimes emphasized to older adults because of the vital role it plays in helping strengthen bones. In addition, new research hints that there may yet be another reason of equal importance: Balance. It appears that vitamin D supplementation (800 IUs a day) may reduce falls in the elderly by as much as 20 percent.[807] Anything that could limit falls in older adults would have profound effects on extending their lives. The reasons behind this effect are still being investigated. This intriguing finding about vitamin D may be particularly important to people in nursing homes as well as those with Alzheimer's disease and other types of senility, who, because of being mostly homebound, have limited exposure to sunlight and may be particularly likely to fall.

Vitamin D and Cancer

Some research finds that there may be a connection between low levels of vitamin D and the development of different types of cancer.[804,806] Vitamin D appears to suppress the unrestricted growth and spread of cells, which is essentially what cancer is. However, strong evidence in support of the low vitamin-D-cancer connection is still lacking. Most of the proof so far is based on laboratory research or studies that look at rates of cancer in large numbers of people. For example, studies sometimes find more cancer in those who get the least sunlight and those who have the lowest vitamin D levels.[805] While this is a very interesting correlation, the real test would be to give vitamin D supplements to thousands of people for several years, compare that to thousands of others who didn't take vitamin D and watch what happens. Until more research is done the connection between vitamin D and cancer remains controversial.

Vitamin D and Sunscreens

Sunscreens are a vital first line defense against skin cancer and premature skin aging. This is especially true for fair-skinned individuals. That being said, sunscreens do reduce the amount of vitamin D made when we are exposed to sunlight. Specifically, sunscreens with an SPF of as little as 8 can reduce vitamin D production by over 90%.[806] Fortunately, it doesn't take much sun to supply us with vitamin D. Only 10-20 minutes of sunlight on the face and arms a few times a week is all that's needed to give us our daily requirement of this nutrient.

Side Effects and Concerns

In amounts commonly found in food and in multivitamins, vitamin D is considered safe. The amount past which the potential for side effects might start to occur is currently thought to be 2000 IUs for adults. Common side effects of too much vitamin D include nausea, constipation, alterations in the way the heart beats and ironically, bone loss.[805] These side effects do not occur when vitamin D is made naturally from sunlight. However, too much sun exposure is definitely connected to skin wrinkling and skin cancer. Thus, even if vitamin D is proven beyond a doubt to reduce the risk of some diseases, this is not an invitation to bake in the sun all day.

Many of the concerns over vitamin D supplements are derived from their potential to raise calcium levels too much, which could be harmful for some people. Calcium is indispensable for the functioning of all muscle tissue including our most important muscle—the heart. Increased calcium absorption brought about via vitamin D supplements might elevate calcium levels too much, which could interfere with the way the heart works. This could be particularly problematic for those with heart conditions.[806] High blood levels of calcium might also interact with medications used by those with heart disease.[805]

Vitamin D supplements may be helpful in maintaining bone mass in those who use anti-inflammatory steroids like prednisone. A side-effect of long-term prednisone use is bone loss.[805]

Some drugs used to treat obesity might reduce the amount of vitamin D that is absorbed from food. Over time, this, combined with a lack of outside activity might deplete vitamin D reserves. Related to this, long-term use of supplements that block the absorption of fat might, in theory also reduce vitamin D absorption.

My Thoughts

Until recently, vitamin D wasn't considered a very *sexy* supplement and as such tended to receive little attention. Intriguing research, though, is suggesting that this nutrient might not just be for bones anymore. Specifically, studies are suggesting that vitamin D may help regulate a number of conditions ranging from cancer and multiple sclerosis to diabetes. The amounts of vitamin D that might impact these disorders is still being studied. For the moment, a daily multivitamin, getting 10-20 minutes of sun a few times a week, coupled with eating foods that contain vitamin D is probably good insurance.

Vitamin E

First discovered in the early 1920s in green leafy vegetables, vitamin E, quickly became and continues to be, one of the most popular of all vitamins used today. Vitamin E is a fat soluble compound that appears to help the body in a number of ways. For example, as an antioxidant, vitamin E acts as one of our defenses against free radicals, which are thought to contribute to disease. In fact, its antioxidant activity is probably the most well known and best researched aspect of this nutrient. Almost as popular as its antioxidant ability is vitamin E's reputation as an *aphrodisiac.* One reason for this may stem from research finding that a lack of vitamin E (in rats) can lead to sterility. In men, vitamin E has been shown to improve the swimming ability of sperm and as such may be of some help to couples who are trying to have children. Despite its inclusion in some over-the-counter aphrodisiacs and love potions, vitamin E's impact on sex drive in healthy people is probably minimal at best.

Because it is a fat soluble vitamin, deficiency in this nutrient is unlikely. Barring any absorption problems, people eating a healthy diet usually store enough vitamin E to last for several years.

The adult RDA for vitamin E is 33 IUs a day for synthetic vitamin E and 22 IUs for all-natural vitamin E.

Good food sources of this vitamin include green leafy vegetables, vegetable oils, wheat germ, and nuts. Other names that also refer to vitamin E include *alpha tocopherol, dl alpha tocopherol, d alpha tocopherol* and *RRR-alpha tocopherol.*

The Different Types of Vitamin E

While usually thought of as a single nutrient, vitamin E really refers to two classes of compounds, which each contain four different varieties of vitamin E. The two big classes of vitamin E are called *tocopherols* and *tocotrienols*.[809] Each of these contains four different and distinct versions called, *alpha, beta, gamma* and *delta*. So there are really eight different types of vitamin E! Of all of these types, *alpha tocopherol* is thought to be the most powerful and is the form that is found in the greatest amount in the body. So, for this reason, most supplements contain alpha tocopherol. That being said, evidence is accumulating that the other types of vitamin E may also have merit. For example, some research hints that gamma tocopherol may slow the growth of prostate cancer and protect blood vessels from the ravages of heart disease.[808]

One possible downside of using mega doses of alpha tocopherol is that it might interfere with the absorption of these other important versions of vitamin E. Because of the possible importance of theses other types of vitamin E, some products may include all of them. These all-encompassing vitamin E products can usually be identified by the term *mixed tocopherols*, which generally means that the product contains various amounts of the different vitamin E types.

Vitamin E and Heart Disease

Vitamin E is very popular among older adults because of a belief that it can reduce heart disease. For example, vitamin E acts like a natural blood thinner, keeping blood moving freely though the blood vessels. Vitamin E has also been shown to protect the breakdown of bad cholesterol (also called LDL), which studies find can contribute to plaque buildup and thus, heart disease. When scientists look at large numbers of people, they tend to find that those who use vitamin E supplements (up to 100 IU a day), have a lower rate of heart disease.[809] Interestingly, this pattern is not seen when vitamin E supplements (400 IU a day) are given to thousands of people who are then followed for several years.[808,809] So, while on the surface, it makes sense that vitamin E might lower heart disease, the evidence is mixed and the use of vitamin E for this purpose continues to be controversial. As always, our best defense against heart disease is prevention. This includes, among other things, regular exercise, not smoking, eating healthy and limiting as much as possible the long-term harmful stresses in our lives.

Vitamin E and Cancer

Studies investigating the impact of Vitamin E on reducing cancer tend to be mixed, which causes this nutrient to be viewed with an eye of skepticism by many in the medical community. Some research finds vitamin E may lower cancer risk while other research shows no effect.[808,809] Some research also suggests that 50 mg per day of vitamin E may be effective for lowering the risk of prostate cancer but more research is needed to confirm this.[810] Conversely, some evidence suggests that 400 IUs of vitamin E might promote the reoccurrence of head and neck cancer.[812] The bottom line is that cancer is complex and many different types of cancer are known to exist. Research to date suggests that vitamin E may not be equally effective against all forms of this disease.

Natural Vs. Synthetic Vitamin E

It is well known that natural vitamin E is more potent than synthetic vitamin E. It turns out that there is a pretty good reason for this. Just as there are right-and left-handed people in the world, so too are there right- and left-handed molecules. Our bodies, being the picky little devils that they are, can only use the right-handed version of this nutrient. When synthetic vitamin E is made in the laboratory it is really a mixture of both right- and left-handed molecules. Natural vitamin E on the other hand is all right-handed molecules. So, if you had 100 IUs of synthetic vitamin E, in theory, only 50 IUs could be used by the body. A 100 IU natural vitamin E supplement would pack more punch so to speak, because in theory it would be made of only the useable, right-handed molecules. The right-handed version is often labeled "D" and the left-handed (synthetic) version is called "L". These letters give rise to the often observed name "DL alpha tocopherol" which adorns the ingredients list of many vitamin labels.

Vitamin E and Arthritis

While not widely studied, some research suggests that 1200 IUs of natural vitamin E acetate used for 12 weeks may help reduce pain levels associated with rheumatoid arthritis.[842] How vitamin E seems to work in this regard is not well understood. Any pain relief achieved appears to be small and individual results will probably vary. Vitamin E does not appear to help the more widespread form, osteoarthritis.

Vitamin E and Alzheimer's Disease

There is some intriguing evidence that vitamin E may slow the progression of Alzheimer's disease.[813] Currently, only a small amount of studies have been done on this topic and many questions still need to be resolved but based on what is known now, encouraging results have been observed with 2000 IU of vitamin E. This is a rather high amount and probably best undertaken while under the supervision of a doctor.

How to Convert from IUs to Milligrams

In the US, the concentration of Vitamin E is usually listed as international units (IUs). In other countries however the concentration of this nutrient may be in milligrams (mg). With a little math, it's easy to translate IUs to mgs and vice versa. For example, 1 IU of natural vitamin E (d alpha tocopherol) equals 0.67 milligrams. So, to covert IUs of natural vitamin E to milligrams, just multiply the IUs by 0.67. For example, 400 IUs of natural vitamin E equals 400 X 0.67 = 268 mg. To convert back to IUs, just divide the milligrams by 0.67.

With respect to synthetic ("dl") vitamin E, 1 IU equals 0.45 milligrams. To convert synthetic vitamin E to milligrams, multiply the IUs by 0.45. In the example used above, 400 IUs of synthetic vitamin E equals 400 X 0.45 =180 mg.

Vitamin E and the Skin

Our skin is the largest organ of the entire body and is in constant contact with our external environment.

Ultraviolet rays from the sun can damage the skin and can contribute to fine lines and wrinkles as well as skin cancer. Ultraviolet rays damage the skin because they produce free radicals. Because vitamin E is an antioxidant, it is often found in skin-care products. While controversial, some evidence does hint that the combination of vitamin E (1000 IU) and vitamin C (2 grams) may help protect the skin from damage if you take them orally.[843] The effectiveness of this compared to traditional sunscreens needs more study. The effectiveness of topically applying these vitamins to the skin's surface also needs more study. Vitamins, whether they are taken orally or applied directly to the skin's surface should not take the place of sunscreens that contain accepted SPF ingredients.

Side Effects and Concerns

Vitamin E is generally considered one of the safer supplements on the market with side effects rarely occurring. Seldom-reported effects from using too much vitamin E include muscle weakness and blurred vision. The amount past which significant side effects might start to occur is currently set at 1500 IUs for natural vitamin E and 1100 IUs for synthetic vitamin E.

Some evidence has linked vitamin E to heightened death rates among those who used 400 IUs daily.[811] More studies are needed to confirm this finding and persons using vitamin E supplements are encouraged to see their physician for the most up-to-date information on this topic.

Because vitamin E has blood thinning properties, it might interact with medications and supplements that also effect blood clotting.

My Thoughts

Vitamin E continues to be as popular as it is controversial. While well researched, it appears that the more we know, the more questions we have. Vitamin E is certainly an essential nutrient; but, its exact roles in maintaining optimal health and prevention of disease are still under investigation.

Whey Protein

Little miss Muffet sat on a tuffet eating her curds and whey... To many, this was a popular nursery rhyme that some reading these words may have recited in their youth or, to their own children today. While curds and whey may have been a popular treat for children at one time, *whey* has taken on an entirely new meaning to the tens of millions of people who exercise regularly.

Whey refers to the watery, protein-rich portion of milk that forms during the process of making cheese. Because it is high in protein, whey is incorporated into a multitude of protein supplements the world over. Beyond this, whey may also have other properties that are only now starting to be understood. Whey protein is usually called "whey protein" or just *whey* for short.

What is Whey Protein?

Whey protein is one of the two main proteins found in milk (the other being the much more abundant protein, casein). Because of this, whey, like all protein from animal sources, is referred to as a *complete protein* which means it contains all of the essential amino acids that we need in the right combinations.

While normally thought of as a single protein, whey is in reality composed of several different types of compounds, many of which appear to have unique properties. Some of the more well known of whey's constitute parts include *lactoferrin*, an antioxidant and immune system stimulator and *cysteine*, an amino acid that's involved in the production of *glutathione*, another antioxidant. Whey also contains a number of antibodies which might also impact human immunity.

The Different Types of Whey Protein

Three general categories of whey protein are usually recognized in supplements. Each type differs in the concentration of whey proteins that it contains. The three categories are *whey protein powder*, *whey protein concentrate* and *whey protein isolate*. Of these, whey protein isolate is the most concentrated form, with over 90% whey protein. The isolate form also tends to contain less lactose, making it an attractive option for those who are lactose intolerant. Whey protein concentrate on the other hand, can contain anywhere from 30% to 89% protein.[815] A third type, *whey protein powder*, tends to contain the least whey protein.

By simply looking at the amount of protein, one might conclude that whey protein isolate is the better choice. Maybe, maybe not. As was mentioned previously, whey contains compounds other than protein which might be beneficial to humans. It's theoretically possible that the filtering process that concentrates whey protein may inadvertently leave out whey's other important parts.

Whey Protein and Exercise

There is little doubt that the vast majority of people who use whey protein supplements are those who exercise regularly. Because of this fact, whey is a prominent figure in many protein supplements. Whey is a well-absorbed, highly usable source of protein. In addition, research also notes that whey can indeed improve muscle mass and strength when combined with a healthy diet and strength training program.[818] Marathoners, cyclists and other endurance athletes may also gravitate to whey because it is rich in the branch chain amino acids (valine, leucine and isoleucine) that might play a role in delaying fatigue during exercise and reduce muscle breakdown. Whey might also improve the body's ability to make glycogen, the storage form of carbohydrate that is used during exercise.[819]

The big question that everybody usually asks is how much protein do people really need? To answer this question, let's start with the recommended dietary allowance (RDA) for protein which is 0.8 grams per kilogram of body weight. Based on the RDA, a 91 kg (200 lb.) male should get about 73 grams of protein a day. While the RDA was designed to meet the needs of the majority of adults, some experts feel that it may be inadequate for athletes and those who exercise regularly and intensely. The question now becomes how much protein do athletes and regular exercisers need? Unfortunately, if you ask ten people, you might get ten different answers, a testament to the controversial nature of this issue. The good news, however, is that many of these recommendations are rather similar, advocating levels just a little above the RDA, generally between 1.2 to 1.5 gram per kilogram of body weight. Thus, for a 91 kilogram (200 lb.) man eating 1.4 grams of protein grams per kilogram of body weight, this equals about 127 grams. If the person is eating 5 meals a day, this comes to about 25 grams of protein per meal.

Experts usually put a cap of about 2 grams per kilogram of body weight as the uppermost amount of protein that should be consumed by humans. This is mostly for potential safety reasons and to reduce the exclusion of other healthy foods from the diet. Beyond this, it is also worth mentioning that high protein diets can interfere with exercise performance. During exercise, the body prefers to use carbohydrate and fat with protein providing far less of our energy needs. Because of this, athletes consuming high protein diets and not enough carbohydrates (and fat) may find themselves running out of steam faster when they workout. This might be especially a problem for those involved with aerobic exercise like running, cycling etc.

What About Protein Supplements?

It is generally agreed upon that for most healthy people, getting enough protein from the food they eat shouldn't be a problem. Even so, many people may find it easier to add a protein bar or protein shake to their diet as added insurance to help make up for what they think they may be missing. While there is nothing wrong with this, like all supplements, protein bars, shakes and other products are designed to *supplement* the diet and not take the place of food. Research on whey protein-based supplements have shown them to improve at least some aspects of exercise performance.[850] Whether whey protein is superior to more traditional forms of protein, like turkey or chicken is unknown at this point. The big advantage for protein supplements however is their convenience. While this can be an asset to people with busy schedules, quality-made protein supplements like those derived from whey may also help defend against muscle loss in those who have difficulty eating, like seniors.

People walking into any supermarket or health food store soon notice that a wide assortment of protein bars, protein powders and ready-to-drink protein shakes are available to choose from. Many of these products differ in not only in their protein content but also in calories, fat and other areas. Consumers should do their homework when deciding which protein supplement might be right for them and their specific needs. The following tables provide a comparison of several commercially available protein supplements. For an expanded and updated list of over 100 protein supplements, get the downloadable e-book *Protein Supplements: How They Compare*, available at wwww.Joe-Cannon.com

Ready-To-Drink Protein Shakes

Product	Calories	Protein (g)	Total Fat (g)	Total Carbs (g)	Sugars (g)
ABB Pure RTD Pro Shake Cookies & Cream. (1can=11 oz)	170	35	1	5	2
GNC Pro Performance® Protein 95, Chocolate. (1 can=11 oz)	140	25	1	7	3
EAS Myoplex Carb Sense Rich Dark Chocolate. (1carton= 11oz)	140	25	4	5	<1
MET-Rx® RTD 40™ Chocolate (1 can=15 oz).	240	40	3	16	3

Protein Powders

Product	Calories	Protein (g)	Total Fat (g)	Total Carbs (g)	Sugars (g)
Atkins Advantage, Chocolate (2 scoops = 34 g)	140	15	4	10	2
Body Tech™ Whey Tech Strawberry Flavor (1 scoop = 24 g)	100	17	1.5	3	3
Designer Whey, Optibol™, Milk Chocolate (2 scoops = 70 g)	300	37	9	17	4
EAS™ Myoplex Original Chocolate Peanut Butter (1 pack=78 g)	280	42	3.5	22	2

Protein Bars

Product	Calories	Protein (g)	Total Fat (g)	Total Carbs (g)	Sugars (g)
Balance® Cookie Dough (1 bar=50g)	200	15	6	22	18
EAS Myoplex Deluxe®. Chocolate Fudge (1bar=90g)	340	24	8	45	28
MET-Rx® Big 100 Chocolate Chip Cookie Dough (1bar=100g)	360	27	5	51	26
PowerBar® Protein Plus™ Vanilla Yogurt (1bar=78g)	290	24	5	37	19

How to Calculate YOUR Protein Needs

Let's readdress the example mentioned previously to illustrate how you can estimate your protein needs. There are 2.2 pounds in 1 kilogram. So the 200 lb. person mentioned above is 91 kg (200 ÷ 2.2 = 91 kg). Suppose this person wants to eat 1.4 grams of protein per kilogram of his body weight. This equals 91 kg X 1.4 = 127 grams per day. For many healthy people who don't exercise, the RDA of 0.8 grams per kilogram of body weight is probably appropriate. Exercisers should generally refrain from using more than about 2 grams of protein per kilogram of body weight because of possible ill effects and to prevent protein from overshadowing other valuable nutrients from the diet.

Whey Protein and Weight Loss

Some evidence suggests that whey protein or a component of whey may be of help to some people who are trying to lose weight. For example, animal research suggests that a diet rich in whey protein concentrate appears to reduce body weight more than a diet that consists mostly of red meat.[817] Whey does contain low levels of conjugated linoleic acid (CLA), a supplement reviewed previously in this book, which might promote fat loss. Whey, like protein in general, might also temporarily raise metabolism. For the moment, though, the reasons behind whey's apparent effect on weight loss are open to speculation and based mostly on animal studies.

<u>Whey Protein and Chronic Disease</u>

Some of the most interesting whey protein investigations relate to how it might help people with debilitating disease. For example, some scientists are investigating whether whey may be of value to those with cancer. Emerging research, in both animals and humans suggests that whey protein—or one or more of its constituent ingredients—may be effective at shrinking some types of tumors.[816,844] The reasons underlining this effect are still being investigated, but some speculate it may be in part tied to whey's ability to increase *glutathione*, one of the body's natural antioxidants. While questions such as the types and stages of cancer that might be most impacted by whey protein still need to be better investigated, some research has noted that several months of whey protein concentrate used at a level of 30 grams a day may hold promise for some.[816]

Another intriguing area of whey protein research has focused on whether it might benefit people infected with the HIV virus. One of the hallmarks of HIV/AIDS is weight and muscle loss, a condition that ultimately robs people of their strength and quality of life. Some research hints that whey protein concentrate may be effective at increasing body weight in those with HIV.[815] The reasons behind whey's effect on HIV-related weight loss require more study but, like cancer mentioned previously, may be linked to elevations in glutathione, which have been observed to increase in those with HIV, following whey supplementation.[815] Investigations noting improvements in body weight among people infected with HIV have used between 8 grams and 80 grams of whey protein concentrate a day.[815]

The Case for Casein

Casein is another milk protein and accounts for about 80% of the total protein found in milk. When consumed, casein tends to be absorbed slower than whey, providing an extended time release of amino acids into the body. While more research is needed, this characteristic might make casein superior to whey at stimulating muscle growth over a longer period of time. In fact, some protein supplements may contain a combination of whey and casein for this very reason. Casein, like whey protein, may have uses that go beyond helping build muscle, with some research hinting that it might aid immunity and blood pressure.[845] People who are allergic to dairy might have a problem using casein because of allergic reactions.

Side Effects and Concerns

Whey protein is generally considered safe, with no confirmed drug or supplement interactions. Because whey is derived from milk, those with lactose intolerance might want to avoid whey or choose a product that is lactose free.

High protein diets can promote dehydration which can interfere with the ability to exercise, especially when protein is used at the expense of other healthy foods like complex carbohydrates.

My Thoughts

There is no doubt that whey is a good, well-absorbed form of protein and can help fortify the body's need for raw materials as it makes new muscle tissue. Because it is derived from milk, whey is expected to be as good as protein-containing food. While there isn't much proof that whey is superior to food at building muscle, one advantage of whey is in its convenience for those on the run and others who want to add a protein-dense supplement to their already healthy diet. Whey protein powders might also benefit seniors and others with special needs who may have difficultly chewing. Indeed, those with special needs like cancer and older adults represent a very interesting and ongoing facet of whey protein research.

Whole Food Supplements

"Let medicine be your food and food be your medicine." These words, spoken by the Greek physician, Hippocrates, 400 years before Jesus walked the earth, essentially sums up the philosophy of those who advocate eating food as the best way of getting nutrients into the body. The foundation for this viewpoint is that individual nutrients like beta carotene and vitamin C, for example, tend to work in cooperation with other compounds to provide their beneficial effects. Because not everybody eats a healthy, well-balanced diet, supplement companies started designing a number of nutritional products that are essentially food extracts in capsule, liquid or powdered form. In essence, entire whole foods are ground up, and mixed together with other pulverized foods. Most, if not all, of the water and fiber is usually removed. The idea behind using these food extracts is that they would better mimic the beneficial effects of eating the foods themselves.

Many whole food supplements are based on the extracts of fruits and vegetables because studies tend to find that people who eat these foods are healthier and get fewer diseases. Other supplements may contain additional ingredients like green tea in the hopes of providing additional benefits. Still other variations of whole food supplements may contain more exotic extracts from plants that live under the sea or in remote areas of the world.

The term *whole food supplement* is generic and can refer to a number of proprietary products that are derived from food. Whole food supplements can usually be identified because they may use the term "whole food" in their advertisements and product labels. Ads for such products also tend to tout the benefits of food over individual vitamins, minerals and other supplements.

Why People Use Whole Food Supplements

Because of the evidence linking vegetable and fruit consumption to improved general health and reduced disease risk, some people use whole food supplements in the hopes that these, too, might elicit similar benefits. For the moment, the jury is out as to whether or not these supplements can prevent or reduce the risk of disease in a manner similar to eating fruits and vegetables themselves. This is because many supplements of this type lack rigorous scientific evidence. One product that does have evidence, however, is a supplement called *Juice Plus +®*. Juice Plus + consists of the extracts of 17 different fruits, vegetables and grains in capsule form. Studies conducted on Juice Plus + and published in peer-reviewed clinical journals suggest that it may help lower cholesterol and homocysteine levels, improve the concentration of a number of antioxidants, protect the integrity of genetic material and help reduce the closing of blood vessels that might occur after eating foods that are high in fat.[820,821,822] In theory, these findings might translate into improved long-term general health but for the moment, more research is needed before this can be said with certainty.

Whole Food Supplements and Exercise

The contribution of whole food supplements to exercise ability has not been widely studied. That being said, by adding to the total amount of fruits and vegetables consumed, a quality whole food supplement might potentially be of value to athletes. For example, professional bodybuilders routinely taper off carbohydrates as they get close to a competition. The reason for this is that carbohydrates promote water retention. This can interfere with the lean, muscular appearance that the bodybuilder is trying to convey to the judges of the contest. While staying away from carbs may help their chances of winning a trophy, from a nutrition standpoint, this practice is not healthy and robs the athlete of precious nutrients. For these individuals, a quality whole food supplement might be something to consider.

At the opposite end of the athletic spectrum are marathon runners, cyclists and triathletes. Studies show that these individuals tend to have an increased risk of infections several days following a race. By helping fortify the immune system, a quality whole food supplement may, in theory help reduce this risk. Indeed, while exercise research is currently lacking, some preliminary evidence does suggest that food extracts may be able to protect various immune cells.[822]

Are Whole Food Supplements a Substitute for Food?

Absolutely not. All supplements, whether they be vitamins, minerals, herbs or even those based on foods, are designed to *supplement* the diet and are not meant to replace eating food. While whole food supplements may provide a variety of fruit and vegetable extracts, as a rule, they lack the fiber and water that you'd get if you eat the food itself.

Side Effects and Concerns

Whole food supplements derived from commonly consumed foods are generally considered safe for healthy adults with no known significant side effects or drug interactions.

In theory, the vitamin K content of some whole food supplements might reduce the effectiveness of blood thinner medications. This caveat may also hold true for supplements that are derived from seaweed or other sea dwelling plants.

Grapefruit is known to interact with a wide array of drugs. Persons with health conditions should exercise caution when using whole food supplements that contain grapefruit.

My Thoughts

Studies suggest that the old adage of eating an apple a day to keep the doctor away may hold true for more than just apples, with the regular consumption of a number of fruits and vegetables also being linked to health maintenance and reduction of disease risk. So, in theory, properly manufactured, quality, whole food supplements might also hold promise. The research conducted so far is very intriguing in that it suggests that extracts of fruits and vegetables (phytonutrients) may help support some aspects of long-term health. Thus, for those who don't eat the often recommended "wide variety of fruits and vegetables", or who wish to add to their already healthy diet, such supplements might be something to consider. That being said, while I personally do like this concept, I must stress again that food is always your best choice and we are still a long way off before anyone utters the proverb "An apple *supplement* a day keeps the doctor away."

Yohimbe

Yohimbe comes from the bark of the yohimbe tree, an evergreen tree that grows in Africa. Because it is found in nature, yohimbe is currently classified as an herbal supplement. The active ingredient in yohimbe is believed to be a chemical called *yohimbine*. Thus yohimbe and yohimbine are sometimes used interchangeably but it should be remembered that they are not the same. One of the main reasons men use yohimbe is to improve sexual performance, although the herb may be used for other reasons as well. Other names that also refer to yohimbe include *Pausinystalia yohimbe*, *Corynanthe yohimbi*, *johimbi*, *herbal Viagra* and *yohimbe alkaloids*.

Yohimbe and Erectile Dysfunction

Erectile dysfunction (ED), more commonly called *impotence*, is defined as an inability to produce or sustain an erection strong enough to facilitate sexual intercourse. According to the American Urological Association, ED is thought to affect about 25 million Americans. A number of conditions are known to raise the risk of ED including being older, having diabetes, high blood pressure or heart disease as well as having either too low or too high levels of the male hormone, testosterone. Some medications may also lead to ED as well.

As was mentioned previously, the main active ingredient in yohimbe is believed to be a compound called yohimbine. It is through the actions of yohimbine that yohimbe is thought to work. Yohimbine is also a drug used sometimes to treat men experiencing mild impotence. Yohimbine appears to produce erections by both increasing blood flow to the penis and restricting its exit from the genital area. Yohimbine also appears to alter the levels of various chemicals in the brain which might also help explain its effects.

For centuries, yohimbe bark (sometimes called *Corynanthe yohimbe* or *Pausinystalia yohimbe*) has been used as a general aphrodisiac and to help men who have trouble in the bedroom. Unlike some legends of yore, there does appear to be something to this. Studies conducted on yohimbe extracts for the treatment of ED sometimes show that it works better than using nothing at all.[823] While this may be good news to some, on the downside, yohimbe may not work for everybody. This is because ED may be caused by a number of conditions, all of which may not respond to yohimbe supplements.[823]

Yohimbe is often found in a number of aphrodisiac and male-performance-enhancing products alongside other natural supplements like arginine, pycnogenol and ginseng in the hopes of amplifying its effect. While in theory, various combinations of products might act in synergy, more study is needed on this issue. Based on the research to date, the following points should be considered by those thinking about experimenting with yohimbe supplements for erectile dysfunction:

1. It's important that yohimbe supplements be derived from the bark of the yohimbe tree because this is where yohimbine is found.

2. Yohimbe and yohimbine are not the same thing. Yohimbe bark contains only small amounts of yohimbine. Some estimate that yohimbe bark contains less than 5% yohimbine. For this

reason, yohimbe supplements are usually standardized according to the amount of yohimbine they contain. Supplements should state on their label the percentage of yohimbine contained in the product. This percentage may also be translated into milligrams to make it easier for people to understand.

3. Studies investigating yohimbe for the treatment of ED have noted beneficial effects at dosages of between 5-30 mg a day.[10,399] To reduce the potential of side effects, it may be wise to start at the low end of this range (or less) and see if this works before increasing the amount. The higher the amount used, the greater the risk of unwanted and possibly harmful side effects.

4. Yohimbe may not work immediately for everybody. While some people may notice a difference after an hour or so, in others it may take a few weeks before effects occur. In still others, yohimbe may not work at all.

5. Yohimbe is mostly studied in men. How the herb affects women is less understood.

6. Yohimbe cannot increase the size of a man's penis beyond its natural potential. Any claims to this effect are not to be believed.

Other Supplements Reputed to Improve Sexual Prowess	
• Pycnogenol	• Arginine
• Tribulus Terrestris	• DHEA
• Ginkgo	• Panax Ginseng
• Epimedium	• Glandulars

Yohimbe and Exercise

Yohimbe may sometimes be found in muscle-building supplements. The idea behind this is the thought that the herb might boost testosterone levels. However, there is little evidence to support this.

Yohimbe may also be found in some energy drinks marketed to fitness enthusiasts. Whether or not yohimbe makes a difference in this regard needs more study. If yohimbe is present, it's probable that the amount is small in order to avoid side effects. A quick way to gauge how much yohimbe is in a product is to look at the ingredients list. In the US, ingredients at the end of the list are less plentiful than those at the beginning. Regardless of where yohimbe is listed, it has not been rigorously tested to determine if it significantly improves exercise performance in humans.

Yohimbe and Weight Loss

Only a few quality studies have looked at how yohimbe might impact weight loss. Those that have been conducted tend to have conflicting results.[425] Thus, this area of yohimbe research requires more study. If yohimbe aids weight loss, it most assuredly works best when combined with a reduced-calorie, healthy diet. Because of the conflicting results and because people who are overweight may have other medical issues like high blood pressure or diabetes, yohimbe is not generally recommended for weight loss.

Yohimbe and Depression

Some antidepressant medications work by blocking the action of a brain enzyme called *monoamine oxidase* (MAO).

It's possible that yohimbine may also do this.[10,339] However, research on its effectiveness and safety are lacking. Because of issues such as the quality of yohimbe products as well as side effects and lack of information on how yohimbe interacts with other supplements and medications, this herb should not be used for the self-treatment of depression. See the *Side Effects and Concerns* section for additional information on yohimbe and depression.

Side Effects and Concerns

In healthy adults, when used in low amounts for short periods of time, yohimbe is usually found to be safe. Yohimbe does carry, however some potentially serious complications which may be amplified when used at high doses or when mixed with medications or other supplements. As such, all persons considering using this herb should see their physician first. Side effects that can occur following the use of yohimbe can include sleeplessness, anxiety, heightened blood pressure, flushed skin, vomiting and rapid heart rate.[10,339]

Because yohimbe is a stimulant, it may have an additive effect if combined with other stimulants such as caffeine, ephedra, bitter orange or guarana. This synergistic effect may cause blood pressure to rise too much.[10] Yohimbe should be used with caution by people with blood pressure problems, heart disease, diabetes or kidney disorders.[10] People with liver problems may have difficultly metabolizing yohimbe. This could cause yohimbe to build up to toxic levels.[10]

Yohimbe may alter the levels of various brain chemicals (neurotransmitters) such as monoamine oxidase (MAO) which plays a role in mood and behavior. As such, yohimbe is not appropriate for those who are depressed or using antidepressants like MAO inhibitors, tricyclics or SSRIs. Yohimbe may also exacerbate symptoms of schizophrenia and other psychiatric disorders.[10]

People using antidepressants like MAO inhibitors must avoid certain foods, like aged cheeses and red wine, because they contain an amino acid called *tyramine* which plays a role in blood pressure regulation. Eating tyramine-containing foods while using MAO inhibitors can cause large and dangerous spikes in blood pressure. Because yohimbe may alter MAO activity, those using this supplement should likewise avoid foods that contain tyramine, to be on the safe side.

Little is known about how yohimbe interacts with supplements like St. Johns wort, 5-HTP and others that are also sometimes used for the self-treatment of depression.

Until more is known, yohimbe should be avoided by men with a history of begin prostatic hyperplasia (BPH), as it may promote prostate growth.[30]

Previous investigations by the FDA have found that some "male performance" supplements may in fact be adulterated with prescription drugs like Viagra that are used medically to treat erectile dysfunction.[824,825] These products are illegal and are usually removed from the US market when the FDA is made aware of them.

My Thoughts

Long before there was Viagra, there was yohimbe. Many studies have been performed on yohimbe with some of them hinting that this herb may indeed be of some benefit to men suffering with erection problems.

Less is known about how yohimbe affects other conditions, like depression. Yohimbe does not work as well prescription as drugs like Viagra and other medications of that ilk. For those who do not have ED, keep in mind that the best way to not get it is to reduce its risk factors. Steps that can be taken right now to lower your risk include: not smoking, not abusing alcohol, getting regular exercise, eating healthy and better managing the harmful stresses in your life. For those who suspect that they have ED and are thinking about experimenting with yohimbe, my advice is to see your physician first. Yohimbe side effects not withstanding, keep in mind that erectile dysfunction can be a symptom of a more serious condition, like heart disease. A simple trip to your doctor might save you a lot of pain and suffering down the road.

Zinc

If your body had to choose between gold and zinc, it would choose zinc in a New York minute! Zinc is the second most plentiful trace mineral in the body, taking part in hundreds of diverse and crucial chemical reactions—ranging from the healing of wounds, immune function, the sense of taste and smell, reproduction and the making of proteins to name a few. Some people supplement their diet with an enzyme called *superoxide dismutase* (SOD), an antioxidant made naturally in the body, to help mop up free radicals. To function properly, SOD requires zinc as well as another mineral, copper.[54] Thus, zinc can also help protect our cells from free radical attack. Signs of zinc deficiency can include hair loss, dry skin, vision problems, low sperm count, low testosterone levels, as well as slowed growth and development. The RDA for zinc is currently set at 11 mg a day for adult men and 8 mg a day for adult women. The upper limit past which side effects might start to occur is 40 mg a day. Zinc in supplements can be found in a number of different forms such as *zinc gluconate, zinc acetate, zinc citrate, zinc sulfate* and *zinc picolinate* to name a few. While known to be an essential nutrient since 1934, a recommended dietary allowance (RDA) for zinc was not published until 1974.[54]

Zinc and the Immune System

There is no doubt that zinc is crucial to the optimal functioning of the immune system. Deficiencies in zinc can negatively impact immunity in a number of ways such as by altering the infection-fighting ability of *T cells*, B cells and natural killer cells as well as other components of the immune system.[829] Based on this, some might be tempted to use high doses of zinc to help make their immune systems even stronger. Unfortunately, this doesn't work. In fact, zinc supplements have not only *not* been found to prevent infections but might actually weaken the immune system when used long-term.[829] This may result in more infections! For this reason, it is not recommended that healthy people use zinc supplements on a daily basis to strengthen their immune systems.

While the regular use of zinc has not been shown to help immunity over the long haul in healthy people, what about occasional use? In other words, might using zinc supplements help us when we are sick? Maybe. Some intriguing research has found that zinc, given at the start of a cold, may be effective at reducing the length of time that people experience cold symptoms.[826] This has resulted in several over-the-counter zinc lozenges and other similar products. For those who wish to try zinc to help battle colds, it's important to start using zinc within 24 hours of the start of cold symptoms and continue every few hours thereafter. On average, this strategy might reduce the duration of cold symptoms by about 2 or 4 days. Supplements designed for this purpose usually contain 13.3 mg zinc gluconate, although some investigations have also used zinc acetate. Both types of zinc have some research to validate their use.[826, 828]

How zinc helps battle colds is still under investigation but some think it works by interfering with the replication of cold viruses. In this way, zinc might help limit the spread of an infection and give the immune system more time to mount an effective attack.

It's important to note that not all research finds that zinc supplements help.[826,828] Thus, the use of zinc products is not a slam dunk for beating colds and results may indeed vary from person to person. This discrepancy in research findings could be due to several factors such as different amounts or types of zinc used in studies, or other issues relating to how the research was conducted.

Zinc and HIV Infection

Another controversial area involves persons infected with the HIV virus. Some studies find HIV-infected individuals have low levels of zinc.[826] This, and because of the role zinc plays in immunity, may tempt some with HIV to use zinc supplements. This may not be a good idea because the HIV virus also appears to need zinc.[826] There is some thought that zinc supplements might speed the progression of HIV infection.[826] Because of the seriousness of this possibility and the ever changing nature of information in this field, persons with HIV are highly encouraged to seek the counsel of their personal physician before using zinc or any other supplement.

Zinc and Exercise

Considering its popularity in some exercise circles, zinc receives little research on how it affects exercise ability. Nevertheless, professional athletes as well as those desiring better fitness in general may use zinc supplements because of a belief that this mineral can raise levels of the anabolic hormone, testosterone, which plays a role in strength development. Zinc does participate in the production of testosterone and some research also finds that deficiencies in this mineral may indeed lower the testosterone levels in men.[831] In theory, increasing zinc might boost testosterone in zinc-deficient individuals. For those already consuming adequate amounts of this mineral, zinc supplements might be less beneficial. Zinc is present in many foods as well as most multivitamins and other supplements people may be using.

Cyclists, triathletes and others interested in aerobic fitness may also be attracted to zinc supplements to boost performance. Carbonic anhydrase is an enzyme that helps carry carbon dioxide to the lungs where it is exhaled. This ability is crucial for the continuation of exercise. It turns out that zinc helps carbonic anhydrase work.[846] Thus, lack of dietary zinc could decrease the effectiveness of carbonic anhydrase which, in turn, might reduce aerobic exercise performance. Some research does in fact show that a zinc-deficient diet can decrease aerobic exercise capacity.[830] Whether extra zinc can help those who are not zinc-deficient needs more study.

Foods That Contain Zinc

Food	Serving	Zinc (mg)
Oysters	6 medium	43.4
Fortified Breakfast Cereal with 100% daily value of zinc	3/4 cup	15
Alaskan King Crab	3 oz	6.5
Beef	3 oz	5.8
Baked Beans	8 oz	3.54
Turkey (dark meat)	3 oz	3.5
Chicken (dark meat)	3 oz	2.4
Tofu	4 oz	1.7
Brown Rice	8 oz	1.1
Milk	8 oz	1
Tuna, water packed	3 oz	0.6

The research on the zinc-exercise connection, albeit limited, is interesting. That being said, there is not enough evidence at this point to support loading up on this mineral, especially in exercisers who may already be getting adequate amounts in their diet. At amounts greater than 150 mg a day, zinc might decrease sports performance by inducing fatigue and interfering with coordination.[846] Until more is known, athletes should examine their current zinc status first and then look to a good multivitamin and foods that contain zinc before opting for high-potency zinc supplements.

Zinc and Senior Citizens

It's possible that older individuals in general may be deficient in zinc because of a poor diet. Because zinc plays important roles in a number of areas needed for health, improving the intake of this mineral may be something to consider. Outside of a good quality multivitamin, though, there isn't enough evidence to warrant the use of zinc supplements for older people. High levels of zinc might lower good cholesterol levels (HDL) which can contribute to the progression of heart disease.[828] This might occur when as little as 50 mg of zinc are used on a regular basis.[846] Because older adults may already be experiencing heart disease, high potency-zinc supplements should be avoided by seniors unless prescribed by a physician.

Side Effects and Concerns

Zinc is a relatively harmless trace mineral when consumed in amounts found in food and when used at the RDA which is 11 mg a day for adult men and 8 mg a day for adult women.[828] The upper limit for zinc intake is 40 mg a day for adult men and women.[828] This means that long-term intakes of zinc past 40 mg a day might increase the potential risk of negative side effects occurring. Side effects from consuming too much zinc can include abdominal pain, queasiness, vomiting and a metallic taste in the mouth. Other signs include fever and fatigue.

Zinc deficiency may affect the swimming ability of sperm. This might impact couples who are trying to have children. However, consuming too much zinc might interfere with sperm quality as well.

Strict vegetarians may be zinc deficient.[828] Zinc from non-meat sources tends be less well absorbed because of the presence of compounds called phytates. In addition, the high fiber diet that's characteristic of a vegetarian lifestyle may also hinder zinc absorption. Thus, vegetarians may want to consider a quality multivitamin that contains zinc and other valuable nutrients.

Zinc may interfere with the absorption of some antibiotics. This might decrease their effectiveness.[826]

Zinc can reduce the absorption of copper, iron and magnesium.[826] Copper, like zinc, is required for the functioning of the enzyme SOD, a natural antioxidant. Thus, in theory, consuming too much zinc from supplements, might diminish our ability to battle free radicals. Likewise, by interfering with iron absorption, zinc might lead to anemia.

Zinc, when used in excess of 50 mg per day, may reduce levels of good cholesterol (HDL).[828,846] Long-term, this might contribute to heart disease.

The prostate gland tends to contain high concentrations of zinc, suggesting that this mineral may play a role in prostate health. In spite of this, men with a history of prostate cancer, should see their physician before using zinc supplements. While controversial, some evidence suggests that 100 mg of zinc used long term (10 years) may increase prostate cancer risk.[827]

Zinc and Libido

Oysters are generally thought of as the quintessential aphrodisiac. This reputation probably stems from the very high levels of zinc that oysters contain. While zinc is needed for the production of testosterone and may improve the quality of sperm produced, there is little proof that oysters or zinc in general, can improve libido or sexual prowess, especially in people who are not zinc-deficient.

My Thoughts

No question about it, zinc is indispensable for all of us if we are going to maintain optimal health. That being said, for those who are already getting adequate zinc in their diet, there currently isn't enough evidence to recommend a daily high potency zinc supplement for most people. The RDA is low enough that healthy people should be able to obtain enough zinc easily through their diet, multivitamin and other supplements that they may already be using.

The Big Picture

It is likely that many people who are reading these words are taking supplements for a number of reasons and conditions. For the most part, this is perfectly fine and depending on the supplement used, may even have long-term health benefits. It is important however to keep in mind that any positive effects derived from the use of nutritional supplements will be magnified when they are combined with other, equally important aspects of a healthy lifestyle. This includes not smoking, getting regular exercise, limiting the bad stresses in your life and yes, eating a healthy, balanced diet that is low in bad fats and high in fruits, vegetables and whole grains. Failing to take these other steps significantly limits the effectiveness of all supplements. Supplements alone, like most things in life, are not a short cut to reaching your goals but rather can be thought of as the *bottom left-hand corner of the big picture*. I understand that many of these other steps to success may seem overwhelming to some. The good news is that you do not have to make the decision to do them all today. Remember, the journey of a thousand miles begins with the first step. For some, the decision to add a quality nutritional supplement to their daily life *is* that first step. If that in turn leads you to making other healthy choices in your life, then the decision was a wise one and you are indeed on the road to a longer, healthier, happier life—which in the end, is what's really important...

404

References

1. Office of Dietary Supplements web site. http://ods.od.nih.gov accessed December 21, 2003.
2. Adebowale AO et. al. (2000). Analysis of glucosamine and chondroitin sulfate content in marketed products and the caco-2 permeability of chondroitin sulfate raw materials. Journal of the American Nutraceutical Association, 3, 1, 37-44.
3. Garvan, C. et al. (2000). Drug-Grapefruit Juice Interactions. Mayo Clinic Proceedings, 75, 933-943.
4. Harkness, R. et al. (2000). Drug-Herb-Vitamin Interactions Bible. Prima Publishers.
5. Gauthier, G.M. et al. (2003). The association of homocysteine and coronary artery disease. Clinical Cardiology, 26,12, 563-568.
6. Temple, M.E. (2000). Homocysteine as a risk factor for atherosclerosis. Annals of Pharmocotherapy, 34,1, 57-65.
7. Stein, J.H. (1998). Hyperhomocysteinemia and atherosclerotic vascular disease: pathophysiology, screening, and treatment. Archives of Internal Medicine, 158,12, 1301-1306.
8. Racette, S.B. Creatine supplementation and athletic performance. Journal of Orthopedic and Sports Physical Therapy, 33,10, 615-621.
9. Hall, W.L et al. (2003). Physiological mechanisms mediating aspartame-induced satiety. Physiology & Behavior, 78, 4-5, 557-562.
10. Fetrow, CW & Avila, JR (2000). The Complete Guide to Herbal Medicines. Springhouse.
11. Consumer Reports on Health, April 2003. Page 10, Speeding the Heart for Weight Loss.
12. McGuffin M, Hobbs C, Upton R, Goldberg A, eds. (1998) American Herbal Products Association's Botanical Safety Handbook. Boca Raton, FL: CRC Press.
13. Penzak SR, et al. (2001). Seville (sour) orange juice: synephrine content and cardiovascular effects in normotensive adults. Journal of Clinical Pharmacology, 41, 10, 1059-1063.
14. Blumenthal M, (1998). The Complete German Commission E Monographs: Therapeutic Guide to Herbal Medicines. American Botanical Council.
15. Malhotra S, et al. (2001) Seville orange juice-felodipine interaction: comparison with dilute grapefruit juice and involvement of furocoumarins. Clinical Pharmacology and Therapeutics, 69,14-23.
16. Blumenthal M, et al. (2000). Herbal Medicine Expanded Commission E Monographs. Newton, MA: Integrative Medicine Communications.
17. Shekelle PG, et al. (2003). Efficacy and safety of ephedra and ephedrine for weight loss and athletic performance: a meta-analysis. JAMA, 289, 1537-45.
18. Review of Natural Products by Facts and Comparisons (1999). St. Louis, MO: Wolters Kluwer Co.
19. Jochimsen EM, et al. (2003). Liver failure and death after exposure to microcystins at a hemodialysis center in Brazil. New England Journal of Medicine, 338, 873–878.
20. Gilroy DJ, et al. (2000). Assessing potential health risks from microcystin toxins in blue-green algae dietary supplements. Environmental Health Perspectives, 108, 435–439.
21. Blue Green Algae. Health Canada Online (May 1999). www.hc-sc.gc.ca/ (accessed January 6 2004).

22. Becker EW, et al. (1986). Clinical and biochemical evaluations of the alga Spirulina with regard to its application in the treatment of obesity. A double-blind cross-over study. Nutrition Reports International, 33, 565–574.

23. FDA Consumer Alert. FDA Plans Regulation Prohibiting Sale of Ephedra-Containing Dietary Supplements and Advises Consumers to Stop Using These Products. P03106. December 30 2003. Food and Drug Administration homepage. http://www.fda.gov. (accessed January 15, 2004).

24. Boozer CN, et al. (2002). Herbal ephedra/caffeine for weight loss: a 6-month randomized safety and efficacy trial. International Journal of Obesity and Related Metabolic Disorders, 26, 593-604.

25. Massey LK. (2001) Is caffeine a risk factor for bone loss in the elderly? American Journal of Clinical Nutrition, 74, 569-70.

26. Lloyd T. et al. (2000). Bone status among postmenopausal women with different habitual caffeine intakes: a longitudinal investigation. Journal of the American College of Nutrition, 19, 256-261.

27. Schulz V, et al. (1998). Rational Phytotherapy: A Physician's Guide to Herbal Medicine. Berlin, GER: Springer.

28 CSPI Press Release, July 31, 1997. Label Caffeine Content of Foods, Scientists, Tell FDA. CSPI web site. www.cspinet.org (accessed February 1, 2004).

29. Guy G (2000). For Dieter, Nearly The Ultimate Loss. Washington Post March 19 p.A23.

30. Brinker F. (1998) Herb Contraindications and Drug Interactions. 2nd edt. Eclectic Medical Publications.

31. Maish WA (1996). Influence of grapefruit juice on caffeine pharmacokinetics and pharmacodynamics. Pharmacotherapy. 16, 6, 1046-1052.

32. American Physiological Society. Press release April 9 2003. American Physiological Society: ttp://www.the-aps.org/press/conference/eb03/5.htm (accessed February 1 2004).

33. Vandenberghe, K et al. (1996). Caffeine counteracts the ergogenic action of muscle creatine loading. Journal of Applied Physiology, 80, 2, 452-457.

34. Heaney, RP (2002). Calcium and Weight: Clinical Studies. Journal of the American College of Nutrition, 21, 2, 152S-155S.

35. Zhang QG et al. (2004). No Effect of Dietary Calcium on Body Weight of Lean and Obese Mice and Rats. American Journal of Physiology. Regulatory, Integrative and Comparative Physiology, 286,4, R669-R677.

36. Supplement Industry Trade Association Urges Crackdown on Coral Calcium Claims. Counsel for Responsible Nutrition.Press release May 16 2003. www.crnusa.org

37. Ishitani K, et al. (1999). Calcium absorption from the ingestion of coral-derived calcium by humans. Journal of Nutritional Science and Vitaminology, 45, 5, 509-517.

38. Bo-Linn GW et al. (1983). Starch blockers--their effect on calorie absorption from a high-starch meal. New England Journal of Medicine, 307, 23, 1413-1416.

39. Hollenbeck CB et al. (1983). Effects of a commercial starch blocker preparation on carbohydrate digestion and absorption: in vivo and in vitro studies. American Journal of Clinical Nutrition, 38,4, 498-503.

40. Umoren J. et al. (1992). Commercial soybean starch blocker consumption: impact on weight gain and on copper, lead and zinc status of rats. Plant Foods for Human Nutrition, 42, 2, 135-142.

41. Consumerlab.com. Product review: Calcium. Consumerlab.com (accessed February 2 2004).

42. Schmidt-Sommerfeld E et al. (1990). Carnitine and total parenteral nutrition of the neonate. Biology of the Neonate, 58, 1, 81-88.
43. Villani, RG et al. (2000). L carnitine supplementation combined with aerobic training does not promote weight loss in moderately obese women. International Journal of Sports Nutrition, 10, 199-207.
44. Brandsch C et al. (2002). Effect of L-carnitine on weight loss and body composition of rats fed a hypocaloric diet. Annals of Nutrition and Metabolism, 46,5, 205-210.
45. Hongu, N et al. (2000). Caffeine, Carnitine and Choline Supplementation of Rats Decreases Body Fat and Serum Leptin Concentration as Does Exercise. Journal of Nutrition, 130,1,152-157.
46. Jellin JM et al. (2003). Natural Medicines Comprehensive Database. Therapeutic Research Foundation.
47. Pittler MH, et al. (1999). Randomized, double-blind trial of chitosan for body weight reduction. European Journal of Clinical Nutrition, 53, 5, 379-81.
48. Ho, SC et al. (2001). In the absence of dietary surveillance, chitosan does not reduce plasma lipids or obesity in hypercholesterolemic obese Asian subjects. Singapore Medical Journal, 42,6-10.
49. Wuolijoki E et al. (1999). Decrease in serum LDL cholesterol with microcrystalline chitosan. Methods and Findings in Clinical and Experimental Pharmacology, 21,5,357-361.
50. Gades, MD (2002). Chitosan supplementation does not affect fat absorption in healthy males fed a high-fat diet, a pilot study. International Journal of Obesity and Related Metabolic Disorders, 26,1,119-122.
51. Barroso, AJ. et al. (2002). Efficacy of a novel chitosan formulation on fecal fat excretion: a double-blind, crossover, placebo-controlled study. Journal of Medicine, 33,1-4,209-225.
52. Tsujikawa T et al. (2003). Supplement of a chitosan and ascorbic acid mixture for Crohn's disease: a pilot study. Nutrition, 19,2,137-139.
53. Rizos, I (2000). Three-year survival of patients with heart failure caused by dilated cardiomyopathy and L-carnitine administration. American Heart Journal, 139, S 120-S123.
54. Groff, JL (1995). Advanced Nutrition and Human Metabolism, 2nd etd. West Publishing Company.
55. Williams, M. (1998). The Ergogenics Edge. Human Kinetics.
56. Trent, LK (1995). Effects of chromium picolinate on body composition. Journal of Sports Medicine and Physical Fitness, 35, 4,273-280.
57. Lawrence ME (2002). Nutrition and sports supplements: fact or fiction. Journal of Clinical Gastroenterology, 35,4, 299-306.
58. Vincent, JB (2003). The potential value and toxicity of chromium picolinate as a nutritional supplement, weight loss agent and muscle development agent. Sports Medicine, 3,3,213-230.
59. Campbell WW et al. (2002). Effects of resistive training and chromium picolinate on body composition and skeletal muscle size in older women. International Journal of Sport Nutrition and Exercise Metabolism, 12,2,125-135.
60. Wayne W et al. (1999). Effects of resistance training and chromium picolinate on body composition and skeletal muscle in older men. Journal of Applied Physiology, 86, 1, 29-39.
61. Hallmark MA et al. (1996). Effects of chromium and resistive training on muscle strength and body composition. Medicine and Science in Sports and Exercise, 28,1,139-144.
62. Livolsi JM et al. (2001). The effect of chromium picolinate on muscular strength and body composition in women athletes. Journal of Strength and Conditioning Research, 15,2,161-166.

63.   Anderson RA et al. (1997). Elevated intakes of supplemental chromium improve glucose and insulin variables in individuals with type 2 diabetes. Diabetes, 46,11,1786-1791.

64.   Grant KE et al. (1997). Chromium and exercise training: effect on obese women. Medicine and Science in Sports and Exercise, 29, 8, 992-998.

65.   Wasser WG, et al. (1997). Chronic renal failure after ingestion of over-the-counter chromium picolinate. [letter] Annals of Internal Medicine, 126,410.

66.   Stearns, DM et al. (1995), Chromium(III) picolinate produces chromosome damage in Chinese hamster ovary cells. FASEB Journal,9,15,1643-8.

67.   Stearns, D.M. (2002). Chromium(III) tris (picolinate) is mutagenic at the hypoxanthine (guanine) phosphoribosyltransferase locus in Chinese hamster ovary cells. Mutagenic Research, 15, 513(1-2):135-142.

68.   Speetjens JK et al. (1999). The nutritional supplement chromium(III) tris(picolinate) cleaves DNA. Chemical Research in Toxicology, 12, 6, 483-487.

69.   Hepburn DD et al. (2003). Nutritional supplement chromium picolinate causes sterility and lethal mutations in Drosophila melanogaster. Proceedings of The National Academy of Sciences of the United States of America,100,7,3766-3771.

70.   Vincent JB (2000). The biochemistry of chromium. Journal of Nutrition 130,4, 715-718.

71.   O'Brien TJ et al. (2003). Complexities of chromium carcinogenesis: role of cellular response, repair and recovery mechanisms. Mutation Research,10, 533,1-2,3-36.

72.   Reading SA (1996). Chromium picolinate. Journal of the Florida Medical Association,83,1,29-31.

73.   McLeod MN et al. (1999). Chromium potentiation of antidepressant pharmacotherapy for dysthymic disorder in 5 patients. Journal of Clinical Psychiatry, 60,4,237-240.

74.   Althuis MD et al. (2002). Glucose and insulin responses to dietary chromium supplements: a meta-analysis. American Journal of Clinical Nutrition, 76,1,148-155.

75.   Crawford V et al. (1999). Effects of niacin-bound chromium supplementation on body composition in overweight African-American women. Diabetes, Obesity and Metabolism, 1, 6, 331-337.

76.   Product Review: Weight Loss, Slimming and Diabetes Management Supplements (Chromium, CLA and Pyruvate. Consumerlab.com (accessed 2/10/04).

77.   Noone EJ et al. (2002). The effect of dietary supplementation using isomeric blends of conjugated linoleic acid on lipid metabolism in healthy human subjects. British Journal of Nutrition, 88,3,243-251.

78.   Blankson H et al. (2001). Stakkestad JA, Fagertun H, et al. Conjugated linoleic acid reduces body fat mass in overweight and obese humans. Journal of Nutrition, 130, 2943-2950.

79.   Benito P et al. (2001). The effect of conjugated linoleic acid on plasma lipoproteins and tissue fatty acid composition in humans. Lipids, 36,8, 229-236.

80.   Larsen TM (2003). Efficacy and safety of dietary supplements containing CLA for the treatment of obesity: evidence from animal and human studies. Journal of Lipid Research, 44, 12, 2234-2241.

81.   Kreider RB et al. (2003). Effects of conjugated linoleic acid supplementation during resistance training on body composition, bone density, strength, and selected hematological markers. Journal of Strength and Conditioning Research, 16, 3, 325-334.

408

82. Smedman A et al. (2001). Conjugated linoleic acid supplementation in humans:metabolic effects. Lipids, 36,8,773-781.
83. Thom E et al. (2001). Conjugated linoleic acid reduces body fat in healthy exercising humans. The Journal of International Medical Research, 29,5, 392-396.
84. Zambell KL et al. (2000). Conjugated linoleic acid supplementation in humans: effects on body composition and energy expenditure. Lipids, 35,7,777-782.
85. Johnson, LW. (2001). Conjugated linoleic acids for body fat mass reduction. Integrative Medicine Consult, 3,3,17-21.
86. Riserus U et al. (2002) Treatment with dietary trans10cis12 conjugated linoleic acid causes isomer-specific insulin resistance in obese men with the metabolic syndrome. Diabetes Care, 25,1516-1521.
87. Belury, M (2002). Not all trans-fatty acids are alike: What consumers may lose when we oversimplify nutrition facts. Journal of the American Dietetic Association,102,11,1606-1607.
88. Baulieu, E. (1996). Dehydroepiandrosterone (DHEA): A fountain of youth? Journal of Clinical Endocrinology and Metabolism, 81,9, 3147-3151.
89. Cleary, M.P. (1990). The role of DHEA in obesity. In M. Kalimi and W. Regelson (Ed.), The Biologic Role of Dehydroepiandrosterone (DHEA). 207-230). Walter de Gruyter & Co., Berlin.
90. Maccario M et al. (1999). Relationships between dehydroepiandrosterone-sulphate and anthropometric, metabolic and hormonal variables in a large cohort of obese women. Clinical Endocrinology,50,5,595-600.
91. Mazza E et al. (1999). Dehydroepiandrosterone sulfate levels in women. Relationships with age, body mass index and insulin levels. Journal of Endocrinological Investigation,22,9, 681-687.
92. Saruc M et al. (2003). The association of dehydroepiandrosterone, obesity, waist-hip ratio and insulin resistance with fatty liver in postmenopausal women--a hyperinsulinemic euglycemic insulin clamp study. Hepato-Gastroenterology, 50,51,771-774.
93. Clore, J. N. (1995). Dehydroepiandrosterone and body fat. Obesity Research, 3, 4, 613s-616s.
94. Morales, AJ et al. (1994). Effects of replacement dehydroepiandrosterone in men women of advancing age. Journal of Clinical Endocrinology and Metabolism, 78,6,1360-1367.
95. Kline MD et al. (1999). Mania onset while using dehydroepiandrosterone (letter). American Journal of Psychiatry,156:971.
96. Dean CE (2000). Prasterone (DHEA) and mania. Annals of Pharmacotherapy,34, 12, 1419-1422.
97. Markowitz JS, et al. (1999). Possible dihydroepiandrosterone-induced mania. Biological Psychiatry, 45,2,241-242.
98. Frye RF, et al. (2000). Effect of DHEA on CYP3A-mediated metabolism of triazolam. Clinical Pharmacology and Therapeutics, 67,109 (abstract PI-82).
99. Skolnick AA. (1996).Scientific verdict still out on DHEA. Journal of the American Medical Association, 276,1365-1367.
100. Ng MK et al. (2003). Dehydroepiandrosterone, an adrenal androgen, increases human foam cell formation: a potentially pro-atherogenic effect. Journal of the American College of Cardiology,42,11, 1967-1974.
101. McCrohon JA et al. (1999). Androgen exposure increases human monocyte adhesion to vascular endothelium and endothelial cell expression of vascular cell adhesion molecule-1, Circulation, 99,17,2317-2322.

102. Remer, T et al. (1998). Short-Term Impact of a Lactovegetarian diet on adrenocortical activity and adrenal androgens. The Journal of Clinical Endocrinology & Metabolism,83,6, 2132-2137.

103. Williams, M. (1998). The Ergogenics Edge. Human Kinetics.

104. Rapuri, PB et al. (2001). Caffeine intake increases the rate of bone loss in elderly women and interacts with vitamin D receptor genotypes. American Journal of Clinical Nutrition, 74,5, 694-700.

105. Heller HJ, et al. (2000). Pharmacokinetic and pharmacodynamic comparison of two calcium supplements in postmenopausal women. Journal of Clinical Pharmacology, 40, 1237-1244.

106. Rizos I. Three-year survival of patients with heart failure caused by dilated cardiomyopathy and L-carnitine administration. American Heart Journal, 139, S120-S123.

107. Schofield RS (2001). Role of metabolically active drugs in the management of ischemic heart disease. American Journal of Cardiovascular Drugs, 1,1,23-35.

108. Hurot JM et al. (2002). Effects of L-carnitine supplementation in maintenance hemodialysis patients: a systematic review. Journal of the American Society of Nephrology, 13,708-714.

109. Vicari E, et al. (2002). Antioxidant treatment with carnitines is effective in infertile patients with prostatovesiculoepididymitis and elevated seminal leukocyte concentrations after treatment with nonsteroidal anti-inflammatory compounds. Fertility and Sterility, 78,1203-1208.

110. Barker, GA et al. (2001). Effect of propionyl-L-carnitine on exercise performance in peripheral arterial disease. Medicine and Science in Sport and Exercise, 33,9, 1415-1422.

111. Vecchiet L et al. (1990). Influence of L-carnitine administration on maximal physical exercise. European Journal of Applied Physiology, 61,486-490.

112 Marconi C et al. (1985). Effects of L-carnitine loading on the aerobic and anaerobic performance of endurance athletes. European Journal of Applied Physiology, 54,131-135.

113. Colombani P et al. (1996). Effects of L-carnitine supplementation on physical performance and energy metabolism of endurance-trained athletes" a double-blind crossover field study. European Journal of Applied Physiology 73,434-439.

114. Van Oudheusden LJ et al. (2002). Efficacy of carnitine in the treatment of children with attention-deficit hyperactivitydisorder. Prostaglandins, Leukotrienes and Essential Fatty Acids, 67,1,33-38.

115. Krahenbuhl S et al. (1997). Carnitine metabolism in chronic liver disease. Life Sciences, 59,19,1579-1599.

116. Thal LJ et al. (1996). A 1-year multicenter placebo-controlled study of acetyl-L-carnitine in patients with Alzheimer's disease. Neurology, 47,705–711.

117. Thal LJ, Calvani M, Amato A, et al. (2000). A 1-year controlled trial of acetyl-l-carnitine in early-onset AD. Neurology, 55, 805–810.

118. Benvenga S et al. (2000). Carnitine is a naturally occurring inhibitor of thyroid hormone nuclear uptake. Thyroid, 10, 1043–1050.

119. Bokura H et al. (2003). Chitosan decreases total cholesterol in women: a randomized, double-blind, placebo-controlled trial. European Journal of Clinical Nutrition, 57, 721-725.

120. Ho SC et al. (2001). In the absence of dietary surveillance, chitosan does not reduce plasma lipids or obesity in hypercholesterolemic obese Asian subjects. Singapore Medical Journal, 42, 6–10.

121. Yang CY et al. (2002). Effects of habitual chitosan intake on bone mass, bone-related metabolic markers and duodenum CaBP D9K mRNA in

410

ovariectomized SHRSP rats. Journal of Nutritional Science and Vitaminology, 48,5,371/378.

122.   Deuchi K (1995). Continuous and massive intake of chitosan affects mineral and fat-soluble vitamin status in rats fed on a high-fat diet. Bioscience, Biotechnology, and Biochemistry, 59,7,1211-1216.

123.   Caraccio, TR. (2002). Chronic arsenic (As) toxicity from Chitosan® supplement [Abstract]. Clinical Toxicology, 644.

124.   Institute of Medicine. Dietary Reference Intakes for Vitamin A, Vitamin K, Arsenic, Boron, Chromium, Copper, Iodine, Iron, Manganese, Molybdenum, Nickel, Silicon, Vanadium, and Zinc. Washington DC: National Academy of Sciences; 2001.

125.   Percheron G, et al. (2003). Effect of 1-year oral administration of dehydroepiandrosterone to 60- to 80-year-old individuals on muscle function and cross-sectional area: a double-blind placebo-controlled trial. Archives of Internal Medicine, 163, 720-727.

126.   Brown GA et al. (1999). Effect of oral DHEA on serum testosterone and adaptations to resistance training in young men. Journal of Applied Physiology, 87,6,2274-2283.

127.   Allolio, B. Arlt, W. (2002). DHEA treatment : myth or reality? Trends in Endocrinology & Metabolism, 13, 7, 288-295.

128.   Kuritzky L. (1998). DHEA: Science or Wishful Thinking? Hospital Practice,33,85-86.

129.   Meston CM et al. (2002). Acute dehydroepiandrosterone effects on sexual arousal in premenopausal women. Journal of Sex & Marital Therapy, 28,53-60.

130.   Hackbert L et al. (2002). Acute dehydroepiandrosterone (DHEA) effects on sexual arousal in postmenopausal women. Journal of Women's Health & Gender-Based Medicine, 11,155-162.

131.   Reiter WJ et al. (2001) Dehydroepiandrosterone in the treatment of erectile dysfunction in patients with different organic etiologies. Urological Research, 29,278-281.

132.   Baulieu EE et al. (2002). Dehydroepiandrosterone (DHEA), DHEA sulfate, and aging:contribution of the DHEAge Study to a sociobiomedical issue. Proceedings of the National Academy of Sciences, 97,8,4279-4284.

133.   Shekelle PG et al. (2003).Efficacy and safety of ephedra and ephedrine for weight loss and athletic performance: a meta-analysis. JAMA, 289,1537-1545.

134.   Shekelle PG et al. (2003). Ephedra and ephedrine: Modest short-term weight loss, with a price. The Journal of Family Practice, 52,7.

135.   Shekelle, PG et al. (2003). Evidence Report/Technology Assessment Number 76. Ephedra and Ephedrine for Weight Loss and Athletic Performance Enhancement: Clinical Efficacy and Side Effects. AHRQ Publication No. 03-E022. www.ahrq.gov.

136.   Bent, S et al. (2003). The relative safety of ephedra compared with other herbal products. Annals of Internal Medicine, 138,6,468-471.

137.   The Natural Pharmacist.

138.   Gurley BJ et al. (2000).Content versus label claims in ephedra-containing dietary supplements. American Journal of Health Systems Pharmacy, 57, 963–969.

139.   Gurley BJ et al. (1998). Ephedrine-type alkaloid content of nutritional supplements containing Ephedra sinica (Ma-huang) as determined by high performance liquid chromatography. Journal of Pharmaceutical Sciences, 87,12,1547-1553.

140.   Morgenstern LB. et al. (2003). Use of Ephedra-containing products and risk for hemorrhagic stroke. Neurology, 14, 60,1,132-135.

141. Walton R et al. (2003). Psychosis related to ephedra-containing herbal supplement use. The Southern Medical Journal, 96,718-720.
142. Robbers JE (1999). Herbs of Choice: The Therapeutic Use of Phytomedicinals. New York, NY: The Haworth Herbal Press.
143. Powell T et al. (1998). Ma-huang strikes again: ephedrine nephrolithiasis. American Journal of Kidney Disorders, 32,153-159.
144. McBride BF et al. (2004). Electrocardiographic and hemodynamic effects of a multicomponent dietary supplement containing ephedra and caffeine: a randomized controlled trial. JAMA, 291, 216-221.
145. Memorial Sloan-kettering Cancer Center. http://www.mskcc.org
146. Stryer, L (1988). Biochemistry, 3rd edt W.H. Freeman and Company.
147. Tran MT (2001). Role of coenzyme Q10 in chronic heart failure, angina, and hypertension. Pharmacotherapy,21,7,797-806.
148. Laaksonen R et al (1995). Ubiquinone supplementation and exercise capacity in trained youg and older men. European Journal of Applied Physiology and Occupational Therapy, 72,1-2,95-100.
149. Porter, DA (1995). The effect of oral coenzyme Q10 on the exercise tolerance of middle-aged, untrained men. International Journal of Sport Nutrition, 16, 421-430.
150. Folkers K, et al. (1991). Coenzyme Q10 increases T4/T8 ratios of lymphocytes in ordinary subjects and relevance to patients having the AIDS related complex. Biochemical and Biophysical Research Communications, 176,786-791.
151. Hodgson JM (2003). Can coenzyme Q10 improve vascular function and blood pressure? Potential for effective therapeutic reduction in vascular oxidative stress. Biofactors, 18,1-4,129-316.
152. Burke BE (2001). Randomized, double-blind, placebo-controlled trial of coenzyme Q10 in isolated systolic hypertension. Southern Medical Journal, 94, 11, 1112-1117.
153. Singh RB et al. (2003). Effect of coenzyme Q10 on risk of atherosclerosis in patients with recent myocardial infarction. Molecular and Cellular Biochemistry,246,75-82.
154. Hodgson JM et al. (2002). Coenzyme Q (10) improves blood pressure and glycemic control: a controlled trial in subjects with type 2 diabetes. European Journal of Clinical Nutrition, 56,1137-1142.
155. Henriksen JE et al. (1999).Impact of ubiquinone (coenzyme Q10) treatment on glycemic control, insulin requirement and well-being in patients with Type 1 diabetes mellitus. Diabetes Medicine, 16,312-318.
156. Muller T et al. (2003).Coenzyme Q(10) supplementation provides mild symptomatic benefit in patients with Parkinson's disease. Neuroscience Letters, 341, 201–204.
157. Shults CW et al. (2002). Effects of coenzyme Q10 in early Parkinson disease: evidence of slowing of the functional decline. Archives of neurology,59,10,1541-1550.
158. Watts TL. (1995). Coenzyme Q$_{10}$ and periodontal treatment: Is there any beneficial effect? British Dental Journal, 178, 209–213.
159. Lister RE (2002). An open, pilot study to evaluate the potential benefits of coenzyme Q10 combined with Ginkgo biloba extract in fibromyalgia syndrome. Journal of International Medical Research, 30,2,195-199.
160. Passi S et al. (2002). Lipophilic antioxidants in human sebum and aging. Free Radical Research, 36,4, 471-477.
161. Kamikawa T et al. (1985). Effects of coenzyme Q10 on exercise tolerance in chronic stable angina pectoris. American Journal of Cardiology, 56, 247-251.
162. Spigset O. (1994). Reduced effect of warfarin caused by ubidecarenone [letter]. Lancet, 344,1372–1373.

412

163.   Engelsen J et al. (2003). Effect of Coenzyme Q10 and Ginkgo biloba on warfarin dosage in patients on long-term warfarin treatment. A randomized, double-blind, placebo-controlled cross-over trial] Ugeskrift for laeger, 165, 18,1868-1871.

164.   Coombes JS et al. (2002). Dose effects of oral bovine colostrum on physical work capacity in cyclists. Medicine and Science in Sports and Exercise, 34,7,1184-1188.

165.   Antonio J et al. (2001). The effects of bovine colostrum supplementation on body composition and exercise performance in active men and women. Nutrition, 17,3,243-247.

166.   Brinkworth GD et al. (2002). Oral bovine colostrum supplementation enhances buffer capacity but not rowing performance in elite female rowers. International Journal of Sport Nutrition and Exercise Metabolism, 12,3,349-363.

167.   Brinkworth GD et al. (2004). Bovine colostrum supplementation does not affect plasma buffer capacity or hemoglobin content in elite female rowers. European Journal of Applied Physiology, 91,2-3,353-356.

168.   Lilius EM et al. (2001). The role of colostral antibodies in prevention of microbial infections. Current Opinions in Infectious Diseases, 14,3,295-300.

169.   Hofman Z et al. (2002). The effect of bovine colostrum supplementation on exercise performance in elite field hockey players. International Journal of Sport Nutrition and Exercise Metabolism, 12,4,461-469.

170.   Sarker SA et al. (2001). Randomized, placebo-controlled, clinical trial of hyperimmunized chicken egg yolk immunoglobulin in children with rotavirus diarrhea. Journal of pediatric gastroenterology and nutrition, 32,1, 19-25.

171.   FDA Press Release Jan 26,2004. Press Release number 301-827-6242. Expanded "Mad Cow" Safeguards Announced to Strengthen Existing Firewalls Against BSE Transmission. http://www.fda.gov/bbs/topics/news/2004/hhs_012604.html (accessed March 5 2004).

172.   Hammarqvist F et al. (1991). Alpha-ketoglutarate preserves protein synthesis and free glutamine in skeletal muscle after surgery. Surgery, 109, 1, 28-36.

173.   DeGroot, L.J. (1995). Endocrinology, Volume 3, 3rd edition. W.B. Saunders.

174.   Broeder CE et al. (2000). The Andro Project: physiological and hormonal influences of androstenedione supplementation in men 35 to 65 years old participating in a high-intensity resistance training program. Archives of Internal Medicine, 160, 20,3093-3104.

175.   Broeder CE (2003). Oral andro-related prohormone supplementation: do the potential risks outweigh the benefits? Canadian Journal of Applied Physiology, 28,1,102-116.

176.   King DS et al. (1999). Effect of oral androstenedione on serum testosterone and adaptations to resistance training in young men: a randomized controlled trial. JAMA, 281,21,2020-2028.

177.   Brown GA et al. (2000). Effects of anabolic precursors on serum testosterone concentrations and adaptations to resistance training in young men. International Journal of Sport Nutrition and Exercise Metabolism, 10, 3,340-359.

178.   Brown GA et al. (2001). Effects of androstenedione-herbal supplementation on serum sex hormone concentrations in 30- to 59-year-old men. International Journal of Vitaminology and Nutrition Research, 71,5,293-301.

179. King DS (2002). Anabolic Prohormones: Superheroes or Superhype? Gatorade Sports Science Institute, www.gssiweb.com (accessed March-6-04).
180. Wallace MB et al. (1999). Effects of dehydroepiandrosterone vs androstenedione supplementation in men. Medicine and Science in Sports and Exercise, 31,12,1788-1792.
181. Ballantyne CS et al. (2000). The acute effects of androstenedione supplementation in healthy young males. Canadian Journal of Applied Physiology, 25,1,68-78.
182. van Weerden WM, et al. (1992) Effects of adrenal androgens on the transplantable human prostate tumor PC-82. Endocrinology, 131,2909-2913.
183. Weber B et al. (2000). Estosterone, androstenedione and dihydrotestosterone concentrations are elevated in female patients with major depression. Psychoneuroendocrinology, 25.8.765-771.
184. Herbert, V (1994). The antioxidant supplement myth. American Journal of Clinical Nutrition, 60,157-158.
185. Food and Drug Administration. November 1-3. 1993. FDA Conference on Antioxidant Vitamins and Cancer and Cardiovascular Disease. Washington. DC: Office of Special Nutritionals. 1993 (transcript).
186. Chromiak JA et al. (2002). Use of amino acids as growth hormone-releasing agents by athletes. Nutrition, 18,7-8,657-661.
187. Rector TS et al. (1996). Randomized, double-blind, placebo-controlled study of supplemental oral L-arginine in patients with heart failure. Circulation, 93,2135-2141.
188. Hambrecht R et al. (2000). Correction of endothelial dysfunction in chronic heart failure: additional effects of exercise training and oral L-arginine supplementation. Journal of the American College of Cardiology, 35,3,706-713.
189. Maxwell AJ et a (2002). Randomized trial of a medical food for the dietary management of chronic, stable angina. Journal of the American College of Cardiology, 39,1,37-45.
190. Blum A et al. (1999). Clinical and inflammatory effects of dictary L-arginine in patients with intractable angina pectoris. American Journal of Cardiology, 83,10,1488-1490.
191. Andres A, et al. (1997). L-arginine reverses the antinatriuretic effect of cyclosporin in renal transplant patients. Nephrology, Dialysis, Transplantation, 12,7,1437-1440.
192. Clark RH et al. (2000). Nutritional treatment for acquired immunodeficiency virus-associated wasting using beta-hydroxy beta-methylbutyrate, glutamine, and arginine: a randomized, double-blind, placebo-controlled study. Journal of Parenteral and Enteral Nutrition, 24,3,133-1339.
193. May PE et al. (2002). Reversal of cancer-related wasting using oral supplementation with a combination of beta-hydroxy-beta-methylbutyrate, arginine, and glutamine. American Journal of Surgery, 183,4,471-479.
194. Metabolic Technologies homepage http://www.mettechinc.com/ (accessed March 17, 2004).
195. Chen J, et al. (1999). Effect of oral administration of high-dose nitric oxide donor L-arginine in men with organic erectile dysfunction: results of a double-blind, randomized, placebo-controlled study. BJU International 83,269-273.
196. Klotz T et al. (1999). Effectiveness of oral L-arginine in first-line treatment of erectile dysfunction in a controlled crossover study. Urologia internationalis, 63,4, 220-223.

414

197. Sandrini G, et al. (1998).Effectiveness of ibuprofen-arginine in the treatment of acute migraine attacks. International Journal ofClinical Pharmacology Research, 18,3,145-150.

198. Maxwell AJ et al. (2000). Nutritional therapy for peripheral arterial disease: a double-blind, placebo-controlled, randomized trial of HeartBar. Vascular Medicine, 5,1,11-19.

199. Oomen CM et al. (2000). Arginine intake and risk of coronary heart disease mortality in elderly men. Arteriosclerosis, Thrombosis, and Vascular Biology, 20,9,2134-2139.

200. Venho B et al. (2002). Arginine intake, blood pressure, and the incidence of acute coronary events in men: the Kuopio Ischaemic Heart Disease Risk Factor Study. American Journal of Clinical Nutrition, 76,2,359-364.

201. Ohtsuka Y et al. (2000). Effect of oral administration of L-arginine on senile dementia. American Journal of Medicine, 108,439.

201. Senkal M et al. (1995). Modulation of postoperative immune response by enteral nutrition with a diet enriched with arginine, RNA, and omega-3 fatty acids in patients with upper gastrointestinal cancer. European Journal of Surgery, 161,115-122.

202. Kemen M et al. (1995). Early postoperative enteral nutrition with arginine-omega-3 fatty acids and ribonucleic acid-supplemented diet vs placebo in cancer patients: an immunologic evaluation of impact. Critical Care Medicine, 23,652-659.

203. Tepaske R et al. (2001). Effect of preoperative oral immune-enhancing nutritional supplement on patients at high risk of infection after cardiac surgery: a randomized placebo-controlled trial. Lancet, 358,696-701.

204. Griffith RS et al. (1981). Relation of arginine-lysine antagonism to herpes simplex growth in tissue culture. Chemotherapy. 27,209–213.

205. Maughan RJ et al. (1982). Effects of pollen extract upon adolescent swimmers. British Journal of Sports Medicine, 16,142-145.

206. Williams MH (1992). Ergogenic and ergolytic substances. Medicine and Science in Sport and Exercise, 24, (9 Suppl), S344-S348.

207. Steben RE et al. (1978). The effects of pollen and protein extracts on selected blood factors and performance of athletes. Journalof Sports Medicine and Physician Fitness, 18,3,221-226.

208. Geyman JP. (1994). Anaphylactic reaction after ingestion of bee pollen. Journal of the American Board of Family Practice, 7,250–252.

209. Albert S et al. (1999). The family of major royal jelly proteins and its evolution. Journal of Molecular Evolution, 49,290-297.

210. Inoue S et al. (2003). Royal Jelly prolongs the life span of C3H/HeJ mice: correlation with reduced DNA damage. Experimental Gerontology, 38,9, 965-969.

211. Vittek J. (1995). Effect of royal jelly on serum lipids in experimental animals and humans with atherosclerosis. Experimentia, 51,9-10,927-935.

212. Davis, JL (2001). The Buzz About Bee Jelly: Beware, It Could Do More Harm Than Good. www.webmd.com accessed March 29, 2004.

213. Gibala MJ et al. (2000). Amino acids, proteins and exercise performance. Gatorade Sports Science Institute. www.gssiweb.com/ accessed March 29 2004.

214. Blomstrand E et al. (1997) Influence of ingesting a solution of branched-chain amino acids on perceived exertion during exercise. Acta Physiologica Scandinavica, 159,41-49.

215. Pripps Bryggerier et al. (1991). Administration of branched-chain amino acids during sustained exercise--effects on performance and on plasma concentration of some amino acids. European Journal of Applied Physiology and Occupational Physiology. 63,2, 83-88.

216.   Blomstrand E. (2001). Amino acids and central fatigue. Amino Acids. 2001;20,1,25-34.
217.   Hiroshige K et al. (2001). Oral supplementation of branched-chain amino acid improves nutritional status in elderly patients on chronic haemodialysis. Nephrology, Dialysis, Transplantation, 16,9,1856-1862.
218.   Cangiano C et al. (1996). Effects of administration of oral branched-chain amino acids on anorexia and caloric intake in cancer patients. Journal of the National Cancer Institute, 88,550-552.
219.   Gatorade Sports Science Institute. Ergogenic Aids Create Controversy in Athletic Performance. http://www.gssiweb.com/ (accessed April 5 2004).
220.   MacLean DA et al. (1996). Stimulation of muscle ammonia production during exercise following branched-chain amino acid supplementation in humans. Journal of Applied Physiology, 493, 3,909-922.
221.   Richardson MA et al. (2003). Efficacy of the branched-chain amino acids in the treatment of tardive dyskinesia in men. American Journal of Psychiatry, 160,1117-1124.
222.   Richardson MA, et al. (1999). Branched chain amino acids decrease tardive dyskinesia symptoms. Psychopharmacology,143,4,358-64.
223.   Richardson MA, et al. (2004). Branched chain amino acid treatment of tardive dyskinesia in children and adolescents. Journal of Clinical Psychiatry, 65,1,92-96.
224.   Robertson DRC et al. (1991)The influence of protein containing meals on the pharmacokinetics of levodopa in healthy volunteers. British Journal of Clinical Pharmacology, 31,413-417.
225.   van Loon LJ et al. (2003). Amino acid ingestion strongly enhances insulin secretion in patients with long-term type 2 diabetes. Diabetes Care 26,625-630.
226.   Scarna Aet al. (2003). Effects of a branched-chain amino acid drink in mania. British Journal of Psychiatry, 182,210-213.
227.   Plaitakis A (1988). Pilot trial of branched-chain amino acids in amyotrophic lateral sclerosis. Lancet, 1,1015-1018.
228.   Tandan Ret al. (1996).A controlled trial of amino acid therapy in amyotrophic lateral sclerosis: I. Clinical, functional, and maximum isometric torque data. Neurology, 47,1220-1226.
229.   Kleiner, S (1998). Power Eating. Human kinetics.
230.   Marcus, A (2003). FDA ban doesn't block cancer causing plant extract. Health on The Net. http://www.hon.ch/News/HSN/515540.html (Accessed April 15 2004.)
231.   Gillerot G et al. (2004). Aristolochic acid nephropathy in a Chinese patient: time to abandon the term "Chinese herbs nephropathy"? American Journal of Kidney Diseases, 38,5, 1141-1142.
232.   Braslavsky A (2001). FDA: Chinese Herb Causes Kidney Failure, Cancer. WebMD.com (accessed April 15 2004).
233.   Nortier JL et al. (2000). Urothelial carcinoma associated with the use of a Chinese herb (Aristolochia fangchi). New England Journal of Medicine, 342,1686-1692.
234.   Unknown authors. Dangerous Supplements: Still At Large. Consumer Reports. (May 2004).
235.   Nortier JL et al. (2002). Renal interstitial fibrosis and urothelial carcinoma associated with the use of a Chinese herb (Aristolochia fangchi). Toxicology, 181-182,577-580.
236.   Cosyns JP et al. (2003). Urothelial lesions in Chinese-herb nephropathy. American Journal of Kidney Diseases, 33,6,1171-1173.
237.   Beattie JH et al. (1993). The influence of a low-boron diet and boron supplementation on bone, major mineral and sex steroid metabolism in postmenopausal women. British Journal of Nutrition, 69,3,871-384.

416

238.   Green NR et al. (1994). Plasma boron and the effects of boron supplementation in males. Environmental Health Perspectives, 102 Suppl 7,73-77.

239.   Ferrando, AA et al. (1993). The effect of boron supplementation on lean body mass, plasma testosterone levels, and strength in male bodybuilders. International Journal of Sport Nutrition, 3,2,140-149.

240.   Williams, (1993). Sports Science Exchange. Nutritional supplements for strength trained athletes. Gatorade Sports Science Institute. www.gssiweb.com/ Accessed April 16 2004.

241.   Newnham RE. (1994). Essentiality of boron for healthy bones and joints. Environmental Health Perspectives, 102,83-85.

242.   Naghii MR. (1997). The effect of boron supplementation on its urinary excretion and selected cardiovascular risk factors in healthy male subjects. Biological Trace Element Research, 56,273-286.

243.   Penland JG. (1994). Dietary boron, brain function, and cognitive performance. Environmental Health Perspectives, 102,65-72.

244.   Nielsen FH et al. (1987). Effect of dietary boron on mineral, estrogen, and testosterone metabolism in postmenopausal women. FASEB Journal, 1, 5, 394-397.

245.   Meacham SL et al. (1994). Effects of boron supplementation on bone mineral density and dietary, blood, and urinary calcium, phosphorus, magnesium, and boron in female athletes. Environmental Health Perspectives, 102,(suppl 7), 79-82.

246.   Cui Y et al. (2004). Dietary boron intake and prostate cancer risk. Oncology Reports, 11,4, 887-892.

247.   Szajewska H et al. (2001). Efficacy of Lactobacillus GG in prevention of nosocomial diarrhea in infants. Journal of Pediatrics, 138,361-365.

248.   Oberhelman RA et al. (1999).A placebo-controlled trial of Lactobacillus GG to prevent diarrhea in undernourished Peruvian children. Journal of Pediatrics, 134,15-20.

249.   Hilton E, Kolakowski P, Singer C, et al. (1997). Efficacy of Lactobacillus GG as a Diarrheal Preventative in Travelers. Journal of Travel Medicine, 4,41-43.

249.   Oksanen PJ et al. (1990). Prevention of travellers' diarrhoea by Lactobacillus GG. Annals of Medicine, 22, 1, 53-56.

250.   Xiao SD et al. (2003). Multicenter, randomized, controlled trial of heat-killed Lactobacillus acidophilus LB in patients with chronic diarrhea. Advances in Therapy, 20,5,253-260.

251.   Simakachorn N et al. (2000). Clinical evaluation of the addition of lyophilized, heat-killed Lactobacillus acidophilus LB to oral rehydration therapy in the treatment of acute diarrhea in children. Journal of pediatric gastroenterology and nutrition, 30,1,68-72.

252.   Konturek JW (2003). Discovery by Jaworski of Helicobacter pylori and its pathogenetic role in peptic ulcer, gastritis and gastric cancer. Journal of Physiology and Pharmacology, 54 (Suppl 3)23-41.

253.   Canducci F et al. (2000). A lyophilized and inactivated culture of Lactobacillus acidophilus increases Helicobacter pylori eradication rates. Alimentary pharmacology & therapeutics, 14,1625-1629.

254.   Halpern GM et al. (1996). Treatment of irritable bowel syndrome with Lacteol Fort: a randomized, double-blind, cross-over trial. American Journal of Gastroenterology 91,1579-1585.

255.   Nobaek S et al. (2000). Alteration of intestinal microflora is associated with reduction in abdominal bloating and pain in patients with irritable bowel syndrome. American Journal of Gastroenterology 95,1231-1238.

256.   Urinary Tract Infections in Teens and Adults. WebMD.com (accessed April 26 2004).

257. Reid G et al. (1992). Influence of three-day antimicrobial therapy and lactobacillus vaginal suppositories on recurrence of urinary tract infections. Clinical Therapeutics, 14,1,11-16.

258. Bruce AW et al. (1988). Intravaginal instillation of lactobacilli for prevention of recurrent urinary tract infections. Canadian Journal of Microbiology, 34,3,339-343.

259. Baerheim A et al. (1994). Vaginal application of lactobacilli in the prophylaxis of recurrent lower urinary tract infection in women. Scandinavian Journal of Primary Health Care, 12,4, 239-243.

260. Sheih YH et al. (2001). Systemic immunity-enhancing effects in healthy subjects following dietary consumption of the lactic acid bacterium Lactobacillus rhamnosus HN001. Journal of the American College of Nutrition, 20,149-156.

261. Gill HS et al. (2001). Probiotic supplementation to enhance natural immunity in the elderly: effects of a newly characterized immunostimulatory strain of Lactobacillus rhamnosus HN001 (DR20) on leucocyte phagocytosis. Nutrition Research,21:183-189.

262. El-Nezami H et al.(1998). Ability of dairy strains of lactic acid bacteria to bind a common food carcinogen, aflatoxin B1. Food and Chemical Toxicology,36,321-326.

263. MacGregor G et al. (2002). Yoghurt biotherapy: contraindicated in immunosuppressed patients? Postgraduate Medical Journal, 78,366–367.

264. FDA. Press release (1997). FDA proposes safety measures for ephedrine dietary supplements. FDA.gov (accessed April 28 2004).

265. Consumerlab.com (accessed April 28 2004).

266. Cancer.gov homepage. Mistletoe Extracts. www.cancer.gov (accessed April 28 2004).

267. Product Review: Probiotic Supplements and Foods (Including Lactobacillus acidophilus and Bifidobacterium). Consumerlab.com (accessed April 30 2004).

268. Wernerman J (1990). Alpha-ketoglutarate and postoperative muscle catabolism. Lancet, 335,(8691), 701-703.

269. Riedel E, Nundel M, Hampl H. (1996). Alpha-Ketoglutarate application in hemodialysis patients improves amino acid metabolism. Nephron, 74,2,261-265.

270. Nutrition News Focus, *Antioxidant Vitamins Not Good for Heart*. www.nutritionnewsfocus.com/ (accessed May 5 2004).

271. Mirkin G. Can bee pollen benefit health? *JAMA* 1989;262:1854-1858.

272. Matsuoka H et al. (1997). Lentinan potentiates immunity and prolongsthe survival time of some patients. Anticancer Research, 17,2751-755.

273. Yoshino S et al. (2000). Immunoregulatory effects of the antitumor polysaccharide lentinan on Th1/Th2 balance in patients with digestive cancers. Anticancer Research, 20,6C,4707-4711.

274. Borchers AT, Stern JS, Hackman RM, et al. (1999). Mushrooms, tumors, and immunity. Proceedings of the Society for Experimental Biology and Medicine, 221,4,281-293.

275. Okamura K et al. (1986). Clinical evaluation of schizophyllan combined with irradiation in patients with cervical cancer. A randomized controlled study. Cancer, 58,4,865-872.

276. Kimura Y et al. (1994). Clinical evaluation of sizofilan as assistant immunotherapy in treatment of head and neck cancer. Acta oto-laryngologica. Supplementum, 511,192-195.

277. Gordon M et al. (1998).A placebo-controlled trial of the immune modulator, lentinan, in HIV-positive patients: a phase I/II trial. Journal of Medicine, 29,5-6,305-330.

418

278. Gordon M et al. et al. (1995). A phase II controlled study of a combination of the immune modulator, lentinan, with didanosine (ddI) in HIV patients with CD4 cells of 200-500/mm3. Journal of Medicine, 26, 5-6,193-207.

279. Nicolosi R et al. (1999). Plasma lipid changes after supplementation with beta-glucan fiber from yeast. American Journal of Clinical Nutrition, 70,2,208-121.

280. Sherwood ER et al.(1987). Enhancement of interleukin-1 and interleukin-2 production by soluble glucan. International journal of immunopharmacology, 9,3,261-267.

281. Browder W, Williams D, Pretus H, et al. Beneficial effect of enhanced macrophage function in the trauma patient. Annals of Surgery, 211,5,605-612.

282. McIntosh GH et al. (1991). Barley and wheat foods: influence on plasma cholesterol concentrations in hypercholesterolemic men. American Journal of Clinical Nutrition, 53,5,1205-1209.

283. New Health Claim Approved for Whole Oat Products. FDA Consumer (April 1997). http://www.fda.gov/fdac/departs/1997/397_upd.html (accessed May 6, 2004).

284. Dellinger EP et al. (1999). Effect of PGG-glucan on the rate of serious postoperative infection or death observed after high-risk gastrointestinal operations. Betafectin Gastrointestinal Study Group. Archives of Surgery, 134,9, 997-983.

285. Hidgon J (2004). Carotenoids. Linus Pauling Institute. http://lpi.oregonstate.edu/infocenter/phytochemicals/carotenoids/index.html (accessed May 9 2004).

286. Age-related macular denegation. Webmd.com. (accessed May 9 2004).

287. Bressler NM et al. (2003). Age-Related Eye Disease Study Research Group. Potential public health impact of age-related eye disease study results: AREDS report no. 11. Archives of Ophthalmology,121,1621-1624.

288. Ambati J et al. (2001). Age-Related Eye Disease Study Research Group. A randomized, placebo-controlled, clinical trial of high-dose supplementation with vitamins C and E, beta carotene, and zinc for age-related macular degeneration and vision loss. AREDS report no. 8. Archives of Ophthalmology, 119, 1417-1436.

289. Seddon JM et al. (1994). Dietary carotenoids, vitamins A, C, and E, and advanced age-related macular degeneration. JAMA, 272,1413-1420.

290. Stahl W et al. (2000). Carotenoids and carotenoids plus vitamin E protect against ultraviolet light-induced erythema in humans. American Journal of Clinical Nutrition, 71,795-798.

291. Garmyn M et al. (1995). Effect of β-carotene on the human sunburn reaction. Experimental Dermatology, 4,101-111.

292. Green A et al. (1999). Daily sunscreen applications and beta-carotene supplementation in prevention of basal-cell and squamous-cell carcinomas of the skin: a randomized controlled trial. Lancet, 354,723-729.

293. Frieling UM et al. (2000). A randomized, 12-year primary-prevention trial of beta carotene supplementation for nonmelanoma skin cancer in the physicians' health study. Archives of Dermatology, 136,179-184.

294. Flagg EW et al. (1995). Epidemiologic studies of antioxidants and cancer in humans. Journal of the American College of Nutrition, 14,149-127.

295. Byers T et al. (1992). Dietary carotenes, vitamin C, and vitamin E as protective antioxidants in human cancers. Annual Review of Nutrition, 12:139-59.

296.   Albanes D et al. (1995). Effects of alpha-tocopherol and beta-carotene
         supplements on cancer incidence in the Alpha-Tocopherol Beta-
         Carotene Cancer Prevention Study. American Journal of Clinical
         Nutrition, 62,(6 suppl), 1427S-1430S.

297.   The Alpha-Tocopherol, Beta Carotene Cancer Prevention Study Group.
         The effect of vitamin E and beta carotene on the incidence of lung
         cancer and other cancers in male smokers. New England Journal of
         Medicine (1994), 330,1029-1035.

298.   Blot WJ et al. (1993). Nutritional intervention trials in Linxian, China:
         supplementation with specific vitamin/mineral combinations, cancer
         incidence, and disease-specific mortality in the general population.
         Journal of the National Cancer Institute, 85,1483-1492.

299.   Lee IM et al. (1999). Beta-carotene supplementation and incidence of
         cancer and cardiovascular disease: the Women's Health Study. Journal
         of the National Cancer Institute, 91,2102-2106.

300.   Hennekens CH, Buring JE, Manson JE, et al. Lack of effect of long-term
         supplementation with beta-carotene on the incidence of malignant
         neoplasms and cardiovascular disease. New England Journal of
         Medicine, 334,1145-1149.

301.   Virtamo J et al. (1998). Effect of vitamin E and beta carotene on the
         incidence of primary nonfatal myocardial infarction and fatal coronary
         heart disease. Archives of Internal Medicine, 158,668-675.

302.   Brown BG et al. (2001). Simvastatin and niacin, antioxidant vitamins, or
         the combination for the prevention of coronary disease. New England
         Journal of Medicine, 345,1583-1593.

303.   Rapola JM et al. (1997). Randomised trial of alpha-tocopherol and beta-
         carotene supplements on incidence of major coronary events in men with
         previous myocardial infarction. Lancet, 349,1715-1720.

304.   Greenberg ER et al. (1996). Mortality associated with low plasma
         concentration of beta carotene and the effect of oral supplementation.
         JAMA, 275,699-703.

305.   Ahn WS et al. (2003). Protective effects of green tea extracts
         (polyphenon E and EGCG) on human cervical lesions. European Journal
         of Cancer Prevention, 12,383-390.

306.   Chantre P et al. (2002). Recent findings of green tea extract AR25
         (Exolise) and its activity for the treatment of obesity. Phytomedicine, 9,3-
         8.

307.   Zheng G et al. (2004). Anti-obesity effects of three major components of
         green tea, catechins, caffeine and theanine, in mice. In Vivo, 18,1,55-62.

308.   Bushman JL. (1998). Green tea and cancer in humans: a review of the
         literature. Nutrition and Cancer, 31,151-159.

309.   Mitscher LA et al. (1997). Chemoprotection: a review of the potential
         therapeutic antioxidant properties of green tea (Camellia sinensis) and
         certain of its constituents. Medicinal Research Reviews,17,327-65.

310.   Wakai K et al. (1993). Prognostic significance of selected lifestyle factors
         in urinary bladder cancer. Japanese Journal of Cancer Research,
         84,1223-1229.

311.   Ohno Y et al. (1985). Case-control study of urinary bladder cancer in
         metropolitan Nagoya. National Cancer Institute Monograph, 69,229-234.

312.   Inoue M et al. (2001). Regular consumption of green tea and the risk of
         breast cancer recurrence: follow-up study from the Hospital-based
         Epidemiologic Research Program at Aichi Cancer Center (HERPACC),
         Japan. Cancer Letters, 167,175-182.

313.   Kaegi E. (1998). Unconventional therapies for cancer: 2. Green tea. The
         Task Force on Alternative Therapies of the Canadian Breast Cancer
         Research Initiative. Caniadian Medical Association Journal, 158,1033-
         1035.

420

314.   Ahn WS et al. (2003). Protective effects of green tea extracts
         (polyphenon E and EGCG) on human cervical lesions. European Journal
         of Cancer Prevention, 12,383-390.
315.   Tsubono Y et al. (2001). Green tea and the risk of gastric cancer in
         Japan. New England Journal of Medicine, 344,632-636.
316.   Jatoi A et al. (2003). A phase II trial of green tea in the treatment of
         patients with androgen independent metastatic prostate carcinoma.
         Cancer, 97, 1442-1446.
317.   Inoue M et al. (1998). Tea and coffee consumption and the risk of
         digestive tract cancers: data from a comparative case-referent study in
         Japan. Cancer, Causes and Control, 9,209-216.
318.   Geleijnse JM et al. (2002). Inverse association of tea and flavonoid
         intakes with incident myocardial infarction: the Rotterdam Study.
         American Journal of Clinical Nutrition, 75, 880-886.
319.   Hergot MG et al. (1993). Dietary antioxidant flavonoids and risk of
         coronary heart disease: the Zutphen Elderly Study. Lancet.
         23,342,8878,1007-1011.
320.   Ascherio A et al. (2001). Prospective study of caffeine consumption and
         risk of Parkinson's disease in men and women. Annals of Neurology,
         50,1,56-63.
321.   Taylor JR et al. (1999). Probable antagonism of warfarin by green tea.
         Annals of Pharmacotherapy, 33,426–428.
322.   Lasswell WL et al. (1984). In vitro interaction of neuroleptics and tricylic
         antidepressants with coffee, tea, and gallotannic acid. Journal of
         Pharmacy Science, 73,8,1056-1058.
323.   Ali M et al. (1987). A potent inhibitor of thrombin stimulated platelet
         thromboxane formation from unprocessed tea. Prostaglandins,
         Leukotrienes, and Medicine, 27,1,9-13.
324.   Watson JM et al. (2000). Influence of caffeine on the frequency and
         perception of hypoglycemia in free-living patients with type 1 diabetes.
         Diabetes Care. 23,4,455-9.
325.   Bell DG et al. (2001). Effect of caffeine and ephedrine ingestion on
         anaerobic exercise performance. Medicine and Science in Sports and
         Exercise, 33,8,1399-4403.
326.   Ross GW et al. (2000) Association of coffee and caffeine intake with the
         risk of Parkinson's disease. JAMA, 283,2674-2679.
327.   Heymsfield SB et al. (1998). Garcinia cambogia (hydroxycitric acid) as a
         potential antiobesity agent: a randomized controlled trial. JAMA,
         280,1596-1600.
328.   Greenwood MR. et al. (1981) Effect of (-)-hydroxycitrate on development
         of obesity in the Zucker obese rat. American Journal of Physiology, 240,
         E72-E78.
329.   Sergio W. (1988). A natural food, the malabar tamarind, may be effective
         in the treatment of obesity. Medical Hypothesis. 27,39–40.
330.   Mattes RD et al. (2000). . Effects of (-)-hydroxycitric acid on appetitive
         variables. Physiology and Behavior,71,87–94.
331.   Kovacs EM et al. (2001). The effects of 2-week ingestion of (--)-
         hydroxycitrate and (--)-hydroxycitrate combined with medium-chain
         triglycerides on satiety, fat oxidation, energy expenditure and body
         weight. International Journal of Obesity and Related Metabolic Disorders,
         25,1087-1094.
332.   Westerterp-Plantenga MS et al. (2002). The effect of (-)-hydroxycitrate
         on energy intake and satiety in overweight humans. International Journal
         of Obesity, 26,870-872.
333.   Liske E et al. (2002) Physiological investigation of a unique extract of
         black cohosh (Cimicifugae racemosae rhizma): a 6-month clinical study

demonstrates no systemic estrogenic effect. Journal of Women's Health & Gender-Based Medicine, 11,163-174.

334. Mahady GB et al. (2002). Black cohosh: an alternative therapy for menopause? Nutrition in Clinical Care, 5,6,283-289.

335. Boyles S (2002). Herb Fights Menopause Symptoms. WebMD.com (accessed 6/30/04).

336. Mahady GB et al. (2002). Black cohosh: an alternative therapy for menopause? Nutrition in Clinical Care, 5,6,283-290.

337. Whiting PW et al. (2002). Black cohosh and other herbal remedies associated with acute hepatitis. Medical Journal of Australia, 177,440–443.

338. Thomsen M et al. (2003). Hepatotoxicity from Cimicifuga racemosa? Recent Australian case report not sufficiently substantiated. Journal of Alternative and Complementary Medicine,9,3,337-340.

339. Black cohosh may make breast cancer drug more toxic. Posted April 7 2003. American Society of Clinical Oncology web site. (accessed 7/5/04).

340. Jones TK et al. (1998). Profound neonatal congestive heart failure caused by maternal consumption of blue cohosh herbal medication. Journal of Pediatrics, 132, 3 Pt 1, 550-552.

341. Haskell CM et al. (1996). Phase I trial of extracellular adenosine 5'-triphosphate in patients with advanced cancer. Medical and Pediatric Oncology, 27, 165-173.

342. Agteresch HJ (2000). Randomized clinical trial of adenosine 5'-triphosphate in patients with advanced non-small-cell lung cancer. Journal of the National Cancer Institute, 92,321-328.

343. Agteresch HJ et al. (2002). Beneficial effects of adenosine triphosphate on nutritional status in advanced lung cancer patients: a randomized clinical trial. Journal of Clinical Oncology, 20,371-378.

344. Alexander N et al. (2004). Effects of oral ATP supplementation on anaerobic power and muscular strength. Medicine and Science in Sports and Exercise, 36,6,983-990.

345. Philips, B. Sports Supplement Review, 3rd issue. Mile High Publishing, Golden CO.

346. Parcell, AC et al. (2004). Cordyceps sinensis (Cordy Max Cs-4) supplementation does not improve endurance exercise performance. International Journal of Sport Nutrition and Exercise Metabolism, 14, 2, 236-242.

347. Warner J (April 2004). Chinese Mushroom May Offer Energy Lift. WebMd.com (accessed 7/24/04).

348. Xu RH, et al. (1992). Effects of cordyceps sinensis on natural killer activity and colony formation of B16 melanoma. Chinese Medical Journal, 105,2,97-101.

349. Chen GZ et al. (1991) Effects of Cordyceps sinensis on murine T lymphocyte subsets. Chinese Medical Journal, 104,1,4-8.

350. Chen YJ et al. (1997). Effect of Cordyceps sinensis on the proliferation and differentiation of human leukemic U937 cells. Life Science, 60,25,2349-2359.

351. Yamaguchi N et al. (1990). Augmentation of various immune reactivities of tumor-bearing hosts with an extract of Cordyceps sinensis. Biotherapy, 2,3,199-205.

352. Li, Y. et. al. (1993). Effect of Cordyceps sinensis on erythropoiesis in mouse bone marrow. Chinese Medical Journal (Engl). 106,4,313-316.

353. Zhu JS et al. (1998). The scientific rediscovery of an ancient Chinese herbal medicine: Cordyceps sinensis: part I. Journal of Alternative and Complementary Medicine, 4,289-303.

422

354.   Bosco C et al. (1997) Effect of oral creatine supplementation on jumping and running performance. International Journal of Sports Medicine, 18,369-372.
355.   McNaughton LR et al. (1998)The effects of creatine supplementation on high-intensity exercise performance in elite performers. European Journal of Applied Physiology, 78,236-240.
356.   Kreider RB et al. (1998). Effects of creatine supplementation on body composition, strength, and sprint performance. Medicine and Science in Sport and Exercise, 30,73-82.
357.   Williams H et al. (1999). Creatine: The Power Supplement. Human Kinetics
358.   Rawson ES et al. (2003). Scientifically debatable: Is creatine worth its weight? Gatorade Sports Science Institute web site. Sports Science Exchange # 91 vol 14,4. www.gssiweb.com (accessed 8/2/04).
359.   Burke LM et al. (1995). Oral creatine supplementation does not improve sprint performance in elite swimmers. Medicine and Science in Sports and Exercise, 27, S146.
360.   Mujika I et al. (1996). Creatine supplementation does not improve sprint performance in competitive swimmers. Medicine and Science in Sports and Exercise, 28,1435-1441.
361.   Odland LM et al. (1997). Effect of oral creatine supplementation on muscle [PCr] and short-term maximum power output Medicine and Science in Sports and Exercise, 29,216-219.
362.   Rawson ES et al. (2000). Acute creatine supplementation in older men. International Journal of Sports Medicine, 21,71-75.
363.   Bermon S, Venembre P, Sachet C, et al. Effects of creatine monohydrate ingestion in sedentary and weight-trained older adults. Acta Physiologica Scandinavica, 165,147-155.
364.   Hultman Eet al. (1996). Muscle creatine loading in men. Journal of Applied Physiology, 81,232-237.
365.   Juhn MS et al. (1998). Potential side effects of oral creatine supplementation: a critical review. Clinical Journal of Sports Medicine, 8,298-304.
366.   Koshy KM (1999). Interstitial nephritis in a patient taking creatine. New England Journal of Medicine, 340,814-815.
367.   Yu PH et al. (2000). Potential cytotoxic effect of chronic administration of creatine, a nutrition supplement to augment athletic performance. Medical Hypotheses, 54,726–728.
368.   Green AL, Simpson EJ, Littlewood JJ, et al. Carbohydrate ingestion augments creatine retention during creatine feeding in humans. Acta Physiologica Scandinavica, 158,195-202.
369.   Steenge GR et al. (2000). Protein- and carbohydrate-induced augmentation of whole body creatine retention in humans. Journal of Applied Physiology, 89, 3,1165-1171.
370.   Heinanen K et al. (1999). Creatine corrects muscle 31P spectrum in gyrate atrophy with hyperornithinaemia. European Journal of Clinical Investigation, 29,1060-1065.
371.   Andrews R et al. (1998). The effect of dietary creatine supplementation on skeletal muscle metabolism in congestive heart failure. European Heart Journal, 19,617-622.
372.   Gordon A et al. (1995). Creatine supplementation in chronic heart failure increases skeletal muscle creatine phosphate and muscle performance. Cardiovascular Research, 30,413-418.
373.   Earnest CP et al. (1996). High-performance capillary electrophoresis-pure creatine monohydrate reduces blood lipids in men and women. Clinical Science (London), 91,113–118.

374.   Walter MC et al. (2000). Creatine monohydrate in muscular dystrophies: A double-blind, placebo-controlled clinical study. Neurology, 54,1848-1850.

375.   Walter MC et al. (2002). Creatine monohydrate in myotonic dystrophy: a double-blind, placebo-controlled clinical study. Journal of Neurology, 249,12,1717-1722.

376.   Chrubasik S et al. (2002). Comparison of outcome measures during treatment with the proprietary Harpagophytum extract doloteffin in patients with pain in the lower back, knee or hip. Phytomedicine, 9,181-194.

377.   Wegener T et al. (2003). Treatment of patients with arthrosis of hip or knee with an aqueous extract of devil's claw (Harpagophytum procumbens DC.). Phytotherapy Research, 17,10,1165-1172.

378.   Leblan D et al. (2000). Harpagophytum procumbens in the treatment of knee and hip osteoarthritis. Four-month results of a prospective, multicenter, double-blind trial versus diacerhein. Joint Bone and Spine, 67,5,462-467.

379.   Laudahn D et al. (2001). Efficacy and tolerance of Harpagophytum extract LI 174 in patients with chronic non-radicular back pain. Phytotherapy Research, 15,7,621-624.

380.   Devils Claw (Harpagophytum procumbens). Aetna Intellihealth homepage. www.intellihealth.com (accessed 8/8/04).

381.   The wrinkle cure. Pericone N. WebMd.com. (accessed 8/9/04).

382.   Uhoda I et al. (2002).Split face study on the cutaneous tensile effect of 2-dimethylaminoethanol (deanol) gel. Skin Research and Technology, 8,164-167.

383.   Alzheimer's, Disease. topic Overview. Webmd.com (accessed 8/9/07).

384.   Fisman M et al. (1981). Double-blind trial of 2-dimethylaminoethanol in Alzheimer's disease. American Journal of Psychiatry, 138,970-972.

385.   Ferris SH et al. (1977). Senile dementia: treatment with deanol. Journal of the American Geriatrics Society, 25,241-244.

386.   About 3M Pharmaceuticals. www.3m.com web site (accessed 8/10/04).

387.   Re' O (1974). 2-Dimethylaminoethanol (deanol). a brief review of its clinical efficacy and postulated mechanism of action. Current Therapeutic Research, Clinical and Experimental, 16,1338-1242.

388.   Knobel M. (1974). Approach to a combined pharmacologic therapy of childhood hyperkinesis. Behavioral Neuropsychiatry. 6,87-90.

389.   Lewis JA (1975). Deanol and methylphenidate in minimal brain dysfunction. Clinical pharmacology and therapeutics. 17,534-540.

390.   Dimpfel W et al. (2003). Efficacy of dimethylaminoethanol (DMAE) containing vitamin-mineral drug combination on EEG patterns in the presence of different emotional states. European Journal of Medical, Research, 30,8,183-191.

391.   Casey DE. (1979). Mood alterations during deanol therapy. Psychopharmacology (Berl), 62,187-191.

392.   de Montigny C et al. (1979).Ineffectiveness of deanol in tardive dyskinesia: a placebo controlled study. Psychopharmacology (Berl), 65,219-223.

393.   Haug BA et al. (1991). Orofacial and respiratory tardive dyskinesia: potential side effects of 2-dimethylaminoethanol (deanol). European Neurology, 31,423-425.

394.   Personal communication 3M Pharmaceuticals August 12 2004.

395.   Hirata JD et al. (1997) Does dong quai have estrogenic effects in postmenopausal women? A double-blind, placebo-controlled trial. Fertility and sterility, 68,981-996.

396. Heck AM et al. (2000). Potential interactions between alternative therapies and warfarin. American Journal of Health-System Pharmacy,57,1221-1227.

397. Amato P, Christophe S, Mellon PL. Estrogenic activity of herbs commonly used as remedies for menopausal symptoms. Menopause 2002;9:145-50.

398. Maltin L (2002). Some herbs Boost Breast Cancer Risk. WebMD.com (accessed 8/14/04).

399. Tyler V (1993). The Honest Herbal. Pharmaceutical Press.

400. Schulten B et al. (2001). Efficacy of Echinacea purpurea in patients with a common cold. A placebo-controlled, randomised, double-blind clinical trial. Arzneimittel-Forschung,51,563-568.

401. Melchart D et al. (2000). Echinacea for preventing and treating the common cold. Cochrane Database Systematic Review, 2, CD000530.

402. Giles JT et al. (2000). Evaluation of echinacea for treatment of the common cold. Pharmacotherapy. 20,6,690-697.

403. Lee AN et al. (2004). Activation of autoimmunity following use of immunostimulatory herbal supplements. Archives of Dermatology, 140,6,723-727.

404. Taylor JA et al. (2003). Efficacy and safety of echinacea in treating upper respiratory tract infections in children: a randomized controlled trial. JAMA, 290,21,2824-2830.

405. Sperber SJ et al. (2004). Echinacea purpurea for prevention of experimental rhinovirus colds. Clinical infectious diseases, 38,10,1367-1371.

406. Grimm W, et al. (1999). A randomized controlled trial of the effect of fluid extract of Echinacea purpurea on the incidence and severity of colds and respiratory infections. American Journal of Medicine, 106,2,138-143.

407. Stimpel M et al. (1984). Macrophage activation and induction of macrophage cytotoxicity by purified polysaccharide fractions from the plant Echinacea purpurea. Infection and Immunity, 46,845-849.

408. Luettig B et al. (1989). Macrophage activation by the polysaccharide arabinogalactan isolated from plant cell cultures of Echinacea purpurea. Journal of the National Cancer Institute, 81,669-675.

409. Schwarz E et al. (2002). Oral administration of freshly expressed juice of Echinacea purpurea herbs fail to stimulate the nonspecific immune response in healthy young men: results of a double-blind, placebo-controlled crossover study. Journal of Immunotherapy, 25,413-420.

410. Product Review: Echinacea. Consumerlab.com (accessed 8/29/04).

411. Goldberg, B. (1993). Alternative Medicine: the Definitive Guide. Future Medicine Publishing.

412. Enzyme Supplements. University of California Berkley Wellness Letter, November 2002.

413. Deitrick RE. (1965). Oral proteolytic enzymes in the treatment of athletic injuries: a double-blind study. Pennsylvania medicine, 68,35-37.

414. Mann D (2004). Supplement Use in Sickness and in Health. Webmd.com (accessed 9/3/04).

415. No authors listed. Headache triggers. Webmd.com. (accessed 9/5/04).

416. Rapuri PB et al. (2001). Caffeine intake increases the rate of bone loss in elderly women and interacts with vitamin D receptor genotypes. American Journal of Clinical Nutrition, 74,694-700.

417. Heaney RP (2002). Effects of caffeine on bone and the calcium economy. Food and Chemical Toxicology, 40,9,163-1270.

418. Terry E. Graham et al. (1996). Caffeine and exercise performance. Gatorade Sports Science Institute homepage. SSE#60, Volume 9, Number 1. ww.gssiweb.com (accessed 6/5/04).

419.   McNaughton LR (1986). The influence of caffeine ingestion on incremental treadmill running. British Journal of Sports Medicine, 20,3,109-112.

420.   Birnbaum LJ et al. (2004). Physiologic effects of caffeine on cross-country runners. Journal of Strength and Conditioning Research, 18,3,463-465.

421.   Cole KJ et al. (1996). Effect of caffeine ingestion on perception of effort and subsequent work production. International Journal of Sports Nutrition, 6,1,14-23.

422.   Warner J (2003). Caffeine May Ease the 'Ouch' of Exercise. WebMd.com. (accessed 9/5/04).

423.   JJ Barone et al. (1996) Caffeine Consumption. Food Chemistry and Toxicology,34, 119-129 and information provided by National Coffee Association, National Soft Drink Association, Tea Council of the USA.

424.   Saldanha Aoki M (2004). arnitine supplementation fails to maximize fat mass loss induced by endurance training in rats. Annals of Nutrition and Metabolism, 48,2,90-94.

425.   Pittler MH et al. (2004). Dietary supplements for body weight reduction: a systematic review. American Journal of Clinical Nutrition, 79, 4, 529-536.

426.   Jing SB, Li L, Ji D, et al. Effect of chitosan on renal function in patients with chronic renal failure. The Journal of Pharmacy and Pharmacology,49,721-723. 427.

428.   Guerciolini R et al. (2001). Comparative evaluation of fecal fat excretion induced by orlistat and chitosan. Obesity Research, 9,364-367.

429.   Wilburn AJ et al. (2004). The natural treatment of hypertension. Journal of Clinical Hypertension. 6,5, 242-248.

430.   Lund E, el al. (1998). Effect of radiation therapy on small-cell lung cancer is rreduces by ubiquinone. Folia Microbiologica, 4,505-506.

431.   Singh RB, Niaz MA, Rastogi SS, et al. (1999). Effect of hydrosoluble coenzyme Q10 on blood pressures and insulin resistance in hypertensive patients with coronary artery disease. Journal of Human Hypertension, 13,208-208.

432.   Henriksen JE, et al. (1999). Impact of ubiquinone (coenzyme Q10) treatment on glycaemic control, insulin requirement and well-being in patients with Type 1 diabetes mellitus. Diabetes Medicine, 16,312-218.

433.   National Cancer Institute web site. Coenzyme Q_{10} Questions and Answers. www.cancer.gov (accessed 9/12/04).

434.   Lockwood K et al. (1994). Partial and complete regression of breast cancer in patients in relation to dosage of coenzyme Q10. Biochemical and Biophysical Research Communications, 199,3,1504-8.

435.   Morisco C et al. (1993). Effect of coenzyme Q10 therapy in patients with congestive heart failure: A long-term, multicenter, randomized study. Clinical Investigations, 71, S134-S136.

436.   Hofman-Bang C et al. (1995). Coenzyme Q10 as an adjunctive in the treatment of chronic congestive heart failure. The Q10 Study Group. Journal of Cardiac Failure, 1,2,101-7.

437.   Khatta M et al. (2000). The effect of coenzyme Q10 in patients with congestive heart failure. Archives of Internal Medicine, 133, 9,745-746.

438.   Soja AM et al. (1997). Treatment of congestive heart failure with coenzyme Q10 illuminated by meta-analyses of clinical trials. Molecular Aspects of Medicine, 18, Suppl:S159-S168.

439.   Watson PS et al. (1999). Lack of effect of coenzyme Q on left ventricular function in patients with congestive heart failure. Journal of the American College of Cardiology, 33,1549-1552.

440. Buckley JD (2003). Effect of bovine colostrum on anaerobic exercise performance and plasma insulin-like growth factor I. Journal of Sport Sciences, 21,577-588. 441.

442. Kamphuis MM et al. (2003). Effect of conjugated linoleic acid supplementation after weight loss on appetite and food intake in overweight subjects. European Journal of Clinical Nutrition, 57,1268-1274.

443. Aro A et al. (2000). Inverse association between dietary and serum conjugated linoleic acid and risk of breast cancer in postmenopausal women. Nutrition and Cancer, 38,151-157.

444. McCann SE et al. (2004). Dietary Intake of Conjugated Linoleic Acids and Risk of Premenopausal and Postmenopausal Breast Cancer, Western New York Exposures and Breast Cancer Study (WEB Study). Cancer Epidemiology, Biomarkers & Prevention, 13,9,1480-1484.

445. Voorrips LE et al. (2002). Intake of conjugated linoleic acid, fat, and other fatty acids in relation to postmenopausal breast cancer: the Netherlands Cohort Study on Diet and Cancer. American Journal of Clinical Nutrition, 76,4,873-782.

446. Field CJ et al. (2004). Evidence for potential mechanisms for the effect of conjugated linoleic acid on tumor metabolism and immune function: lessons from n-3 fatty acids. American Journal of Clinical Nutrition, 79,(6 Suppl),1190S-1198S.

447. Masters N et al. (2002). Maternal supplementation with CLA decreases milk fat in humans. Lipids, 37,2,133-8.

448. Miner JLet al. (2001). Conjugated linoleic acid (CLA), body fat, and apoptosis. Obesity Research, 9,129-134.

449. Mihic S et al. (2000). Acute creatine loading increases fat-free mass, but does not affect blood pressure, plasma creatinine, or CK activity in men and women. Medicine and Science in Sports and Exercise, 32,291-296.

450. Calhoun KE et al. (2003). Dehydroepiandrosterone sulfate causes proliferation of estrogen receptor-positive breast cancer cells despite treatment with fulvestrant. Archives of Surgery, 138,879-883.

451. Stoll BA. (1999). Dietary supplements of dehydroepiandrosterone in relation to breast cancer risk. European Journal of Clinical Nutrition, 53,771-775.

452. Orner GA et al. (1995). Dehydroepiandrosterone is a complete hepatocarcinogen and potent tumor promoter in the absence of peroxisome proliferation in rainbow trout. Carcinogenesis, 16,2893-2898.

453. Orner GA, et al. (1998). Modulation of aflatoxin-B1 hepatocarcinogenesis in trout by dehydroepiandrosterone: initiation/post-initiation and latency effects. Carcinogenesis, 19,1,161-167.

454. Araghiniknam M et al. (1996). Antioxidant activity of dioscorea and dehydroepiandrosterone (DHEA) in older humans. Life Sciences, 59,11, PL147-P157.

455. Roger PP et al. (1990). Regulation of dog thyroid epithelial cell cycle by forskolin, an adenylate cyclase activator. Experimental Cell Research, 172,282-292.

456. Christenson JT et al. (1995). The effect of forskolin on blood flow, platelet metabolism, aggregation and ATP release. Journal of Vascular Disease, 24,56-61.

457. Roy S et al. (2004). Body weight and abdominal fat gene expression profile in response to a novel hydroxycitric acid-based dietary supplement. Gene Expression, 11,(5-6):251-262.

458. Kengo Ishihara et al. (2000). Chronic (-)-Hydroxycitrate Administration Spares Carbohydrate Utilization and Promotes Lipid Oxidation during Exercise in Mice, Journal of Nutrition, 130, 2990-2995.

459.   Lim K, et al. (2002). Short-term (-)-hydroxycitrate ingestion increases fat oxidation during exercise in athletes. Journal of Nutritional Science and Vitaminology, 48(2):128-33.

460.   Tomita K et al. (2003). (-)-hydroxycitrate ingestion increases fat oxidation during moderate intensity exercise in untrained men. Bioscience, Biotechnology, and Biochemistry, 67, 9, 1999-2001.

461.   Cirigliano MD et al. (2001). Horny goat weed for erectile dysfunction. Alternative Medical Alert. 4,19-22.

462.   Frick L. Gale Encyclopedia of Alternative Medicine. (accessed 9/18/04).

463.   Kruger MC, et al. (1998). Calcium, gamma-linolenic acid and eicosapentaenoic acid supplementation in senile osteoporosis. Aging (Milano), 10,385-394.

464.   Bassey EJ et al. (2000). Lack of effect of supplementation with essential fatty acids on bone mineral density in healthy pre- and postmenopausal women: two randomized controlled trials of EfacalW v. calcium alone. British Journal of Nutrition, 83, 629–635.

465.   Khoo SK et al. (1990). Evening primrose oil and treatment of premenstrual syndrome. Medical Journal of Australia, 153,4,189-192.

466.   Chenoy R et al. (1994). Effect of oral gamolenic acid from evening primrose oil on menopausal flushing. British Medical Journal, 308,501-503.

467.   Budeiri D et al. (1996). Is evening primrose oil of value in the treatment of premenstrual syndrome? Controlled Clinical Trials, 17,60-68.

468.   Hardy ML (2000). Herbs of special interest to women. Journal of the American Pharmaceutical Association. 40,2,234-242.

469.   Gateley CA et al. (1992). Drug treatments for mastalgia: 17 years experience in the Cardiff Mastalgia Clinic. Journal of the Royal Society of Medicine, 85,1,12-5.

470.   Pye JK et al. (1985). Clinical experience of drug treatments for mastalgia. Lancet, 2,373-377.

471.   Blommers J et al. (2000). Evening primrose oil and fish oil for severe chronic astalgia: a randomized, double-blind, controlled trial. American Journal of Obstetrics and Gynecology, 187,5,1389-1394.

472.   Belch JJ et al. (1988). Effects of altering dietary essential fatty acids on requirements for non-steroidal anti-inflammatory drugs in patients with rheumatoid arthritis: A double blind placebo controlled study. Annals of the Rheumatic Diseases,47,96-104.

473.   Belch JJ et al. (2000). Evening primrose oil and borage oil in rheumatologic conditions. American Journal of Clinical Nutrition, 71,352S-360S.

474.   Brzeski M et al. (1991). Evening primrose oil in patients with rheumatoid arthritis and side-effects of non-steroidal anti-inflammatory drugs. British Journal of Rheumatology, 30,5,370-372.

475.   Hansen TM et al. (1983). Treatment of rheumatoid arthritis with prostaglandin E1 precursors cis-linoleic acid and gamma-linolenic acid. Scandinavian Journal of Rheumatology. 12,2,85-88.

476.   Zurier RB et al. (1996). Gamma-Linolenic acid treatment of rheumatoid arthritis. A randomized, placebo-controlled trial. Arthritis and Rheumatism, 39,11,1808-1817.

477.   WebMD Homepage. Dean Ornish, MD Q and A. Is the omega-6 supplement harmful? (accessed 9/19/04).

478.   Dove D et al. (1999). Oral evening primrose oil: its effect on length of pregnancy and selected intrapartum outcomes in low-risk nulliparous women. Journal of Nurse-Midwifery, 44,320-324.

479.   Vaddadi KS. (1981). The use of gamma-linolenic acid and linoleic acid to differentiate between temporal lobe epilepsy and schizophrenia. Prostaglandins and Medicine,6,375-379.

428

480.   Holman CP, et al. (1983). A trial of evening primrose oil in the treatment of chronic schizophrenia. *Journal of Orthomolecular Psychiatry*, 12,302-304.
481.   Lee KA et al. (2001). Restless legs syndrome and sleep disturbance · during pregnancy: the role of folate and iron. Journal of Women's Health & Gender-Based Medicine, 10,4,335-341.
482.   Murphy MM et al. (2004). Maternal homocysteine before conception and throughout pregnancy predicts fetal homocysteine and birth weight. Clinical Chemistry, 50,8,1406-1412.
483.   Austin RC et al. (2004). Role of hyperhomocysteinemia in endothelial dysfunction and atherothrombotic disease. Cell Death and Differentiation, 11 Suppl 1:S56-S64.
484.   Graham IM et al. (1997). Plasma homocysteine as a risk factor for vascular disease. The European Concerted Action Project. *JAMA*. 277,1775–1781.
485.   Wald NJ et al. (1998). Homocysteine and ischemic heart disease: results of a prospective study with implications regarding prevention. Archives of Internal Medicine, 158, 862–867.
486.   No author listed. What is homocysteine? American Heart Association. www.americanheart.org (accessed 9/20/04).
487.   Shrubsole MJ et al.(2001). Dietary folate intake and breast cancer risk: results from the Shanghai Breast Cancer Study. Cancer Research, 61,7136-7141.
488.   Fuchs CS et al. (2002). The influence of folate and multivitamin use on the familial risk of colon cancer in women. Cancer epidemiology, biomarkers & prevention, 11,227-234.
489.   Stolzenberg-Solomon RZ et al. (2001). Dietary and other methyl-group availability factors and pancreatic cancer risk in a cohort of male smokers. American Journal of Epidemiology, 153,680-987.
490.   Schroder H et al. (1986). Folic acid supplements in vitamin tablets: a determinant of hematological drug tolerance in maintenance therapy of childhood acute lymphoblastic leukemia. Pediatric Hematology and Oncology, 3,241-247.
491.   Cannon J (2004). Nutrition Essentials. Infinity publishers.
492.   Froscher W et al. (1995) Folate deficiency, anticonvulsant drugs, and psychiatric morbidity. Clinical Neuropharmacology, 18,165-182.
493.   Tonstad S et al. (1996). Low dose colestipol in adolescents with familial hypercholesterolemia. Archives of disease in childhood, 74,157-160.
494.   Morrow LE et al. (1999). Long-term diuretic therapy in hypertensive patients: effects on serum homocysteine, vitamin B6, vitamin B12, and red blood cell folate concentrations. Southern Medical Journal, 92,866-870.
495.   Margen, S (2002). Wellness Foods A to Z. UC Berkley. Rebus.
496.   No author. Folic Acid Fortification. FDA Consumer Magazine. February 1999. www.fda.gov/FDAC/ (accessed 9/20/04).
497.   Bang HO et al. (1973). The composition of food consumed by Greenlandic Eskimos. Acta medica Scandinavica, 200,69-73.
498.   Dallongeville J et al. (2003). Fish consumption is associated with lower heart rates. Circulation, 108,820-825.
499.   Nestel PJ. (2000). Fish oil and cardiovascular disease: lipids and arterial function. American Journal of Clinical Nutrition, 71,228S-231S.
500.   Tavani A et al. (2003). n-3 polyunsaturated fatty acid intake and cancer risk in Italy and Switzerland. International Journal of Cancer, 105, 113-116.
501.   Wigmore SJ et al. (2000). Effect of oral eicosapentaenoic acid on weight loss in patients with pancreatic cancer. Nutrition and Cancer, 36,2, 177-84.

502.　Barber MD et al. (1996). The effect of an oral nutritional supplement enriched with fish oil on weight-loss in patients with pancreatic cancer. British Journal of Cancer, 81,1, 80-6.

503.　Geusens P et al. (1994). Long-term effect of omega-3 fatty acid supplementation in active rheumatoid arthritis. A 12-month, double-blind, controlled study. Annals of Rheumatology, 37,6, 824-829.

504.　Volker D et al. (2000). Efficacy of fish oil concentrate in the treatment of rheumatoid arthritis. Journal of Rheumatology,27,10, 2343-2346.

505.　Vandongen R et al. (1993). Effects on blood pressure of omega 3 fats in subjects at increased risk of cardiovascular disease. Hypertension, 22,371-379.

506.　Toft I, Bonaa KH, Ingebretsen OC, et al. Effects of n-3 polyunsaturated fatty acids on glucose homeostasis and blood pressure in essential hypertension. A randomized, controlled trial. Annals of Internal Medicine, 123,911-918.

507.　von Schacky C et al. (1999). The effect of dietary omega-3 fatty acids on coronary atherosclerosis. A randomized, double-blind, placebo-controlled trial. Annals of Internal Medicine, 130, 554-562.

508.　Mori TA et al. (1999). Dietary fish as a major component of a weight-loss diet: effect on serum lipids, glucose, and insulin metabolism in overweight hypertensive subjects. American Journal of Clinical Nutrition, 70,817-825.

509.　Bao DQ et al. (1998). Effects of dietary fish and weight reduction on ambulatory blood pressure in overweight hypertensives. Hypertension, 32,4, 710-7.

510.　Wander J (2003). The New Heart Alarm. WebMD.com. (accessed 9/21/04).

511.　Jones WL et al. (2002). Pilot study; an emulsified fish oil supplement can significantly improve C-reactive protein, hemoglobin, albumin and urine output in chronic hemodialysis volunteers. Journal of the American Nutraceutical Association, 5,46-50.

512.　Mori TA et al. (2000). Purified eicosapentaenoic and docosahexaenoic acids have differential effects on serum lipids and lipoproteins, LDL particle size, glucose, and insulin in mildly hyperlipidemic men. American Journal of Clinical Nutrition, 71,5,1085-1094.

513.　Meydani SN et al. (1993). Influence of dietary fatty acids on cytokine production and its clinical implications. Nutrition in Clinical Practice, 8,65-72.

514.　Product Review: Omega-3 Fatty Acids (EPA and DHA) from Fish/Marine Oils Consumerlab.com. (accessed 9/22/04).

515.　No author listed. Omega-oil: fish or pills? Consumer Reports, July 2003.

516.　Adapted from: American Heart Association Web site. Fish, levels of mercury and omega-3 fatty acids. www.americanheart.org (accessed 9/22/04).

517.　Colman, E et al. (2002). Sport science exchange roundtable #50. Vol 13, number 4. Herbal supplements and sport performance. Gatorade Sport Science Institute web site. www.gssiweb.com. (accessed 9/23/04).

518.　Fry AC (1997). The effects of gamma-oryzanol supplementation during resistance exercise training. International Journal of Sport Nutrition, 7,4, 318-329.

519.　Williams M (1993). Sport science exchange #47. Vol 6, number 6. Nutritional supplements for strength trained athletes. Gatorade Sport Science Institute web site. www.gssiweb.com (accessed 9/23/04).

520.　Wheeler KB et al. (1991). Gamma oryzanol-plant sterol supplementation: metabolic, endocrine, and physiologic effects. International Journal of Sport Nutrition, 1,170-177.

430

521. Cicero AF et al. (2001). Rice bran oil and gamma-oryzanol in the treatment of hyperlipoproteinaemias and other conditions. Phytotherapy Research, 15,277-289.

522. Seetharamaiah GS et al. (1991). Gamma oryzanol-plant sterol supplementation: metabolic, endocrine, and physiologic effects. International Journal of Sport Nutrition, 1,2,170-177.

523. Koscielny J et al. (1999). The antiatherosclerotic effect of Allium sativum. Atherosclerosis, 144,237-249.

524. Vorberg G et al. (1990). Therapy with garlic: results of a placebo-controlled, double-blind study. British Journal of Clinical Practice Supplement, 69,7-11.

525. Adler AJ, et al. (1997). Effect of garlic and fish-oil supplementation on serum lipid and lipoprotein concentrations in hypercholesterolemic men. American Journal of Clinical Nutrition, 65,2,445-450.

526. Fleischauer AT (2000). Garlic consumption and cancer prevention: meta-analyses of colorectal and stomach cancers. American Journal of Clinical Nutrition, 72,1047-1052.

527. Hsing AW et al. (2002). Allium vegetables and risk of prostate cancer: a population-based study. Journal of the National Cancer Institute, 94,1648-1651.

528. Ide N et al. (1999)> Aged garlic extract attenuates intracellular oxidative stress. Phytomedicine, 6,125-131.

529. Ankri S et al. (1999). Antimicrobial properties of allicin from garlic. Microbes and infection, 1,125-129.

530. Josling P. (2001). Preventing the common cold with a garlic supplement: a double-blind, placebo-controlled survey. Advances in Therapy, 18,189-193.

531. Piscitelli SC et al. (2002). The effect of garlic supplements on the pharmacokinetics of saquinavir. Clinical Infectious Diseases, 34,234-238.

532. Schardt, D (2000). Garlic: case unclosed. Nutrition Action Health Letter. www.cspinet.org (accessed 9/26/04).

533. Stevinson C et al. (Oct. 2000). Garlic for treating hypercholesterolemia. A meta-analysis of randomized clinical trials. Annals of Internal Medicine, 133,6,420-429.

534. Ackermann RTet al. (2001). Garlic shows promise for improving some cardiovascular risk factors. Archives of Internal Medicine, 161,813-824.

535. Schardt, D (May 2001). Keeping a lid on blood sugar. Nutrition Action Health Letter www.cspinet.org (accessed 9/26/04).

536. Tschop, M et. al. (2000). Ghrelin induces adiposity in rodents. Nature, 407, 908-913.

537. Wren, A.M. et. al. (2000). The novel hypothalamic peptide ghrelin stimulates food intake and growth hormone secretion. Endocrinology, 141,4325-4328.

538. Mucciloi, G. et. al. (2002). Neuroendocrine and peripheral activities of ghrelin. European Journal of Pharmacology, 440, 2-3, 235-254.

539. Hansen, T.K. (2002). Weight loss increases circulating levels of ghrelin in human obesity. Clinical Endocrinology, 56, 2, 203-206.

540. No author. Research Highlights: the hormone that harms diets. National Institutes of Health. www.nih.gov. (accessed 9/26/04).

541. Kraemer RR et al. (2004). Ghrelin and other glucoregulatory hormone responses to eccentric and concentric muscle contractions. Endocrine, 1,93-98.

542. Moskowitz RW. (2000). Role of collagen hydrolysate in bone and joint disease. Seminars in Arthritis and Rheumatism, 30,87-99.

543. Kiesewetter H et al. (2000). Efficacy of orally administered extract of red vine leaf AS 195 (folia vitis viniferae) in chronic venous insufficiency

(stages I-II). A randomized, double-blind, placebo-controlled trial. Arzneimittelforschung, 50,109-17.

544. Vigna GB et al. (2003). Effect of a standardized grape seed extract on low-density lipoprotein susceptibility to oxidation in heavy smokers. Metabolism. 52,10,1250-1257.

545. Nuttall SL et al. (1998). An evaluation of the antioxidant activity of a standardized grape seed extract, Leucoselect. Journal of clinical Pharmacy and Therapeutics, 23,5,385-389.

546. Pataki T et al. (2002). Grape seed proanthocyanidins improved cardiac recovery during reperfusion after ischemia in isolated rat hearts. American Journal of Clinical Nutrition, 75,5,894-899.

547. Sato M et al. (1999). Cardioprotective effects of grape seed proanthocyanidin against ischemic reperfusion injury. Journal of Molecular and Cellular Cardiology, 31,6,1289-1297.

548. Sharma G et al. (2004). Synergistic anti-cancer effects of grape seed extract and conventional cytotoxic agent doxorubicin against human breast carcinoma cells. Breast Cancer Research and Treatment, 85,1,1-12.

549. Vayalil PK, et al. (2004). Proanthocyanidins from grape seeds inhibit expression of matrix metalloproteinases in human prostate carcinoma cells, which is associated with the inhibition of activation of MAPK and NF kappa B. Carcinogenesis, 25,5,987-995.

550. Singh RP et al. (2004). Grape seed extract inhibits advanced human prostate tumor growth and angiogenesis and upregulates insulin-like growth factor binding protein-3. International journal of Cancer, 108,5,733-740.

551. Gehm BD et al. (1997). Resveratrol, a polyphenolic compound found in grapes and wine, is an agonist for the estrogen receptor. Proceedings of the National Academy of Sciences, 94,25,14138-14143.

552. Kozuki Y et al. (2001). Resveratrol suppresses hepatoma cell invasion independently of its anti-proliferative action. Cancer Lett 2001;167:151-6. Cancer Letters, 167,151-156.

553. Bertelli AA, et al. (1995). Antiplatelet activity of synthetic and natural resveratrol in red wine. International Journal of Tissue Reactions, 17,1,1-3.

554. Rai GS et al. (1991). A double-blind, placebo-controlled study of Ginkgo biloba extract ('tanakan') in elderly outpatients with mild to moderate memory impairment. Current Medical Research and Opinion, 12, 350-355.

555. Rigney U et al. (1999). The effects of acute doses of standardized Ginkgo biloba extract on memory and psychomotor performance in volunteers. Phytotherapy Research, 13,5, 408-415.

556. Le Bars PL et al. (1997). Berman N, et al. A placebo-controlled, double-blind, randomized trial of an extract of Ginkgo biloba for dementia. North American EGb Study Group. JAMA, 278,1327–1332.

557. Solomon PR et al. (2002). Ginkgo for memory enhancement: a randomized controlled trial. JAMA, 288,835-840.

558. Kennedy DO et al. (2000). The dose-dependent cognitive effects of acute administration of Ginkgo biloba to healthy young volunteers. Psychopharmacology, 151,416-423.

559. Brautigam MR et al. (1998). Treatment of age-related memory complaints with Gingko biloba extract: a randomized double blind placebo-controlled study. Phytomedicine 1998;5:425-34.

560. Diamond BJ et al. (2000). Ginkgo biloba extract: mechanisms and clinical indications. Archives of Physician Medicine and Rehabilitation, 81,668-678.

432

561. Paick J et al. (1996). An experimental study of the effect of ginkgo biloba extract on the human and rabbit corpus cavernosum tissue. Journal of Urology, 156,1876-1880.
562. Kanowski S et al. (1996). Proof of efficacy of the ginkgo biloba special extract EGb 761 in outpatients suffering from mild to moderate primary degenerative dementia of the Alzheimer type or multi-infarct dementia. Pharmacopsychiatry, 29,2,47-56.
563. van Dongen M (2003). Ginkgo for elderly people with dementia and age-associated memory impairment: a randomized clinical trial. Journal of Clinical Epidemiology, 56,4,367-376.
564. Oken BS et al. (1998). The efficacy of Ginkgo biloba on cognitive function in Alzheimer disease. Archives of Neurology, 55,1409-1415.
565. Cohen AJ, et al. (1998). Ginkgo biloba for antidepressant-induced sexual dysfunction. Journal of Sex and Marital Therapy, 24,2,139-143.
566. Granger AS. (2001). Ginkgo biloba precipitating epileptic seizures. Age and Ageing, 30,6,523-525.
567. Kudolo GB (2000). The effect of 3-month ingestion of Ginkgo biloba extract on pancreatic beta-cell function in response to glucose loading in normal glucose tolerant individuals. Journal of Clinical Pharmacology, 40,6,647-654.
568. Kudolo GB (2001). The effect of 3-month ingestion of Ginkgo biloba extract (EGb 761) on pancreatic beta-cell function in response to glucose loading in individuals with non-insulin-dependent diabetes mellitus. Journal of Clinical Pharmacology, 41,6, 600-611.
569. Benjamin J et al. (2001). A case of cerebral haemorrhage-can Ginkgo biloba be implicated? Journal of Postgraduate Medicine, 77,904,112-113.
570. Kiple KF (2000). The Cambridge World History of Food. Cambridge University Press, Cambridge.
571. Wang X et al. (1999). Determination of ginsenosides in plant extracts from Panax ginseng and Panax quinquefolius L. by LC/MS/MS. Analytical Chemistry, 71,8,1579-1584.
572. Vuksan V et al. (2000). American ginseng (Panax quinquefolius L) reduces postprandial glycemia in nondiabetic subjects and subjects with type 2 diabetes mellitus. Archives of Internal Medicine, 160,1009-1013.
573. Vuksan V et al. (2001). American ginseng (Panax quinquefolius L.) attenuates postprandial glycemia in a time-dependent but not dose-dependent manner in healthy individuals. American Journal of Clinical Nutrition, 73,4, 753-758.
574. Vuksan V et al. (2000). Similar postprandial glycemic reductions with escalation of dose and administration time of American ginseng in type 2 diabetes. Diabetes Care, 23,1221-1226.
575. Sotaniemi EA et al. (1995). Ginseng therapy in non-insulin-dependent diabetic patients. Diabetes Care, 18,1373–1375.
576. Vuksan V et al. (2000). American ginseng improves glycemia in individuals with normal glucose tolerance: effect of dose and time escalation. Journal of the American College of Nutrition, 19,6,738-744.
577. Morris AC et al. (1996). No ergogenic effect on ginseng ingestion. International Journal of Sports Nutrition, 6,263-271.
578. Allen JD et al. (1998). Ginseng supplementation does not enhance healthy young adults' peak aerobic exercise performance. Journal of the American College of Nutrition, 17,5, 462-466.
579. Coleman et al. (2002). Herbal supplements and sport performance. Sports Science Exchange Roundtable 50. Vol 13 Number 4 Gatorade Sport Science Institute www.gssiweb.com. (accessed October 19 2004).

433

580.   Yuan CS et al. (1999). Panax quinquefolium L. inhibits thrombin-induced endothelin release in vitro. American Journal of Chinese Medicine, 27,331-338.
581.   Chan LY et al. (2003). An in-vitro study of ginsenoside Rb(1)-induced teratogenicity using a whole rat embryo culture model. Human Reproduction And Genetic Ethics,18,2166-2168.
582.   Yuan CS, et al. (2004). Brief Communication: American Ginseng reduces Warfarin's effect in healthy patients. Annals of Internal Medicine, 141,23-27.
583.   Yun TK et al. (2001). Epidemiological study on cancer prevention by ginseng: are all kinds of cancers preventable by ginseng? Journal of Korean Medical Science, 16 Suppl:S19-27.
584.   Yun TK et al. (1998). Non-organ specific cancer prevention of ginseng: a prospective study in Korea. International Journal of Epidemiology, 27,3,359-364.
585.   Food and Drug Administration. Center for Food Safety and Applied Nutrition. Products that Consumers Inquire About. http://vm.cfsan.fda.gov/~dms/ds-prod.html (accessed October 22 2004).
586.   Food and Drug Administration. Information Paper on L-tryptophan and 5-hydroxy-L-tryptophan. February 2001.www.fda.gov. (accessed October 22 2004),
587.   Clarkson PM. Sport Sciences Library. Will ginseng get my energy up for races? Gatorade Sport Science institute. www.gssiweb.com (accessed 10/25/04)
588.   Lieberman HR (2001). The effects of ginseng, ephedrine, and caffeine on cognitive performance, mood and energy. Annual Review of Nutrition, 59,4,91-102.
589.   Kennedy DO et al. (2003). Electroencephalograph effects of single doses of Ginkgo biloba and Panax ginseng in healthy young volunteers. Pharmacology, Biochemistry, and Behavior, 75,3,701-709.
590.   Sorensen H et al. (1996). A double-masked study of the effects of ginseng on cognitive functions. Current Therapeutic Research, 57,959-968.
591.   Persson J et al. (2004). The memory-enhancing effects of Ginseng and Ginkgo biloba in healthy volunteers. Psychopharmacology (Berl),72,4, 430-434.
592.   Hong B et al.(2002). A double-blind crossover study evaluating the efficacy of Korean red ginseng in patients with erectile dysfunction: a preliminary report. Journal of Urology, 168,2070-2073.
593.   Kang HY et al. (2002). Effects of ginseng ingestion on growth hormone, testosterone, cortisol and insulin-like growth factor 1 to acute resistance exercise. Journal of Strength and Conditioning Research, 16,2,179-183.
594.   Engles, HJ et al. (2001). Effect of ginseng supplementation on supramaximal exercise performance and short term recovery. Journal of Strength and Conditioning Research, 15,3,290-295.
595.   Engles HJ et al. (1997). No ergogenic effects of ginseng (Panax ginseng, C.A. Meyer) during graded maximal aerobic exercise. Journal of the American Dietetic Association, 97,1110-1115.
596.   Wiklund IK et al. (1999). Effects of a standardized ginseng extract on quality of life and physiological parameters in symptomatic postmenopausal women: a double-blind, placebo-controlled trial. International Journal of Clinical Pharmacology Research,19,89-99.
597.   Huntley AL et al. (2003). A systematic review of herbal medicinal products for the treatment of menopausal symptoms. Menopause, 10,5,465-476.

598.   Keum YS et al. (2000). Antioxidant and anti-tumor promoting activities of the methanol extract of heat-processed ginseng. Cancer Letters, 150,1,41-48.

599.   Moon J et al. (2000). Induction of G(1) cell cycle arrest and p27(KIP1) increase by panaxydol isolated from Panax ginseng. Advances in Steroid Biochemistry and Pharmacology, 59,9,1109-1116.

600.   Shin HR et al. (2000). The cancer-preventive potential of Panax ginseng: a review of human and experimental evidence. Cancer Causes and Control, 11,565-576. 601.

602.   Yun TK (2003). Experimental and epidemiological evidence on non-organ specific cancer preventive effect of Korean ginseng and identification of active compounds. Mutation Research, 523-524,63-64.

603.   Jeon BH et al. (2000). Effect of Korea red ginseng on the blood pressure in conscious hypertensive rats. General Pharmacology, 35,3, 135-141.

604.   Yun YP et al. (2001). Effects of Korean red ginseng and its mixed prescription on the high molecular weight dextran-induced blood stasis in rats and human platelet aggregation. Journal of Ethnopharmacology, 77,259-264.

605.   Lee Y et al. (2003). A ginsenoside-Rh1, a component of ginseng saponin, activates estrogen receptor in human breast carcinoma MCF-7 cells. Journal of Steroid Biochemistry and Molecular Biology, 84,4,463-468.

607.   Baranov AI (1982). Medicinal uses of ginseng and related plants in the Soviet Union: recent trends in the Soviet literature. Journal of Ethnopharmacology, 6,3,339-353.

608.   Davydov M et al. (2000). Eleutherococcus senticosus (Rupr. & Maxim.) Maxim. (Araliaceae) as an adaptogen: a closer look. Journal of Ethnopharmacology, 72,345-393.

609.   Dowling EA et al. (1996). Effect of Eleutherococcus senticosus on submaximal and maximal exercise performance. Medicine and Science in Sports and Exercise, 28,4, 482-489.

610.   Eschbach LC et al. (2000). The effect of siberian ginseng (Eleutherococcus senticosus) on substrate utilization and performance. International Journal of Sport Nutrition and Exercise Metabolism, 10,444-151.

611.   Asano K, Takahashi T, Miyashita M, et al. (1986). Effect of Eleutherococcus senticosus extract on human physical working capacity. Planta Medica, 3,175-177.

612.   Bucci LR (2000). Selected herbals and human exercise performance. American Journal of Clinical Nutrition, 72, 2, 624S-636s.

613.   Arushanian EB et al. (2003). Effect of eleutherococcus on short-term memory and visual perception in healthy humans. Eksperimental'naia I Klinicheskaia Farmakologiia, 66,5,10-30.

614.   Winther K et al. (1997). Russian root (Siberian Ginseng) improves cognitive functions in middle-aged people, whereas Ginkgo biloba seems effective only in the elderly. Journal of the Neurological Sciences, 150, S90.

615.   Sui DY et al. (1994). [Effects of the leaves of Acanthopanax senticosus (Rupr. et Maxim.) Harms. On myocardial infarct size in acute ischemic dogs]. [Article in Chinese]. China Journal of Chinese Materia Medica, 19,746-764.

616.   Han L et al. (1998). Clinical and experimental study on treatment of acute cerebral infarction with Acanthopanax Injection. Zhongguo Zhong Xi Yi Jie He Za Zhi 18,472-474.

617.   Wang H et al. (2003). Asian and Siberian ginseng as a potential modulator of immune function: an in vitro cytokine study using mouse

macrophages. International Journal of Clinical Chemistry, 327(1-2),123-128.

618. Jeong HJ et al. (2001). Inhibitory effects of mast cell-mediated allergic reactions by cell cultured Siberian Ginseng. Immunopharmacology and Immunotoxicology. 23,1,107-117.

619. Gaffney BT et al. (2001). The effects of Eleutherococcus senticosus and Panax ginseng on steroidal hormone indices of stress and lymphocyte subset numbers in endurance athletes. Basic Life Sciences, 70,4,431-442.

620. Harkey MR. (2001). Variability in commercial ginseng products: an analysis of 25 preparations. American Journal of Clinical Nutrition, 73, 6, 1101-1106.

621. Rundek T et al. (2004). Atorvastatin decreases the coenzyme Q10 level in the blood of patients at risk for cardiovascular disease and stroke. Archives of Neurology, 61,6,889-892.

622. Bargossi AM et al. (1994). Exogenous CoQ10 supplementation prevents plasma ubiquinone reduction induced by HMG-CoA reductase inhibitors. Molecular Aspects of Medicine, 15, Suppl., S187-S193.

623. Hikino H et a; (1986). Isolation and hypoglycemic activity of eleutherans A, B, C, D, E, F, and G: glycans of Eleutherococcus senticosus roots. Journal of Asian Natural Products Research, 49,293-297.

624. McRae S. (1996). Elevated serum digoxin levels in a patient taking digoxin and Siberian ginseng. Canadian Medical Association Journal, 155,293-295.

625. Yun-Choi HS et al. (1987). Potential inhibitors of platelet aggregation from plant sources, III. Journal of Asian Natural Products Research, 50,1059-1064.

626. Kumar M et al. (2003). Radioprotective effect of Panax ginseng on the phosphatases and lipid peroxidation level in testes of Swiss albino mice. Biological & Pharmaceutical Bulletin, 26,3,308-312.

627. Han KH et al. (1998). Effect of red ginseng on blood pressure in patients with essential hypertension and white coat hypertension. American Journal of Chinese Medicine, 26,2,199-209.

628. Neil HA et al. (2001). Randomized controlled trial of use by hypercholesterolaemic patients of a vegetable oil sterol-enriched fat spread. Atherosclerosis, 156,329-337.

629. Vido L et al. (1993). Childhood obesity treatment: double blinded trial on dietary fibres (glucomannan) versus placebo. Padiatrie und Padologie, 28(5):133-6.

630. Cairella M et al. (1995). Evaluation of the action of glucomannan on metabolic parameters and on the sensation of satiation in overweight and obese patients. La Clinica terapeutica, 146,4,269-274.

631. Livieri C et al. (1992). The use of highly purified glucomannan-based fibers in childhood obesity [Article in Italian]. Medical and Surgical Pediatrics, 14,195-198.

632. Vita PM et al. (1992). Chronic use of glucomannan in the dietary treatment of severe obesity [Article in Italian]. Minerva Medica, 83,135-139.

633. Walsh DE et al. (1984). Effect of glucomannan on obese patients: a clinical study. International Journal of Obesity, 8,289-293.

634. Gallaher CM et al. (2000). Cholesterol reduction by glucomannan and chitosan is mediated by changes in cholesterol absorption and bile acid and fat excretion in rats. Journal of Nutrition, 130,2753-2759.

635. Chen HL et al.(2003). Konjac supplement alleviated hypercholesterolemia and hyperglycemia in type 2 diabetic subjects--a randomized double-blind trial. Journal of the American College of Nutrition, 22,36-42.

436

636.   Vuksan V et al. (1999). Konjac-mannan (glucomannan) improves glycemia and other associated risk factors for coronary heart disease in type 2 diabetes. A randomized controlled metabolic trial. Diabetes Care, 22,913-919.

637.   Arvill A, et al. (1995). Effect of short-term ingestion of konjac glucomannan on serum cholesterol in healthy men. American Journal of Clinical Nutrition, 61,3,585-589.

638.   Henry DA et al. (1986). Glucomannan and risk of oesophageal obstruction. British Medical Journal, 1986;292:591–592.

639.   Runkel D et al. (1999). Glucosamine sulfate use in osteoarthritis. American Journal of Health-System Pharmacy, 56,267-269.

640.   Reginster JY et al. (2001). Long-term effects of glucosamine sulfate on osteoarthritis progression: a randomized, placebo-controlled trial. Lancet, 357,251-256.

641.   Wise C (2001). Osteoarthritis. In DC Dale, DD Federman, eds., Scientific American Medicine, vol. 3, part 15, chap. 10, pp. 1–8. New York: Scientific American.

642.   Drovanti A et al. (1980). Therapeutic activity of oral glucosamine sulfate in osteoarthritis: A placebo-controlled double-blind investigation. Clinical Therapeutics, 3, 4, 260-272.

643.   da Camara CC (1998). Glucosamine sulfate for osteoarthritis. Annals of Pharmacotherapy, 32, 580-587.

644.   Braham R et al. (2003). The effect of glucosamine supplementation on people experiencing regular knee pain. British Journal of Sports Medicine, 37,45-49.

645.   Richy F et al. (2003). Structural and symptomatic efficacy of glucosamine and chondroitin in knee osteoarthritis: a comprehensive meta-analysis. Archives of Internal Medicine, 163,1514-1522.

646.   Pavelka K et al. (2002). Glucosamine sulfate use and delay of progression of knee osteoarthritis: A 3-year, randomized, placebo-controlled, double-blind study. Archives of Internal Medicine, 162,2113-2123.

647.   Rindone JP et al. (2000). Randomized, controlled trial of glucosamine for treating osteoarthritis of the knee. Western Journal of Medicine, 172,91-94.

648.   Hughes R et al. (2002). A randomized, double-blind, placebo-controlled trial of glucosamine sulphate as an analgesic in osteoarthritis of the knee. Rheumatology, 41,279-284.

649.   No authors. Glucosamine in arthritis. Gatorade Sport Science Institute Website. www.gssiweb.com . (accessed Nov. 12 2004).

650.   National Institutes of Health news release. Questions and Answers: NIH glucosamine/chondroitin arthritis intervention trial (GAIT). National Center for Complimentary and Alternative Medicine. http://nccam.nih.gov/ (accessed Nov. 12 2004).

651.   Muller-Fassbender H et al. (1994). Glucosamine sulfate compared to ibuprofen in osteoarthritis of the knee. Osteoarthritis Cartilage, 2,1,61-69.

652.   Davis JL (2000). Study raises new questions about glucosamine. WebMd.com. (accessed 11/16 /04).

653.   Rossetti L et al. (1995). In vivo glucosamine infusion induces insulin resistance in normoglycemic but not in hyperglycemic conscious rats. Journal of Clinical Investigation, 96,132-140.

654.   Scroggie DA et al. (2003). The effect of glucosamine-chondroitin supplementation on glycosylated hemoglobin levels in patients with type 2 diabetes mellitus: a placebo-controlled, double-blinded, randomized clinical trial. Archives of Internal Medicine, 163, 1587-1590.

655.   Yu JG et al. (2003). The effect of oral glucosamine sulfate on insulin sensitivity in human subjects. Diabetes Care, 30:523-528.

656.   Gray HC (2004). Is glucosamine safe in patients with seafood allergy
       (letter)? Journal of Allergy and Clinical Immunology, 114,459-460.
657.   Rozenfeld V et al. (2004). Possible augmentation of warfarin effect by
       glucosamine-chondroitin. American Journal of Health System Pharmacy,
       61,306-307.
658.   Tallia AF (2002). Asthma exacerbation associated with glucosamine-
       chondroitin supplement. Journal of the American Board of Family
       Practice, 15, 481-484.
659.   Leeb BF et al. (2000). A meta-analysis of chondroitin sulfate in the
       treatment of osteoarthritis. Journal of Rheumatology, 27,205-211.
660.   Erikson KM et al. (2004). Manganese exposure and induced oxidative
       stress in the rat brain. The Science of the Total Environment, 334-
       335,409-416.
661.   Medina MA. (2001). Glutamine and cancer. Journal of Nutrition, 131,
       2539S-2542S.
662.   Nieman DC (2003). Current perspective on exercise immunology.
       Current Sports Medicine Reports, 2,5, 239-242.
663.   Holecek M (2002). Relation between glutamine, branched-chain amino
       acids, and protein metabolism. Nutrition, 18,2,130-133.
664.   Shabert JK (1999). Wilmore DW. Glutamine-antioxidant supplementation
       increases body cell mass in AIDS patients with weight loss: a
       randomized, double-blind controlled trial. Nutrition, 15,860-864.
665.   Jones C (1999). Randomized clinical outcome study of critically ill
       patients given glutamine-supplemented enteral nutrition. Nutrition,
       15,108-115. 666.
667.   Antonio J et al. (2002). The effects of high-dose glutamine ingestion on
       weightlifting performance. Journal of Strength Condoning Research,
       16,157–160.
668.   Candow DG et al. (2001). Effect of glutamine supplementation combined
       with resistance training in young adults. European Journal of Applied
       Physiology,86,142–149.
669.   Haub MD et al. (1998). Acute L-glutamine ingestion does not improve
       maximal effort exercise. Journal of Sports Medicine and Physical
       Fitness, 38,3,240-244.
670.   Castell LM et al. (1998). Glutamine and the effects of exhaustive
       exercise upon the immune response. Canadian Journal of Physiology
       and Pharmacology. 76,5,524-532.
671.   Castell LM (2002). Can glutamine modify the apparent
       immunodepression observed after prolonged, exhaustive exercise?
       Nutrition, 18,5, 371-375.
672.   Mebane AH. L-Glutamine and mania [letter]. American Journal of
       Psychiatry, 141,1302-1303.
673.   Lamb B. Will taking glutamine prevent me from getting sick after a long
       race? Gatorade Sports Science Institute. www.gssiweb.com (accessed
       Nov. 26 2004).
674.   Chapman AG. (2000). Glutamate and epilepsy. Journal of Nutrition,
       130,1043S-1045S.
675.   Panton LB et al. (2000).Nutritional supplementation of the leucine
       metabolite beta-hydroxy-beta-methylbutyrate (HMB) during resistance
       training. Nutrition, 16,734-739.
676.   Vukovich MD et al. (2001). Body composition in 70-year-old adults
       responds to dietary beta-hydroxy-beta-methylbutyrate similarly to that of
       young adults. Journal of Nutrition, 131,7,2049-2052.
677.   Nissen S (2003). Effect of dietary supplements on lean mass and
       strength gains with resistance exercise: a meta analysis. Journal of
       Applied Physiology.94,651-659.

438

678. Nissen S et al. (1996). Effect of leucine metabolite beta-hydroxy-beta-methylbutyrate on muscle metabolism during resistance-exercise training. Journal of Applied Physiology, 81,5,2095-2104.

679. Thomson JS (2004). Beta-Hydroxy-beta-Methylbutyrate (HMB) supplementation of resistance trained men. Asia Pacific Journal of Clinical Nutrition.

680. Décombaz J (2003). HMB meta-analysis and the clustering of data sources. Journal of Applied Physiology, 95(5):2180-2182; author reply 2182.

681. O'Connor DM et al. (2003). Effects of beta-hydroxy-beta-methylbutyrate and creatine monohydrate supplementation on the aerobic and anaerobic capacity of highly trained athletes. Journal of Sports Medicine and Physical Fitness, 43,1,64-68.

682. Ransone J et al. (2003). The effect of beta-hydroxy beta-methylbutyrate on muscular strength and body composition in collegiate football players. Journal of Strength and Conditioning Research, 17(1):34-9.

683. Slater G et al. (2001). Beta-hydroxy-beta-methylbutyrate (HMB) supplementation does not affect changes in strength or body composition during resistance training in trained men. International Journal of Sport Nutrition and Exercise Metabolism, 11,3,384-396.

684. Slater GJ et al. (2000). Beta-hydroxy-beta-methylbutyrate (HMB) supplementation and the promotion of muscle growth and strength. Sports Medicine, 30,2,105-116.

685. Nissen, SK et al. (1997). Nutritional role of the leucine metabolite B-hydroxy B-methylbutyrate (HMB). Journal of Nutritional Biochemistry, 8, 300-311.

686. Slater GJ, et al. (2000). Beta-hydroxy beta-methylbutyrate (HMB) supplementation does not influence the urinary testosterone: epitestosterone ratio in healthy males. Journal of Science and Medicine in Sport / Sports Medicine Australia, 3,79-83.

687. No Authors listed. New product for treating facial wrinkles. FDA Consumer Magazine. March-April 2004.

688. Boyles S. (2003). Arthritis "Chicken Shots" May Not Work. WebMD.com (accessed 11/29/04).

689. Warning Letter to Hyalogic, LLC. May 5 2004. FDA web site. www.fda.gov (accessed 11/29/04).

690. Lebot, V. (1992). Kava: the Pacific Drug. Yale University.

691. Anke J et al. (2004). Kava Hepatotoxicity: Are we any closer to the truth? Planta Medica, 70(3):193-6.

692. Consumer Advisory (March 25 2002): Kava containing dietary supplements may be associated with severe liver injury. FDA Center for Food Safety and Applied Nutrition. FDA .www.cfsan.fda.gov (accessed 11/30/04).

693. Singh, Y.N. (1992). Kava: an Overview. Journal of Ethnopharmacology, 37, 13-45.

694. Swensen JN. (1996). Man convicted of driving under the influence of kava. Salt Lake City, UT: Desert News.

695. Stannard JN (Oct 28 2000). Kava drinking case in San Bruno ends in mistrial. San Francisco Chronicle p. A.24.

696. Russmann S et al. (2001). Kava hepatotoxicity [letter]. Annals of Internal Medicine, 135,68.

697. Mathews J et al. (1988). Effects of the heavy usage of kava on physical health: summary of a pilot survey in an Aboriginal community. Medical Journal of Australia, 148,548-555.

698. Schelosky L et al. (1995). Kava and dopamine antagonism [letter]. Journal of Neurology, Neurosurgery, and Psychiatry, `58,639-640.

699. Mathews JM et al. (2002). Inhibition of human cytochrome P450 activities by kava extract and kavalactones. Drug Metabolism and Disposition, 30,1153-1157.

700. Zou L et al. (2004). Effects of kava (Kava-kava, 'Awa, Yaqona, Piper methysticum) on c-DNA-expressed cytochrome P450 enzymes and human cryopreserved hepatocytes. Phytomedicine,11,4, 285-294.

701. Volz HP et al. (1997). Kava-kava extract WS 1490 versus placebo in anxiety disorders—a randomized placebo-controlled 25-week outpatient trial. Pharmacopsychiatry,30,1–5.

702. Pittler MH et al. (2000). Efficacy of kava extract for treating anxiety: systematic review and meta-analysis. Journal ofClinical Psychopharmacology,20,1,84-90.

703. Steiner GG. (2000). The correlation between cancer incidence and kava consumption. Hawaii Medical Journal, 59,420-422.

704. Bartlett H et al. (2004). An ideal ocular nutritional supplement? Ophthalmic & Physiological Optics, 24,4,339-349.

705. Alves-Rodrigues A (2004). The science behind lutein. Toxicology Letters, 150,1,57-83.

706. Mozaffarieh M (2004). The role of the carotenoids, lutein and zeaxanthin, in protecting against age-related macular degeneration: A review based on controversial evidence. Journal of Nutrition,2,20. www.nutritionj.com/content/2/1/20 (accessed 121/04)

707. Nkondjock A et al. (2004). Dietary carotenoids and risk of colon cancer: case-control study. International Journal of Cancer, 110,1,110-116.

708. Holden JM et al. (1999). Carotenoid content of US foods: an update to the database. Journal of Food Composition and Analysis, 12,169-196.

709. Donaldson MS (2004). Nutrition and Cancer: a review of the evidence for an anticancer diet. Journal of Nutrition,3,1,3-19.

710. Gionvannucci E. (1999). Tomatoes, tomato-based products, lycopene, and cancer: review of the epidemiological literature. Journal of the National Cancer Institute, 91,317-331.

711. Lu QY et al. (2001). Inverse associations between plasma lycopene and other carotenoids and prostate cancer. Cancer Epidemiology, Biomarkers & Prevention, 10,749-756.

712. Gartner C (1997). Lycopene is more bioavailable from tomato paste than from fresh tomatoes. American Journal of Clinical Nutrition, 66,1,116-122.

713. Adapted from: USDA/NCC Carotenoid Database for U.S. Foods (1998) & Linus Pauling Institute Macronutrient Information Center.

714. Gann PH, Khachik F. Tomatoes or lycopene versus prostate cancer: is evolution anti-reductionist? Journal of the National Cancer Institute, 95,1563-1565.

715. St-onge MP et al. (2002). Physiological Effects of Medium-Chain Triglycerides: Potential Agents in the Prevention of Obesity. Journal of Nutrition, 132,329-332.

716. Coyle EF et al. (1995). Fat metabolism during exercise. Fat metabolism during exercise. Sport Science Exchange SSE #59 Volume 8 number 6 Gatorade Sports Science Institute website. www.gssiweb.com (accessed 12/15/04).

717. Hawley JA et al. (1998). Strategies to enhance fat utilization during exercise. Sports Medicine, 25,4,241-257.

718. Melhorta, S et al. (2004). The therapeutic potential of melatonin: a review of the science. Medscape. General Medicine, 6,2. www.medscape.com (accessed 12/22/04).

719. Regelson W et al. (1987). Melatonin: A rediscovered antitumor hormone? Its relation to surface receptors; sex steroid metabolism,

440

immunologic response, and chronobiologic factors in tumor growth and therapy. Cancer Investigations, 5,379-385.

720. Herxheimer A et al. (2003). Melatonin for preventing and treating jet lag. British Medical Journal, 326,296-297.

721. Edwards BJ et al. (2000). Use of melatonin in recovery from jet-lag following an eastward flight across 10 time-zones. Ergonomics, 43,10, 1501-1513.

722. Leon J et al. (2005). Melatonin mitigates mitochondrial malfunction. Journal of Pineal Research, 38,1,1-9.

723. Zeitzer JM et al. (1999). Do plasma melatonin concentrations decline with age? American Journal of Medicine, 107,432-436.

724. Zhdanova IV et al. (2000).Melatonin treatment attenuates symptoms of acute nicotine withdrawal in humans. Pharmacology, Biochemistry, and Behavior, 67,131-153.

725. Luboshitzky R et al. (2002). Melatonin administration alters semen quality in healthy men. Journal of Andrology, 23,572-578.

726. Cagnacci A, Arangino S, Renzi A, et al. (2001). Influence of melatonin administration on glucose tolerance and insulin sensitivity of postmenopausal women. Clinical Endocrinology, (Oxf). 54, 339–346.

727. Usha PR et al. (2004). Randomised, double-blind, parallel, placebo-controlled study of oral glucosamine, methylsulfonylmethane and their combinations. Clinical Drug Investigations, 24, 353-363.

728. ee SJ et al. (2001). Regulation of myostatin activity and muscle growth. Proceedings of the National Academy of Sciences,98,16, 9306-9311.

729. Whittemore LA et al. (2004). Inhibition of myostatin in adult mice increases skeletal muscle mass and strength. Biochemical and Biophysical Research Communications, 300,4,965-971.

730. Nestor F et al. (1998). Organization of the human myostatin gene and expression in healthy men and HIV-infected men with muscle wasting. Proceedings of the National Academy of Sciences, 95,14938-14943.

731. Ramazanov Z et al. (2003). Sulfated polysaccharides of brown seaweed Cystoseira canariensis bind to serum myostatin protein. Acta Physiologica et Pharmacologica Bulgarica, 27,2-3,101-106.

732. Willoughby DS (2004). Effects of an alleged myostatin-binding supplement and heavy resistance training on serum myostatin, muscle strength and mass and body composition. International Journal of Sport Nutrition and Exercise Metabolism, 14,4,461-472.

733. Walker KS et al. (2004). Resistance training alters plasma myostatin but not IGF-1 in healthy men. Medicine and Science in Sports and Exercise, 36,5,787-793.

734. Elliott RB et al. (1996). A population based strategy to prevent insulin-dependent diabetes using nicotinamide. Journal of Pediatric Endocrinology & Metabolism,9,501-509.

735. Jonas WB et al. (1996)The effect of niacinamide on osteoarthritis: a pilot study. Inflammation Research, 45,330-334.

736. Morgan JM et al. (2004). The effects of niacin on lipoprotein subclass distribution. Preventive Cardiology, 7,4,182-187.

737. Garg R et al. (1999). Niacin treatment increases plasma homocyst(e)ine levels. American Heart Journal, 138,1082-1087.

739. Hornick CA et al. (2003). Inhibition of angiogenic initiation and disruption of newly established human vascular networks by juice from Morinda citrifolia (noni). Angiogenesis, 6(2),143-9.

740. Hiramatsu T et al. (1993). Induction of normal phenotypes in ras-transformed cells by damnacanthal from Morinda citrifolia. Cancer Letters, 73,161-166.

741.   Goheen SC et al. (1981). The prevention of alcoholic fatty liver using dietary supplements: dihydroxyacetone, pyruvate and riboflavin compared to arachidonic acid in pair fed rats. Lipids. 19, 43-51.

742.   Stanko, R et al. (1992). Body composition, energy utilization and nitrogen metabolism with a 4.25-MJ /d diet supplemented with pyruvate. American Journal of Clinical Nutrition, 56, 630-635.

743.   Stanko, R., Tietze, Arch, J.E. (1992b). Body composition, energy utilization and nitrogen metabolism with a severely restricted diet supplemented with dihydroxyacetone and pyruvate. American Journal of Clinical Nutrition, 55, 771-776.

744.   Stanko, R. et. al. (1990). Enhanced leg exercise endurance with a high carbohydrate diet and dihydroxyacetone and pyruvate. Journal of Applied Physiology, 69, 1651-1656.

745.   Renea A et al. (2002). Induction of Apoptosis in Low to Moderate-Grade Human Prostate Carcinoma by Red Clover-derived Dietary Isoflavones. Cancer Epidemiology Biomarkers & Prevention,11, 1689-1696.

746.   Kirchheimer S (2003). Herbal remedies can aid prostate health: A review of supplements finds pros and cons. Webmd.com. (accessed 1/18/05).

747.   Wuttke W et al. (2002). Phytoestrogens for hormone replacement therapy? Journal of Steroid Biochemistry and Molecular Biology, 83, 1-5,133-147.

748.   Tice JA et al. (2003). Phytoestrogen supplements for the treatment of hot flashes: the Isoflavone Clover Extract (ICE) study: a randomized controlled trial. Journal of the American Medical Association, 290, 207-214.

749.   Heber D et al. (1999). Cholesterol-lowering effects of a proprietary Chinese red-yeast-rice dietary supplement. American Journal of Clinical Nutrition, 69,231-236.

751.   Castano G et al. (2001). Effects of policosanol 20 versus 40 mg/day in the treatment of patients with type II hypercholesterolemia: a 6-month double-blind study. International Journal of Clinical Pharmacology Research, 21,1,43-57.

752.   Brilla LR et al. (1992). Effect of magnesium supplementation on strength training in humans. Journal of the American College of Nutrition,11,3, 326-329.

753.   Song Y et al. (2004). Dietary Magnesium Intake in Relation to Plasma Insulin Levels and Risk of Type 2 Diabetes in Women. Diabetes Care, 27:59-65.

754.   Rude RK et al. (2004). Magnesium deficiency and osteoporosis: animal and human observations. Journal of Nutritional Biochemistry, 15,12,710-716.

755.   Linde K, Mulrow CD. St. John's wort for depression. Cochrane Database SystemicReview, 2:CD000448.

756.   Irefin S et al. (2000). A possible cause of cardiovascular collapse during anesthesia: long-term use of St. John's Wort. Journal of Clinical Anesthesia,12,498-499.

757.   Moses EL et al. (2000).St. John's wort: Three cases of possible mania induction. Journal of Clinical Psychopharmacology, 20,115-117.

758.   Shippy RA et al. (2004). S-adenosylmethionine (SAM-e) for the treatment of depression in people living with HIV/AIDS. BioMed Central Psychiatry, 11,4,11;4,1,38.

759.   Jacobsen S et al. (1991). Oral S-adenosylmethionine in primary fibromyalgia. double-blind clinical evaluation. Scandinavian Journal of Rheumatology, 20,294-302.

760.   Volkmann H et al. (1997). Double-blind, placebo-controlled cross-over study of intravenous S-adenosyl-L-methionine in patients with fibromyalgia. Scandinavian Journal of Rheumatology, 26,3,206-211.

442

761.   Najm WI etr al (2004). S-adenosyl methionine (SAMe) versus celecoxib for the treatment of osteoarthritis symptoms: a double-blind cross-over trial. BMC Musculoskeletal Disorders, www.biomedcentral.com/1471-2474/5/6 (accessed 1/20/05).

762.   Fogelholm GM et al. (1993)Low-dose amino acid supplementation: no effects on serum human growth hormone and insulin in male weightlifters. International Journal of Sport Nutrition, 3,290-297.

763.   Wilt TJ et al. (1998). Saw palmetto extracts for treatment of benign prostatic hyperplasia: a systematic review. Journal of the American Medical Association, 280,1604-1609.

764.   Wilt T et al. (2002). Serenoa repens for benign prostatic hyperplasia. Cochrane Database Systematic Review, 3, CD001423.

765.   Tyler V (1994). Herbs of Choice. Pharmaceutical Products Press.

766.   Brooks JD et al. (2001) Plasma selenium level before diagnosis and the risk of prostate cancer development. Journal of Urology, 166,2034-2038.

767.   Miller DRet al. (1998). Phase I/II trial of the safety and efficacy of shark cartilage in the treatment of advanced cancer. Journal of Clinical Oncology, 16,3649-3655.

768.   Barber R, et al. (2001). Oral shark cartilage does not abolish carcinogenesis but delays tumor progression in a murine model. Anticancer Research, 21,1065-1070.

769.   Anderson JW et al. (1995). Meta-analysis of the effects of soy protein intake on serum lipids. New England Journal of Medicine, 333,5,276-282.

770.   Simons LA et al. (2000). Phytoestrogens do not influence lipoprotein levels or endothelial function in healthy, postmenopausal women. American Journal of Cardiology, 85,1297-1301.

771.   Hodgson JM et al. (1998).Supplementation with isoflavonoid phytoestrogens does not alter serum lipid concentrations: a randomized controlled trial in humans. Journal of Nutrition, 128,728-732.

772.   Hidgon J. Soy isoflavonoids. Linus Pauling Institute. www.lpi.oregonstate.edu (accessed 2/24/05).

773.   Setchell D et al. (2003). Dietary phytoestrogens and their effect on bone: evidence from in vitro and in vivo, human observational, and dietary intervention studies. American Journal of Clinical Nutrition, 78, 3, 593S-609S.

774.   Cambria-Kiely JA. (2002). Effect of soy milk on warfarin efficacy. Annals of Pharmacotherapy, 36,1893-1896.

775.   McMichael-Phillips DF et al. (1998). Effects of soy-protein supplementation on epithelial proliferation in the histologically normal human breast. American Journal of Clinical Nutrition, 68,1431S-1435S.

776.   Gardner-Thorpe D et al. (2003). Dietary supplements of soya flour lower serum testosterone concentrations and improve markers of oxidative stress in men. European Journal of Clinical Nutrition, 57,100-106.

777.   Gebbhart, B (2005). Benefit of ribose in a patient with fibromyalgia. . Pharmacotherapy, 24,11,1646-1648.

778.   Kreider RB (2003). Effects of oral D-ribose supplementation on anaerobic capacity and selected metabolic markers in healthy males. International Journal of Sport Nutrition and Exercise Metabolism, 13,76-86.

779.   Berardi JM et al. (2003). Effects of ribose supplementation on repeated sprint performance in men. Journal of Strength and Conditioning Research, 17,1,47-52.

780.   Hellsten Y et al. (2004). Effect of ribose supplementation on resynthesis of adenine nucleotides after intense intermittent training in humans. Journal of Applied Physiology, 286: R182-R188.

781. Pliml W et al.(1992). Effects of ribose on exercise-induced ischemia in stable coronary artery disease. Lancet, 340,507-510.
782. Antonio, J et al. (2000). Effects of tribulus terrestris on body composition and exercise performance in resistance-trained males. International Journal of Sport Nutrition and Exercise Metabolism, 10,2,208-215.
783. Gauthaman K et la (2003). Sexual effects of puncturevine (Tribulus terrestris) extract (protodioscin): an evaluation using a rat model. Journal of Alternative and Complementary Medicine, 9,2,257-265.
784. Shaw K et al. (2002). Tryptophan and 5-hydroxytryptophan for depression. Cochrane Database Systematic Review,1, CD003198.
785. Cangiano C et al. (1998). Effects of oral 5-hydroxy-tryptophan on energy intake and macronutrient selection in non-insulin dependent diabetic patients. International Journal of Obesity and Related Disorders, 22,7,648-654.
786. Birdsall T (1998). 5-hydroxytryptophan: a clinically effective serotonin precursor. Alternative Medicine Review,3,4,271-280.
787. Pfaffenrath V et al. (2002).The efficacy and safety of Tanacetum parthenium (feverfew) in migraine prophylaxis--a double-blind, multicentre, randomized placebo-controlled dose-response study. Cephalalgia, 22,523-532.
788. Ernst E et al. (2000). The efficacy and safety of feverfew (Tanacetum parthenium L.): an update of a systematic review. Public Health Nutrition, 3,(4A,509-14.
789. Edralin A et al. (2002). Flaxseed improves lipid profile without altering biomarkers of bone metabolism in postmenopausal women. Journal of Clinical Endocrinology & Metabolism, 87, 4, 1527-1532.
790. De Stéfani E et al. (2000). α-Linolenic Acid and Risk of Prostate Cancer: A Case-Control Study in Uruguay. Cancer Epidemiology Biomarkers & Prevention 9, 335-338.
791. Lemay A et al. (2002). Flaxseed dietary supplement versus hormone replacement therapy in hypercholesterolemic menopausal women. Obstetrics and Gynecology, 100,3,495-504.
792. Szapary PO et al. (2003). Guggulipid for treatment of hypercholesterolemia: a randomized controlled trial. Journal of the American Medical Association, 290,765-772.
793. Thappa DM et al. (1994). Nodulocystic acne: oral gugulipid versus tetracycline. Journal of Dermatology, 21,729-731.
794. Bianchi A et al. (2004). Rhabdomyolysis caused by Commiphora mukul, a natural lipid-lowering agent. Annals of Pharmacotherapy, 38,7-8,1222-1225.
795. Hadley S et al. (2004). Valerian. American Family Physician, 67,8,1755-1778.
796. Fawcett JP et al. (1996). The effect of oral vanadyl sulfate on body composition and performance in weight-training athletes. International Journal of Sport Nutrition, 6,4,382-390.
797. Hidgon J (2003). Vitamin B12. Linus Pauling Institute. www.lip.origonstate.edu (accessed 4/15/05).
798. Pongchaidecha M et al. (2004). Effect of metformin on plasma homocysteine, vitamin B12 and folic acid: a cross-sectional study in patients with type 2 diabetes mellitus. Journal of the Medical Association of Thailand, 87,7,780-787.
799. Bender DA (1992). The Biochemistry of the Vitamins. Cambridge University Press.
800. Higdon J (2004). Vitamin C. Linus Pauling Institute. www.lip.origonstate.edu (accessed 4/19/05).

444

801.   Laswon S (2000). Is vitamin C harmful to cancer patients? Linus Pauling Institute http://lpi.oregonstate.edu/s-s00/vitaminc.html (accessed 4/19/05).
802.   Hemila H (2004). Vitamin C supplementation and respiratory infections: a systematic review. Military Medicine, 169,11,920-925.
803.   Langolis M et al. (2001). Serum Vitamin C Concentration Is Low in Peripheral Arterial Disease and Is Associated With Inflammation and Severity of Atherosclerosis. Circulation, 103,1863-1869.
804.   Higdon, J (2004).Vitamin D. Linus Pauling Institute. www.lpi.oregonstate.edu(accessed 4/28/05).
805.   No authors listed (2004). Vitamin D fact sheet. Office of Dietary Supplements and National Institutes of Health. www.ods.od.nih.gov (accessed 4/28/05).
806.   Singh YN (2004). Vitamin D part I: are we getting enough? US Pharmacist, 10,66-72. www.uspharmacist.com.
807.   Bischoff-Ferrari HA, et al. (2004). Effect of Vitamin D on falls: a meta-analysis. Journal of the American Medical Association, 291,1999-2006.
808.   Higdon J (2004). Vitamin E. Linus Pauling Institutehttp://lpi.oregonstate.edu (accessed 5/10/05).
809.   No authors listed. Facts about vitamin E. Office of Dietary supplements and National Institutes of Health. www.ods.od.nih.gov (accessed 5/5/05).
810.   Weinstein SJ et al. (2005). Serum alpha-tocopherol and gamma-tocopherol in relation to prostate cancer risk in a prospective study. Journal of the National Cancer Institute, 97,5,396-399.
811.   Miller ER et al. (2005). Meta-analysis: High-dosage vitamin E supplementation may increase all-cause mortality. Annals of Internal Medicine, 142,60520-60553.
812.   Bairati I et al. (2005). A randomized trial of antioxidant vitamins to prevent second primary cancers in head and neck cancer patients. Journal of the National Cancer Institute, 97,481-488.
813.   Tabet N et al. (2000). Vitamin E for Alzheimer's disease. Cochrane Database Systematic Review. 4, CD002854.
814.   Brown EC et al. (2004). Soy versus whey protein bars: Effects on exercise training impact on lean body mass and antioxidant status. Nutrition Journal. www.nutritionj.com (accessed 5/23/05).
815.   Marshall, K (2004). Therapeutic applications of whey protein. Alternative Medicine Review, 9,2,136-156.
816.   Kennedy RS et al. (1995). The use of a whey protein concentrate in the treatment of patients with metastatic carcinoma: a phase I-II clinical study. Anticancer Research, 15,2643-2649.
817.   Belobrajdic DP et al. (2004). A high-whey-protein diet reduces body weight gain and alters insulin sensitivity relative to red meat in wistar rats. Journal of Nutrition, 134,1454-1458.
818.   Burke DG et al. (2001). The effect of whey protein supplementation with and without creatine monohydrate combined with resistance training on lean tissue mass and muscle strength. International Journal of Sport Nutrition and Exercise Metabolism, 11,349-364.
819.   Morifuji M et al. (2005). Dietary whey protein increases liver and skeletal muscle glycogen levels in exercise-trained rats. British Journal of Nutrition, 93,4,439-445.
820.   Samman S et al. (2003). A mixed fruit and vegetable concentrate increases plasma antioxidant vitamins and folate and lowers plasma homocysteine in men. Journal of Nutrition, 133:2188-93.
821.   Plotnick GD et al. (2003). Effect of supplemental phytonutrients on impairment of the flow-mediated brachial artery vasoactivity after a single high-fat meal. Journal of the American College of Cardiology, 41:1744-9.

822. Smith MJ et al. (1999). Supplementation with fruit and vegetable extracts may decrease DNA damage in the peripheral lymphocytes of an elderly population. Nutrition Research 19:1507-18.

823. Ernst E et al. (1998). Yohimbine for erectile dysfunction: a systematic review and meta-analysis of randomized clinical trials. Journal of Urology, 159,433-436.

824. Health Canada warns public not to use Bell Magicc Bullet. Health Canada Online 2003-90. November 26, 2003. www.hc-sc.gc.ca (accessed 7/1/05).

825. FDA Talk Paper. FDA Public Health Advisory: FDA Warns Consumers Against Taking the Following Dietary Supplements-SIGRA, STAMINA Rx and STAMINA Rx for Women, Y-Y, Spontane ES and Uroprin. Food and Drug Administration. TO3-48. June 20 2003www.fda.gov. (accessed 7/1/05).

826. Higdon J (2003). Zinc. Linus Pauling Institute. www.lpi.oregonstate.edu (accessed 7/7/05).

827. Leitzmann MF et al. (2003). Brief Communication. Zinc supplement use and risk of prostate cancer. Journal of the National Cancer Institute 95,13,1004-1007.

828. No authors listed. The facts about dietary supplements: zinc. National Institutes of Health. Office of Dietary Supplements. www.ods.od.nih.gov (accessed 7/7/05).

829. Ibs HK et al. (2003). Zinc-altered immune function. Journal of Nutrition, 133,1452S-1456S.

830. Lukaski HC (2005). Low dietary zinc decreases erythrocyte carbonic anhydrase activities and impairs cardiorespiratory function in men during exercise. American Journal of Clinical Nutrition, 81,5,1045-1051.

831. Prasad AS et al. (1996). Zinc status and serum testosterone levels of healthy adults. Nutrition, 12,5,344-348.

832. Alford, C et al. (2001). The effects of red bull energy drink on human performance and mood. Amino Acids, 21,2,139-150.

833. Laird RD et al. (2001). Psychotic episode during use of St. John's wort. J Herb Pharmacotherapy,1,81-87.

834. Ernst E. (2002).St. John's Wort supplements endanger the success of organ transplantation. Archives of Surgery, 137,316-319.

835. Klier CM (2002). St. John's wort (Hypericum perforatum)--is it safe during breastfeeding? Pharmacopsychiatry,35,1,29-30.

836. Murphy PA et al. (2005). Interaction of St. John's Wort with oral contraceptives: effects on the pharmacokinetics of norethindrone and ethinyl estradiol, ovarian activity and breakthrough bleeding. Contraception, 71,402-408.

837. Delle Chiaie R et al. (2002). Efficacy and tolerability of oral and intramuscular S-adenosyl-Lmethionine 1,4-butanedisulfonate (SAMe) in the treatment of major depression: comparison with imipramine in multicenter studies. American Journal of Clinical Nutrition, 76,1172S-1176S.

838. Bradley JD et al. (1994). A randomized, double blind, placebo controlled trial of intravenous loading with S-adenosylmethionine (SAM) followed by oral SAM therapy in patients with knee osteoarthritis. Journal of Rheumatology, 21,905-911.

839. Alekel DL, St. Germain A, Peterson CT et al. Isoflavone-rich soy protein isolate attenuates bone loss in the lumbar spine of perimenopausal women. American Journal of Clinical Nutrition, 72,844-582.

840. Halberstam M et al. (1996).Oral vanadyl sulfate improves insulin sensitivity in NIDDM but not in obese nondiabetic subjects. Diabetes, 45,659-666.

841.   Kelly G. (2003). The interaction of cigarette smoking and antioxidants. Part III: ascorbic acid. Alternative Medicine Review, 8,43-54.

842.   Edmonds SE et al. (1997). Putative analgesic activity of repeated oral doses of vitamin E in the treatment of rheumatoid arthritis. Results of a prospective placebo controlled double blind trial. Annals of the Rheumatic Diseases, 56,649-655.

843.   Eberlein-Konig B et al. (1998). Protective effect against sunburn of combined systemic ascorbic acid (vitamin C) and d-alpha-tocopherol (vitamin E). Journal of the American Academy of Dermatology, 38,45-48.

844.   Reza Hakkak et al. (2001). Diets Containing Whey Proteins or Soy Protein Isolate Protect against 7,12-Dimethylbenz(a)anthracene-induced Mammary Tumors in Female Rats. Cancer Epidemiology Biomarkers & Prevention, 9, 113-117.

845.   Townsend RR et al. (2004). A randomized, double-blind, placebo-controlled trial of casein protein hydrolysate (C12 peptide) in human essential hypertension. American Journal of Hypertension, 17 (11 pt 1) 1056-1058.

846.   Jackson, K (2005). The Role of Zinc in Men's Health. US Pharmacist,8,29-34.

847.   Ryder KM et al. (2005). Magnesium intake from food and supplements is associated with bone mineral density in healthy older white subjects. Journal of the American Geriatric Association 53,11,1875-1880.

848.   Zhah SP et al. (2004). Xuezhikang, an extract of Cholestin protects endothelial function through anti-inflammatory and lipid lowering mechanisms in patients with coronary heart disease. Circulation, 110, 7, 915-920.

849.   Bottiglieri T. (2002). S-Adenosyl-L-methionine (SAMe): from the bench to the bedside--molecular basis of a pleiotrophic molecule. American Journal of Clinical Nutrition, 76,1151S-1157S.

850.   Lands LC et al. (1999). Effect of supplementation with a cysteine donor on muscular performance. Journal of Applied Physiology, 84,4,1381-1385.

Index

Y

Z

About the Author

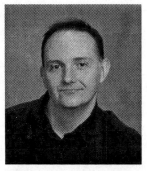

Joe Cannon is an exercise physiologist, health educator, and lecturer. He holds an MS degree in Exercise Science and a BS degree in Chemistry and Biology as well as two certifications from the National Strength and Conditioning Association (NSCA). For over ten years, he has lectured on the topics of nutrition, supplements, exercise, and wellness, for the American Aerobics Association International/International Sports Medicine Association (AAAI/ISMA). He is single and in his spare time enjoys biking, weightlifting, history, politics and *making a difference.*

For more information, or to order additional copies of this book, please visit Joe's official website, www.Joe-Cannon.com